ABORTION IN JUDAISM

Abortion in Judaism presents a complete Jewish legal history of abortion from the earliest relevant biblical references through the end of the twentieth century. For the first time, almost every Jewish text relevant to the abortion issue is explored in detail. These texts are investigated in historical sequence, thereby elucidating the development inherent within the Jewish approach to abortion. Following an examination of the foundational sources, contemporary responses from across the Jewish spectrum are introduced in order to probe their place in this history, as well as to discern the directions in which they would have the law proceed. The impact of Jewish abortion law upon Israeli legislative enactments is evaluated, along with the social outcomes of such legislation. Finally, the work considers the insights that this thematic history provides into Jewish ethical principles, as well as into the role of *halakhah* within Judaism.

DANIEL SCHIFF is the Jewish Education Institute Community Scholar in Pittsburgh, and Rabbi of B'nai Israel in White Oak, Pennsylvania. His articles have appeared in a number of books and journals.

ABORTION IN JUDAISM

DANIEL SCHIFF

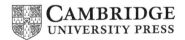

CAMBRIDGE
UNIVERSITY PRESS

CAMBRIDGE
UNIVERSITY PRESS

University Printing House, Cambridge CB2 8BS, United Kingdom

Cambridge University Press is part of the University of Cambridge.

It furthers the University's mission by disseminating knowledge in the pursuit of
education, learning and research at the highest international levels of excellence.

www.cambridge.org
Information on this title: www.cambridge.org/9780521521666

© Daniel Schiff 2002

First published 2002

A catalogue record for this publication is available from the British Library

Library of Congress Cataloguing in Publication data
Schiff, Daniel.
Abortion in Judaism / Daniel Schiff.
p.   cm.
Includes bibliographical references and index.
ISBN 0 521 80622 4 (hardback) ISBN 0 521 52166 1 (paperback)
1. Abortion (Jewish law).   I. Title.
KBM3119.A36.S35   2002
296.3´6976 – dc21   2002067371

ISBN 978-0-521-80622-0 Hardback
ISBN 978-0-521-52166-6 Paperback

Contents

Preface

At the core of Judaism is the legal system known as *halakhah*, from the Hebrew meaning "to go" or "to walk." Originating at Sinai, *halakhah* shapes Jewish life and, ideally, directs Jews towards righteous and exalted conduct. Yet even this legal system, seen to be based in divine revelation, is not exempt from its share of complex questions, uncertainties, and disagreements about the appropriate path to follow. In those occasional circumstances when the correct legal ruling is unclear, *halakhic* authorities formulate responses through the application of precedents and principles to the situation under consideration. This task, accomplished as it is by gifted but fallible human beings, at times produces differing interpretations and rulings such that the law generates various solutions that cannot be neatly reconciled. While, in time, the *halakhah* usually converges on a path that comes to be regarded as normative, this "right way" is rarely so obvious that it can be determined with ease, nor can alternative potential legal options be dismissed without reservation.

The issue of abortion presents the *halakhah* with exactly this type of challenge. While there is fundamental agreement on the broad parameters of the distinctive Jewish attitude to abortion, legal clarity on critical particulars – a low priority for many centuries – has proven to be a difficult goal to attain. This reality makes the thought of the rabbis – as they grapple with a delineated textual tradition, wrenching actual moral dilemmas, and a diversity of developing responses – particularly intriguing.

For this reason I have chosen to write a historical account of the development of the Jewish response to abortion. It is, of course, relatively unusual to explore *halakhic* issues through the lens of historical reflection. The methodical study of history is, after all, essentially a modern enterprise involving analyzing, comparing, and contrasting events from differing epochs. *Halakhic* subjects, conversely, are typically explored according to topic, without regard to time-period. Thus, the examination of a particular *halakhic* question might consider the positions of the Talmudic rabbis, Rashi, Maimonides, Caro, and contemporary figures as if they were all sitting around the same table, rather than spread across two millennia. This approach is useful when trying to fathom the assorted insights that bear upon a discrete legal problem. It does not, however, attempt to survey the broader view of how one generation reacts to a range of issues within a given field, and how subsequent generations deal with the legal inheritance transmitted to them, within altered contextual settings.

This volume, then, provides an account of the Jewish legal response to abortion through the centuries. It is a history replete with unexpected developments. Alongside important ethical insights there are unforeseen prohibitions, significant divisions on pivotal issues, bold departures from inherited assumptions, forgery allegations, and unsettled conundrums. The absorbing saga of the Jewish reaction to abortion unfolds through a succession of vastly different historical conditions, from the wandering in the desert to the contemporary state of Israel, and gives eloquent testimony to the flexibility and the adaptability that appear to be enduring strengths of the *halakhic* system.

Two cautions are in order. First, this is a history of the response of Judaism to abortion, not that of Jews. There is, consequently, no attempt to describe the varied emotions and feelings that Jews have on the delicate matter of abortion. Rather, I have restricted my analysis to those legal statements that have contributed to the *halakhic* picture of abortion, together with those reflective observations that offer commentary on the law and on its coherence and conduciveness.

Second, this work should not be used as a Jewish legal handbook in individual cases. In large measure, this book is a study of the *shèeilot uteshuvot* (questions and answers) literature, the rabbinic responsa, which have been penned through the centuries and apply the law to those specific inquiries that have not received a previous reply that could be considered adequate. Hence, I have encapsulated rabbinic rulings on the suitability of abortions in numerous situations like those that could arise in personal experience. Jewish law, however, counsels that every case is different and must be judged on its own merits. This is particularly so in the matter of abortion, where the consequences of any decision inevitably are weighty. *Halakhah*, it must be stressed, cannot be self-administered from a knowledge of general conclusions. A competent rabbinic authority must be consulted in order to determine the *halakhic* answer to any real-life abortion question.

I am deeply grateful to all those who have provided me with their insights, their thoughtfulness and the strength of their support during the production of this work:

To my colleagues: Mark Washofsky for his encouragement, his academic erudition, and for the time that he devoted to this endeavor; Moshe Zemer, who first sparked my interest in the responsa literature, for his detailed comments on each chapter, and for his keen assistance and eagerness throughout; Aaron Mackler, who offered thoughtful observations on the completed text; Walter Jacob, who greeted my scholarly endeavors with enthusiasm, and who invited me to use the rabbinic libraries and the wonderful responsa collection of Rodef Shalom Congregation.

To those who provided outstanding technical assistance: Kevin Taylor and his expert team at Cambridge University Press, who brought this book to fruition with professionalism; my mother, Judi Schiff, who initially proofread the work, thereby enabling me to correct many imperfections; Lea Black, who added so much through her numerous editorial suggestions; Jan Chapman, who refined the final text with copy-editing that was both thorough and precise; Sarah Barnard of the Hebrew Union College – Jewish Institute of Religion Klau Library in Cincinnati, who smoothed my way by regularly locating sources for me, and sending them to me with prompt dispatch.

To my children, David and Adina Schiff, who have lived with my research throughout their young lives, for all their understanding and patience, and for the great inspiration that each has provided to my life; and to my wife, Anne Schiff, for her love, for the hours she gave as the first one to read and improve each section, and for her unending support and companionship every step of the way.

Words are inadequate to express the fullness of my appreciation to each of these extraordinarily fine individuals. Naturally, any errors, omissions, or deficiencies in the final work are mine alone.

Finally, I give thanks to God for the gift of life itself, for the manifold blessings bestowed upon me, and for having been granted the ability to embark upon and to complete this project.

CHAPTER I

The conundrum takes shape: foundational verses

It all began with a struggle. We will never discover what it was that caused the fight or precisely when it took place. Nor will we ever find out the circumstances under which two men happened to clash in the immediate vicinity of a pregnant woman. All we know is that the tussle ended in disaster. There came a point when the men, engrossed in combat and oblivious to bystanders, collided with the pregnant woman, and loss of life resulted. The Torah, at Exodus 21:22–25, provides two alternative conclusions to the incident:

If men fight, and they push a pregnant woman and she miscarries, but no other injury (*ason*) occurs, the one responsible shall surely be fined, when the husband of the woman shall assess, and he shall pay as the judges shall determine. But if an injury (*ason*) does occur, then you shall award a life for a life, an eye for an eye, a tooth for a tooth, a hand for a hand, a foot for a foot, a burn for a burn, a wound for a wound, a bruise for a bruise.[1]

In relation to either outcome, the aggressor was to be judged on the basis of regulations that appear to be fairly unremarkable. In practice, such cases would have been handled with customary dispatch, and their role in the history of *halakhah* should have been regarded as minor. With the passing generations, however, their obscurity came to be transformed into prominence, owing to the fact that this episode afforded a critical

---

[1] The author's translation from the Hebrew in the *Jewish Publication Society Hebrew–English Tanakh*. Unless otherwise indicated, the author is responsible for all the translations in this work.

Deuteronomy 25:11–12 provides another example of a fight between two men in which the wife of one of the men tries to intervene. It is reasonable to assume, therefore, that such fights were by no means unknown, and that the Torah gives its rulings here in the context of events that would have been within the experience of the Israelites. Rabbi Daniel Sinclair reports the finding of other scholars that " . . . women would often adjudicate in disputes, thereby exposing themselves to blows of this nature. This may also account, to some extent, for the detailed treatment in both the Bible and other ancient Near-Eastern codes, of a situation which does not seem, at first sight, to deserve such extensive attention"; "The Legal Basis for the Prohibition on Abortion in Jewish Law," *Israel Law Review*, volume 15, number 1, 1980: 110, n. 4

I

insight into the Israelite view of the relative values that were to be ascribed to the life of the woman and the fetus.[2] Millennia later, long after
the adjudication of such physical conflicts had become banal, the implications of this distinction between a woman and her unborn child would
continue to be the cause of determined *halakhic* struggle.

In the ancient world, however, this outcome could not even have been
contemplated, much less foreseen. The *Tanakh* (Hebrew Bible) is silent
on the issue of abortion as it is understood in contemporary society: the
intentional termination of a pregnancy resulting in the death of the fetus
by physical or chemical means.[3] Exodus 21:22–25, which is thought
to date back to at least the ninth century BCE,[4] refers to spontaneous
abortion or miscarriage. Given that "[a]bortions were always available"[5]
in antiquity, it is hardly plausible that this silence reflects ignorance of
such practices. Rather, this muteness may be due to the orientation of
the Israelite tradition, which consistently placed a great emphasis on
the *mitzvah* (commandment) of procreation. "Be fruitful and multiply"
(Genesis 1:28) is the very first commandment of the Torah. The instruction is repeated following the flood (Genesis 9:7). The initial barrenness
of three of the four matriarchs, Sarah, Rebecca, and Rachel, which is
overcome through God's "remembering" them, seems to teach that pregnancy cannot be taken as a biological assumption, but is touched by the
Divine. Jacob's rhetorical question of Rachel, "[A]m I in God's stead,
who has withheld from you the fruit of the womb?" is particularly telling

[2] This statement will be further elaborated upon below. Debate often arises surrounding the appro-
     priate word to be used for an unborn, developing human being. Some maintain that the use of the
     term "fetus" provides more of an emotional distance that further opens the door to abortion than
     if the term "baby" is utilized. While this argument should not be dismissed, "fetus" is technically
     a more precise and suitable term for one who is still within the womb. In no way should the use
     of the term "fetus" be comprehended as a diminution of the value of the unborn.
[3] Technically speaking, this definition describes induced abortion. Since the abortion discussion
     focuses particularly on induced abortion, the term "abortion" will be used to refer to induced
     abortions. References to spontaneous abortion or miscarriage utilize the appropriate specified
     term: the unintended expulsion of a non-viable fetus during the first three months of pregnancy
     is usually referred to as "spontaneous abortion," whereas the unintended expulsion of the fetus
     later in pregnancy is usually referred to as "miscarriage."
[4] This is the dating of those who subscribe to the documentary hypothesis of biblical criticism,
     though most would agree that the traditions contained in the text probably existed earlier in
     oral form. According to the documentary hypothesis, the Exodus passage is part of the so-
     called "Covenant Code" (Exodus 21–23), representing the oldest law collection of Israel. Jewish
     tradition ascribes a much earlier date to the giving of the Torah, placing it some time in the 1200s
     BCE. See B.W. Anderson, *Understanding the Old Testament* (3rd edition), New Jersey, Prentice-Hall
     Incorporated, 1975, pp. 18–21.
[5] J. M. Riddle, *Contraception and Abortion from the Ancient World to the Renaissance*, Cambridge, MA,
     Harvard University Press, 1992, p. 7.

in this regard.[6] This emphasis on the centrality of procreation led one scholar of ancient Judaism to observe: "[s]een from this faith perspective, I think that abortion was absolutely inconceivable. This does not mean that forced abortion could not have occurred in Israelite families at all; but the necessity of an explicit legal regulation pertaining to this matter obviously did not exist."[7] It is also possible that the Torah seeks to separate Israelite conduct decisively from abortion by casting it in the category of an unmentionable, repugnant foreign practice. According to either interpretation, it is plausible that the Israelite ideological milieu made abortion sufficiently rare that biblical statements on the subject would have seemed superfluous.

It may be assumed, then, that the judges of the biblical era understood well how the provisions of Exodus 21:22–25 were to be applied in their day. Since that time, however, the meaning of the text has become sufficiently opaque that even its plain sense is no longer clear. Among the issues that require elucidation, the following have the greatest significance: What exactly was meant by the Hebrew term *ason* – translated above as "injury" – to which the account refers? Who was considered to be the victim of the *ason*? Further, what was the precise nature of the penalties that were to be imposed?

Certain biblical scholars, such as Michael Fishbane and Nahum Sarna, consider the answers to these questions to be indeterminable from the Torah passage itself. Fishbane postulates that the text may well have been shaped in the light of some unrecorded interpretative tradition,[8] so that it is no longer possible to perceive the correct biblical intent of these verses and their significance, without employing the spectacles of later generations. He regards the Exodus 21:22–25 legislation as a primary example of a biblical structure that is beyond comprehension without the help of interpretation: "it is quite clear that the present instance of *aberratio ictus* is thoroughly dependent upon legal exegesis for its viability. There is virtually no feature of its present formulation and redaction which is entirely unambiguous and self-sufficient."[9] Both scholars believe it is impossible to state definitively whether the Exodus case is an instance of premature birth, instant miscarriage, delayed stillbirth,

---

[6] See Genesis 16:1–2; 17:15–21; 21:1–2; 25:21; 30:1–2, 22–24.

[7] A. Lindemann, " 'Do Not Let a Woman Destroy the Unborn Babe in Her Belly.' Abortion in Ancient Judaism and Christianity," *Studia Theologica*, volume 49, 1995: 258.

[8] M. Fishbane, *Biblical Interpretation in Ancient Israel*, Oxford, Clarendon Press, 1985, p. 19.

[9] *Ibid.*, p. 94.

or term delivery.[10] Neither scholar finds that the victim of the *ason* is identifiable with any certainty.[11]

However, where Fishbane and Sarna see uncertainty, the biblical linguist Benno Jacob provides definitive answers based on the internal logic of the passage. In contrast to his colleagues, Jacob contends that although the meaning of the Hebrew word *ason* is attested to in many places in the strata of post-biblical Judaism,[12] its correct interpretation can readily be derived from the context of the Torah itself. The term *ason* occurs five times in the Torah: twice in Exodus 21:22–25, as well as three times in the Joseph narrative of Genesis.[13] Jacob holds that a logical reading of verses 23–25 must conclude that an *ason* is "an accident which could lead to any type of injury or even to death."[14] The contention that an *ason* is an accidental, rather than a deliberate, harm is supported by the three references in Genesis to *ason* which depict it as an event which might "happen along the road," and, therefore, includes "overtones of bad luck and misfortune."[15]

Jacob further discerns that the Hebrew term *ve-nagfu* (push) in verse 22 is never employed for the direct act of striking someone, but is adopted in those circumstances where a blow "might unintentionally strike a third party."[16] Hence, the combination of *ve-nagfu* with *ason* reinforces the impression of the passage that the tragic collision with the pregnant woman was an unintentional act. A scholar of Jewish law, Rabbi Daniel Sinclair, asserts that "the term *nagaf* . . . generally refers to a hostile, deliberate act," and that "[a]ccording to several Talmudic sources, the blow was intentional, but was aimed at someone other than the pregnant woman. . ."[17] Sinclair and Jacob are not necessarily in conflict with one another in their understanding of *ve-nagfu*. The blow may well have been "hostile and deliberate" towards the other man, yet unintentionally struck the woman. However, Jacob would contend that there is no need

---

[10] These matters, according to Fishbane, are relevant to the viability of the fetus at the time of the incident, and, therefore, may help to indicate the "legal protection and benefits" to which the fetus is entitled.

[11] Fishbane, *Biblical Interpretation*, and N. Sarna, *Exploring Exodus: The Heritage of Biblical Israel*, New York, Schocken Books, 1986, p. 186.

[12] *Ason* has always been understood by tradition to mean "injury" or "harm." For the rabbinic definition, see J. C. Lauterbach (ed.), *Mekilta de-Rabbi Ishmael*, volume III, *Nezikin*, Philadelphia, 1935, chapter 8, pp. 65–66, and *Sanhedrin* 74a, 79a.

[13] See Genesis 42:4; 42:38; and 44:29.

[14] B. Jacob, *The Second Book of the Bible: Exodus* (translated by W. Jacob), Hoboken, Ktav Publishing House Incorporated, 1992, p. 656.

[15] *Ibid*.   [16] *Ibid*., p. 654.   [17] Sinclair, "Legal Basis," 110–111.

to go to the Talmud for a fuller understanding of the term, since this sense can be derived from the word itself.

A credible reason why the Exodus ruling is set in the context of a conflict between two adversaries may be in order to avoid any suggestion of premeditation, an understanding that supports Jacob's analysis. For the laws promulgated by these verses certainly did not require the presence of more than one aggressor. Precisely the same regulations could have been established had only a sole individual collided with the pregnant woman. It can be seen in the verses immediately preceding the text under consideration that while Exodus 21:18–19 involves two people in its description of the punishments for injuries inflicted in a fight, Exodus 21:20–21 depicts only one individual in its delineation of the penalties for a person who strikes a slave. While either of these two paradigms could have been used for Exodus 21:22–25,[18] it is quite conceivable that the Torah employs the two-person model so that there should be no doubt that "here we had no direct attack, but an accidental injury to a third party..."[19]

Regarding the identity of the assaulted "third party," although the rabbis considered the possibility of various victims of the *ason*,[20] no coherent sense can be made of the Exodus text were the casualty to be anybody but the pregnant woman. For example, Jacob refutes the rabbinic suggestion that the fetus be considered a candidate as the victim of the *ason* in verses 23–25 by pointing out that the fetus could not have been included in the "tooth for a tooth" provision because it possessed no teeth, and hence could not be the subject of the injuries listed! Jacob concludes that the woman must be the injured party by deducing that the Hebrew term *baàl*, which appears in verse 22 as a part of the expression *baàl haïshah* (husband; literally, husband of the woman), always alludes either to the one who has "responsibility for damages which must be borne" or to "a recipient for payment of damages to a dependent."[21] Thus, in this case, the use of *baàl haïshah* implies that the husband was to be paid in his capacity as the recipient of payment for any damages done to his dependent wife. The text, after all, could have simply used *baàlah* (her husband) rather than *baàl haïshah* (husband of the woman). Jacob contends that the term *baàl haïshah* is utilized here so that there should be no doubt that the husband is receiving the money on account

---

[18] Fishbane, *Biblical Interpretation*, p. 92, n. 7.   [19] B. Jacob, *Exodus*, p. 656.
[20] See below, chapter 2, p. 29, n. 9.   [21] B. Jacob, *Exodus*, p. 656.

of his dependent wife's misfortune. Thus, the use of *baʿal haʾishah* indicates that the Exodus text perceived the pregnant woman as the victim of whatever collateral *ason* occurred in connection with the expulsion of the fetus. Consequently, the Torah can be understood as requiring that if the fetus alone were lost, then the one who caused the damage should be fined, but, if the woman were also killed, then it was a matter of *nefesh tachat nefesh*,[22] "a life for a life."[23]

What, though, did these stated punishments actually imply in practice? In the case of the fine for fetal loss, the translation of the Hebrew word *kaʾasher* to mean "as much as" leads to the following confusing reading: "[T]he one responsible shall surely be fined, *as much as* the husband of the woman shall assess, and he shall pay as the judges shall determine."[24] Obviously, if both the husband and the judges had set out to establish the fine, it would have been a recipe for legal chaos. Avoiding this route, some concluded that the text actually provides for the imposition of not one, but two fines.[25] However, as Rashi makes clear, such contortions are unnecessary if the word *kaʾasher* is given its other suitable translation of "when" or "if."[26] This offers the simplest understanding, namely that the fine was not levied automatically by societal demand, but was applied only in circumstances where the aggrieved husband called for it. If the husband requested that the fine be imposed, then the authorities determined the appropriate amount. It follows from this reading of the text that the fetus did not have a fixed value, and the husband would have been recompensed for his "property loss" according to its assessed worth. A comparison with other sources from antiquity supports the notion that the fetus' value was probably arrived at on the basis of sundry criteria such as viability and gender.[27]

---

[22] The Hebrew term *nefesh* refers to a "living soul." E. Urbach, *The Sages: Their Concepts and Beliefs* (translated by Israel Abrahams), Jerusalem, Magnes Press of the Hebrew University, 1979, p. 214, expresses the definition with precision: "In the Bible a monistic view prevails. Man is not composed of two elements – body and soul, or flesh and spirit. In Genesis (ii 7) it is stated 'and man became a living soul [*nefesh*]', but the term *nefesh* is not to be understood in the sense of *psyche, anima*. The whole of man is a living soul. The creation of man constitutes a single act. The *nefesh* is in actuality the living man . . ." Thus, the question of if and when a fetus, or baby, actually becomes a *nefesh* – from a Jewish perspective – will become highly relevant to the abortion issue.

[23] Clearly, if she were not killed, but lost an eye, it would be "an eye for an eye"; if a foot, "a foot for a foot," etc. (see below for the definition of these expressions). Since, however, she had been struck in such a way as to cause her to lose her fetus, the loss of her life was the most likely outcome of the irreversible damages listed.

[24] Some translate: . . . and he shall pay "based on reckoning." See *JPS Hebrew – English Tanakh*, Exodus 21:22.

[25] See below, pp. 18, 22–23.   [26] Rashi to Exodus 21:22 at "*kaʾasher yashit alav.*"

[27] See the four ancient texts mentioned below, p. 9. See also B. Jacob, *Exodus*, p. 657.

The second penalty, that of *nefesh tachat nefesh* if the woman were killed, has a long history of being misunderstood. It is well known that the rabbis interpreted *nefesh tachat nefesh* as requiring financial compensation for the value of a life, rather than capital punishment for the perpetrator.[28] It is, however, less well known that, even without this rabbinic interpretation, financial compensation rather than capital punishment is what was intended in the text originally. Benno Jacob writes with forceful conviction that when Exodus 21:23–25 is described as a law of talion,[29] "we can recognize this to be absolutely wrong, and the words *ne-fesh tahat ne-fesh* could only indicate *compensation through money*, as I have clearly demonstrated through numerous proof texts…"[30] Jacob's two principal arguments that refute the possibility that the Exodus law is an example of talion are founded in the Hebrew words *ve-natatah* and *tachat*. According to Jacob, *ve-natatah*, translated above as "you shall award," always carries with it the sense of "handing over" something which another party can receive. Thus, the punishment cannot mean, "you shall give up" one life for another, because in the "giving up" of a life, the deceased individual is lost and nothing is transmitted to the injured party. Similarly, if an eye were removed as punishment, it could not be "handed over" to anyone, but would be discarded, and *ve-natatah* is not a word that could possibly describe such an activity. The use of the word *ve-natatah*, then, indicates that something tangible was "given over," not "given up."[31] When this understanding is combined with the precise meaning of *tachat*, "in place of" or "something that could function as a substitute," the text actually can be comprehended to communicate: "You shall hand over a life as a substitute for the life that was lost."[32] Jacob demonstrates, furthermore, that *tachat* was regularly used to denote a pecuniary substitution. He writes, "there are not only many places in which *tachat* means 'substitute,' but that there are absolutely no other meanings. Moreover, there are numerous citations in which it signifies a financial restitution…"[33] Thus, a linguistic analysis of this punishment demonstrates that something had to be handed over, something of equivalent value, which could be substituted for a life, an eye, or the

---

[28] *M. Baba Kamma* 8:1, *Baba Kamma* 83b–84a.
[29] "*Lex talionis*." A law of talion demanded that the perpetrator suffer the exact equivalent act – as punishment – to that committed in the crime. However, as will be demonstrated, the law which appears three times in the Torah (Exodus 21:23–25; Leviticus 24:17–22; and Deuteronomy 19:18–19, 21) does not possess the characteristics of talion.
[30] B. Jacob, *Exodus*, p. 657. For a fuller treatment of the subject, see Jacob's comprehensive work: *Auge um Auge: Eine Untersuchung zum Alten und Neuen Testament*, Berlin, Philo Verlag, 1929.
[31] B. Jacob, *Exodus*, p. 657.   [32] *Ibid*.   [33] B. Jacob, *Auge um Auge*, pp. 37–38.

other injuries mentioned, and that "something" was most likely to be money.

This explanation is not only linguistically compelling, but intuitively satisfying as well, given that the common understanding of the text is that it provides for sentences of capital punishment, mutilation, or dismemberment. For if the Torah were actually calling for the death of the one who killed the pregnant woman, this would be an excessive penalty for what is acknowledged to be an inadvertent act and which, at worst, should be considered manslaughter.[34] Indeed, it has been shown that in other ancient codes, a true law of talion, actually insisting on the taking of a life for a life, is only prescribed in cases where the resulting harm was committed intentionally.[35] Unintentional acts never resulted in the death of the perpetrator in any comparable ancient source,[36] and thus it stretches credibility to assert that the Torah presents a highly exceptional or blatantly disproportionate case here. Hence, the Torah's plain meaning yields a position that calls for monetary payment, albeit on wholly different scales, for the loss of either the fetus or the mother.[37]

This statement is controversial. The biblical scholar, Umberto Cassuto, for example, was undoubtedly referring to those of a similar mind to Jacob when he wrote about what he described as *talio*:

This principle implies, according to the Rabbis, that one who takes a life, and one who blinds an eye must pay the value of the eye, and so forth, and the apologetically inclined commentators have endeavoured to show that this was the meaning of the formula even in ancient Hebrew. But this is impossible. It is not feasible that the meaning of the word "eye" should be "the value of the eye..."[38]

Cassuto maintains that this *talio* is an example of a formula which was meant literally at first, and only at some later point came to signify financial restitution. Sarna agrees that the wording was formulaic, rather than specific to a particular circumstance, but seems to concur with Jacob that it had already come to signify monetary compensation in the Bible itself: "Thus in Israelite law ... unlike its Near Eastern predecessors, the

---

[34] This, however, did not prevent some later rabbinic interpreters from continuing to view this as a capital offense. See below, chapter 2, p. 30.
[35] B. Jacob, *Exodus*, pp. 658–659.
[36] The Ancient Near Eastern texts cited below call for the death penalty in the context of what are considered to be intentional attacks. Exodus is the only text that avoids the inference of an intentional act by way of the two-man approach.
[37] B. Jacob, *Exodus*, p. 662.
[38] U. Cassuto, *A Commentary on the Book of Exodus* (translated by I. Abrahams), Jerusalem, The Magnes Press, 1967, p. 275.

'eye for an eye' formula was stripped of its literal meaning and became fossilized as the way in which the abstract legal formula of equivalent restitution was expressed."[39]

Jacob, however, makes a powerful case that the principle was designed to exact punishment, although not capital punishment, for this unintentional act. The perpetrator could not be allowed to avoid penalty, as the Code of Hammurabi (see below) provided, but neither could his physical disfigurement be intended. Jacob almost seems to be replying to Cassuto when he writes:

> For the Hebrew it must have been impossible to extract a sentence of bodily crippling *talion* from *ne-fesh ta-hat ne-fesh*, but also the English "eye *for* an eye" is not appropriate linguistically, nor was it original. This was transmitted to us through the Greek and Latin translators as well as the New Testament; through them it entered medieval law and eventually the various modern languages. The unbelievable tenacity with which this interpretation has been preserved, as well as the reluctance to admit error, has its roots in the feeling that *talion* was the simplest and most primitive path of justice. But the Torah had left the primitive world far behind . . .[40]

The *ason*, then, was regarded by the Jewish tradition as an accidental injury to the pregnant woman. If the fetus died but no *ason* occurred, then only the fine for the fetus' value had to be paid. If an *ason* leading to the woman's death did occur, then full financial compensation for the lost *nefesh* was required. The significance of these conclusions can be comprehended by comparing Exodus 21:22–25 with the four sources of ancient Near Eastern law that contained similar passages concerning injury to a pregnant woman: the Sumerian Laws, a text from approximately the nineteenth century BCE,[41] the Babylonian Code of Hammurabi, parts of which may date back to the eighteenth century BCE,[42] the Middle Assyrian Laws, which could be as old as the fifteenth century BCE,[43] and the Hittite Laws from around the fourteenth century BCE.[44] Each one has telling differences from the biblical text, which serve to amplify features of the deliberate wording found in the *Tanakh*.

---

[39] Sarna, *Exploring Exodus*, p. 189.   [40] B. Jacob, *Exodus*, p. 662.

[41] "Sumerian Laws" translated by J. J. Finkelstein, as found in J. B. Pritchard, *Ancient Near Eastern Texts Relating to the Old Testament* (3rd edition), Princeton, Princeton University Press, 1969, p. 525.

[42] "The Code of Hammurabi" translated by Theophile J. Meek, as found in Pritchard, *Ancient Near Eastern Texts*, p. 175, sections 209–214.

[43] "The Middle Assyrian Laws" translated by Theophile J. Meek, as found in Pritchard, *Ancient Near Eastern Texts*, pp. 181, 184–185, sections 21, 50–53.

[44] "The Hittite Laws" translated by Albrecht Goetze, as found in Pritchard, *Ancient Near Eastern Texts*, p. 190, sections 17–18.

What emerges from juxtaposing Exodus 21:22–25 with these other ancient legal texts is a picture that makes the biblical source appear consistent and advanced. The biblical outlook shares some features with these texts, while yet articulating profound differences from the attitudes of neighboring cultures. Where, for example, the other texts differentiate on the basis of social standing, the Exodus text does not. Although Israelite society allowed for a relatively benign form of slavery and at times applied divergent damage laws to citizens and slaves,[45] there is no hint in Exodus of an attempt to impose some alternate punishment for the loss of a woman or a fetus from a lower social stratum. Where the biblical words do draw a distinction, it is between existent maternal life and the potential life of the unborn. Indeed, a close analysis reveals that the Exodus text is unique and represents a truly progressive drive for legal impartiality in considering all maternal life to be of similar worth and all fetal life to be of similar worth, while yet creating a substantive differentiation between the value of the two, a differentiation that brooked no exceptions. Moreover, in Exodus, neither the loss of the fetus nor that of the mother could be recompensed through the payment of a fixed fine; both had to be compensated to the fullness of their worth. That compensation, furthermore, had to come from the one responsible for the injury, and, unlike some of the parallel texts of the ancient Near East, there is no intimation in Exodus that punishment could be inflicted on any other party.[46]

Perhaps of greatest significance, however, the Exodus legislation is without peer insofar as it is does not merely depict the mother's life as being of a higher value, but it ascribes to her a status that is on a qualitatively different plane. It stands alone in requiring that the compensation for her loss be appropriate to the loss of a *nefesh*, while the compensation for the fetus is evaluated simply on the basis of its features. Moshe Greenberg has demonstrated, by comparing the laws of homicide, that

---

[45] See, for example, Exodus 21:26–27, immediately after the section under discussion. Here a slave receives his freedom for the loss of his eye or his tooth, but the financial penalty of "an eye for an eye, a tooth for a tooth" is not imposed upon the assailant. The rabbis held that this was the case for heathen slaves, but not for Hebrew slaves, for whom the same punishments as for Hebrew citizens would have been exacted. See *Kiddushin* 24a, *Baba Kamma* 74a. From a plain reading of Exodus, however, all that is certain is that citizens and slaves were not treated identically in this regard.

[46] The *Tanakh* scholar, Moshe Greenberg, contrasts the readiness of the ancient Near Eastern law codes to punish relatives of the perpetrator for crimes committed, with the biblical attitude that only the instigator could be punished. Greenberg is of the view that "In this...there is doubtless to be seen the effect of the heightened stress on the unique worth of each life that the religious-legal postulate of man's being the image of God brought about"; M. Greenberg, "Some Postulates of Biblical Criminal Law," in M. Haran (ed.), *Sefer HaYovel LeYehezkel Kaufmann*, Jerusalem, Magnes Press, 1960, pp. 20–27.

there is a dramatic gap in the relative values ascribed to "life" and "property" between the *Tanakh* and the other ancient Near Eastern sources. The other texts, with their lodestars of social status and the strength of the community, could legislate for a homicide to be financially compensated, or a property offense to be paid for with a life. But not the *Tanakh*:

[I]n biblical law life and property are incommensurable; taking of life cannot be made up for by any amount of property, nor can any property offense be considered as amounting to the value of a life. Elsewhere the two are commensurable: a given amount of property can make up for life, and a grave enough offense against property can necessitate forfeiting life . . . [A] basic difference in the evaluation of life and property separates the one from the others. In the biblical law a religious evaluation; in non-biblical law, an economic and political evaluation, predominates.[47]

From Greenberg's analysis, it can be seen that the *nefesh tachat nefesh* formula of Exodus 21:23 serves as a powerful reminder that, although the involuntary nature of the incident allowed for a financial restitution for the loss of the woman's life, this restitution actually represented a sizable legal compromise. According to the value system of the *Tanakh*, a singular and supreme human life had been lost for which no amount of property could adequately compensate. Conversely, the fact that the loss of the fetus could be calculated readily and a fine imposed without such considerations being involved demonstrates that, from the biblical point of view, the fetus did not possess a status equivalent to that of its mother. As Exodus presents it, then, fetal expulsion represented the loss of property, the value of which had to be repaid; the death of the woman, on the other hand, represented the loss of a life, an unquestionably living soul, which deserved a full restitution, the amount of which could not be preordained, but had to befit the extinguishing of a unique, extant human being.

The historic role of these Exodus verses vis-à-vis abortion should, therefore, have been simple. In their specification of the mother as a *nefesh*, as opposed to the fetus, they appear to convey the sense that the status of maternal life is superior to that of the fetus. This suggests that in circumstances where mother and fetus are in a competition for life the Torah might advise saving the life of the mother over that of the fetus. The ramifications of this ranking for the issue of abortion are, of course, dramatic. Since the *Tanakh* does not address the topic of abortion directly, it might be assumed from these verses that any abortion performed with the express purpose of saving the mother's life would be permitted.

47 *Ibid.*, pp. 18–19.

This conclusion, of course, presupposes, as most authorities agree, that feticide contravenes no other laws of the Torah.[48] Such a conclusion could open the door to abortion within the limited range of instances in which the fetus is directly threatening its mother's existence. However, even before the full implications of Exodus 21:22–25 could become the subject of analysis by later rabbis and codifiers, a variant understanding of the meaning of the passage's words arose. Although this alternative rendering sprang from Jewish roots, it ultimately would provide the basis for deep divisions in Western thought. This effectively ensured the positioning of these Exodus sentences at the core of a controversy that would refuse to be dismissed easily.

The Exodus verses transmitted through history belong to the Hebrew Masoretic (received) text of the *Tanakh*, finalized some time in the second century CE from the various proto-Masoretic texts which had been in circulation in the centuries before.[49] However, already in the third century BCE, the prominent Jewish community of Alexandria in Egypt[50] had begun the production of a *Tanakh* translation into Greek to be used for public recitation and study. This first ever translation of the *Tanakh*, the Septuagint,[51] was far from just an attempt at the conversion of Hebrew words into their Greek equivalents:

The Septuagint was not simply a literal translation. In many passages, the translators used terms from Hellenistic Greek that made the text more accessible to Greek readers, but they also subtly changed its meaning. Elsewhere, the translators introduced Hellenistic concepts into the text. At times, they translated from Hebrew texts that differed from those current in Palestine, a matter now made clearer through the evidence of the biblical scrolls from Qumran. At other points, the Septuagint reflects knowledge of Palestinian interpretative traditions enshrined in rabbinic literature.[52]

[48] See chapter 2, generally.
[49] L. H. Schiffman, *Reclaiming the Dead Sea Scrolls*, Philadelphia, The Jewish Publication Society, 1994, pp. 161–173.
[50] Immediately after the founding of Alexandria in 332 BCE, the city became an instant magnet for Jews, so that by the first century BCE its Jewish population was said to be of the order of four hundred thousand. It was indubitably the largest Jewish community of its time, even compared with those of Judea. See J. Alpher (ed., English edition), *Encyclopedia of Jewish History* (translated by Haya Amir et al.), Ramat Gan, Israel, Massada Publishers, c. 1986, pp. 58–59.
[51] "Septuagint" – also abbreviated as "LXX" – means "seventy." The name derives from a legend to be found in the Letter of Aristeas (a Greek work thought to be from the late second century BCE) and in the Talmud, claiming that the translation was produced in seventy-two days by seventy-two elders brought from Jerusalem to Alexandria by Ptolemy II Philadelphus (285–246 BCE). See "Introduction" in *The Septuagint Version of the Old Testament and Apocrypha*, Grand Rapids, Zondervan Publishing House, 1972, pp. i–ii.
[52] Schiffman, *Dead Sea Scrolls*, p. 212.

The Septuagint, then, represents a work that coalesced from the interpretation of particular groupings of *Tanakh* texts (the specific texts used depending on the given translator), which had been filtered through the lens of Hellenistic terminology and thought. In reality, given that several centuries would pass before the Septuagint would be standardized, it is probably more accurate, before the Common Era, to speak of the work in progress as "Septuagintal-type manuscripts."[53] Even though there were numerous places where these manuscripts deviated from the meaning of the Hebrew that would ultimately comprise the Masoretic text, their use became widespread among Jews, not just in Alexandria, but in the Hellenistic world generally and remained so until rabbinic times.

Characteristic of the Septuagint, the phrasing that was finally enshrined in the standardized version cast Exodus 21:22–25 in a quite different light from the view presented by the Masoretic text. A literal translation from the Greek produces the following reading:

And if two men strive and smite a woman with child, and her child be born imperfectly formed, he shall be forced to pay a penalty: as the woman's husband may lay upon him, he shall pay with a valuation. But if it be perfectly formed, he shall give life for life . . .[54]

In understanding the word *ason* as "form" rather than "accidental injury," the Greek reading totally changed the meaning of the text. The Septuagint effectively removed the matter of the woman's death from consideration and, instead, based the severity of punishment upon whether or not the fetus was fully formed. If the fetus was not yet formed, then a fine was to be paid to the husband in recompense for the loss; if it was formed, then capital punishment was the appropriate penalty.

How did the Septuagint arrive at this widely variant rendering? In each of the three Genesis occurrences of the Hebrew term *ason*, the Septuagint employs a form of the Greek noun *malakia*, generally translated as "affliction," for *ason*.[55] Had the Septuagint utilized *malakia* in Exodus 21:22–25, it would have conveyed a sufficiently similar sense to the original Hebrew that it would have been highly unlikely to have become the cornerstone of a wholly divergent approach to the status of the fetus. But, in Exodus 21:22–25, instead of *malakia*, the Septuagint twice

[53] S. Sandmel, *Philo of Alexandria*, New York, Oxford University Press, 1979, pp. 168–169. See also S. Daniel, "Bible Translations," in *Encyclopaedia Judaica*, Jerusalem, Keter Publishing House, volume IV, pp. 851–856.
[54] *The Septuagint Version*, Exodus 21:22–23, p. 98.   [55] *The Septuagint Version*, pp. 57, 58, 61.

uses the Greek participle *exeikonismenon* to translate *ason*.[56] A scholar of
Hellenistic Judaism, Richard Freund, has made the case that the translator of these verses, who either deliberately bypassed or was ignorant
of the translation used elsewhere, arrived at his version through a process of homophonic substitution.[57] This technique was not uncommon
in both Greek and rabbinic texts. According to this explanation, the
translator probably transliterated *ason* into some form of the Greek word
soma, meaning "human life," and then replaced this Greek translitera-
tion with a synonymous term that offered a more profound theological
resonance.[58] This resonance can be readily apprehended through the literal translation of *exeikonismenon*: "made from the image,"[59] which evokes
an immediate connection to the wording of Genesis 1:27, "In the image
of God, God created man." Freund posits that the usage of the verb
exeikonizein in the Septuagint and Philo establishes a strong connection
to the "made from the image" metaphor. This remarkable textual al-
lusion led Freund to conclude that "[i]t is clear from the LXX use of
exeikonizein in Exodus 21.22–23 that the translator had some idea, principle, or presupposition in mind, which made him deliberately violate a
literal translation in favor of a more complex formulation."[60]

It is possible, moreover, to conjecture why this "more complex formulation" was preferred by the translator. Using *exeikonismenon*, the translator's literal rendering of verse 23 would be "If it be made in the image,
he shall give life for life." This implies that one who kills a fetus that is
already "made from the image" deserves death. But the translator must
have been aware of the fact that one of the Torah's six references to
being "made from the image" explicitly calls for the capital punishment
of a murderer on the grounds that he had destroyed a being "made
from the image": "Whoever sheds the blood of man, by man shall his
blood be shed; for in God's image did God make man."[61] It is, therefore, reasonable to deduce that the Septuagint translator, through the
employment of *exeikonismenon*, intended to create a link between feticide
and homicide by way of the "made from the image" formulation.[62]
As a result, "formation" became critical because it was only when the
fetus had attained a form that could be considered to be recognizably

[56] *Ibid.*, p. 98.
[57] R. Freund, "The Ethics of Abortion in Hellenistic Judaism," *Helios*, volume 10, number 2, 1983:
129–131.
[58] *Ibid.*   [59] *Ibid.*, 127–128.   [60] *Ibid.*, 128.   [61] Genesis 9:6.
[62] Freund, "Ethics of Abortion," 128–129. This link also would appear in later rabbinic literature.
See below, chapter 2, p. 52.

"in God's image" that it would be considered sufficiently human that its destruction would become the equivalent of homicide.

The nature of the impact of Hellenistic thought on this section of the Septuagint has been much discussed. The scholar Victor Aptowitzer contends that the Septuagint's portrayal of the status of the fetus effectively compromised between two schools of Greek philosophy, Plato (the Academy) and the Stoics. While the Stoics saw the fetus as being an integral part of the mother's womb, the Academy regarded it as an independent living being. Hence the compromise entailed viewing the fetus either as dependent or as independent, contingent upon formation.[63] Others have pointed to the similarities between the Septuagint's focus on the pivotal role of formation and Aristotelian thought which held that full human status was conferred at formation, since it was at that juncture that the soul was thought to infuse the body.[64]

But perhaps the most significant Hellenistic idea of all was to be found in the notion that the willful abortion of a formed fetus was to be considered one of the most serious transgressions imaginable, deserving of the death penalty. From a range of pagan and Hellenistic sources, Moshe Weinfeld, a prominent thinker in the field, has demonstrated that the Assyrian attitude of determined opposition to the woman who self-aborted was generally dominant in the Hellenistic world.[65] Thus, bringing about the loss of a fetus was cited regularly alongside witchcraft, murder, adultery, and theft as principal societal crimes.[66] In contrast to this strong stance against feticide, however, the Hellenistic world often legitimated a relaxed attitude of "complete lawlessness" to infanticide, especially for children who were in any way defective. Indeed, Aristotle

---

[63] V. Aptowitzer, "Observations on the Criminal Law of the Jews," *The Jewish Quarterly Review*, volume 15, 1924: 115–116.

[64] There was significant philosophical debate as to when formation occurred, with thirty, forty, and ninety days being suggested possibilities (see B. Jacob, *Exodus*, p. 655). Aristotle was of the view that the fetus possessed vegetative life at conception, received an animal soul several days later, and was endowed with a fully rational human soul forty days after conception for the male fetus and eighty days for the female (see D. L. Perry, "Abortion and Personhood: Historical and Comparative Notes," at http://www.home.earthlink.net/~davidlperry/abortion.htm [the publisher has endeavored to ensure that the URLs for external websites referred to in this book are correct and active at the time of going to press. However, the publisher has no responsibility for the websites and can make no guarantee that a site will remain live or that the content is or will remain appropriate]). In this section, however, the Septuagint provides no timing estimates and makes no gender distinctions.

[65] M. Weinfeld, "*Hamitat Ubar: Emdatah Shel Masoret Yisrael BeHashva'ah LeEmdat Amim Acherim*," *Zion*, volume 42, 1977: 129–142. Weinfeld quotes the Septuagint, Aristotle, the Didache (see below, p. 24), an inscription from Philadelphia in Asia Minor, the Hippocratic and other oaths, the letter of Barnabas, and Pseudo-Phocylides as representing this position.

[66] *Ibid.*, p. 134.

openly expressed limited support for infanticide in close proximity to his clearly stated rejection of the killing of the formed fetus.[67] This stark polarity of forceful resistance to the destruction of the formed fetus alongside a measure of acceptance of infanticide, conveys that the pagan and Hellenistic orientation in this regard was not rooted in a moral vision of the value of life, as such a vision might be perceived within contemporary Western civilization, but rather was rooted in a practical approach to the needs of society. The developing fetus needed to be protected for its economic, military, or communal value; the disabled child was a burden to be discarded. According to this understanding, despite the Septuagint's theological concerns with being "created in the image," opposition to abortion in the Hellenistic world had little ethical motivation, but saw fetal destruction as a "crime against state and society: [it represented] the loss of manpower and the diminution of community and family, and, for that reason, society was determined to punish transgressors."[68]

The Septuagint did not absorb all these aspects of Hellenistic philosophy. However, to ignore the remarkable resemblances between the Septuagint and the Greek philosophical setting and thereby to judge the difference between the Septuagint and the Masoretic texts as being simply the result of mistranslation or of chance interpretation is not intellectually tenable.[69] As in numerous other places, the Septuagint Hellenized the Exodus 21:22–25 text, in accordance with its goal of making biblical concepts more comprehensible to those who lived within an essentially Greek *Weltanschauung*. Small wonder, then, that one of the foremost Jewish scholars in this area would observe that the Septuagint "is not genuinely Jewish but must have originated in Alexandria under Egyptian-Greek influence."[70]

But if the Septuagintal-type manuscripts were not "genuinely Jewish" then this would have been genuinely startling to the dominant

---

[67] Aptowitzer, "Criminal Law," 99. Weinfeld, "*Hamitat Ubar*," xvi, 136. See especially Aristotle, *The Politics*, edited by S. Everson, Cambridge, Cambridge University Press, 1988, VII. 14, p. 182, who states: "As to the exposure and rearing of children, let there be a law that no deformed child shall live. But as to an excess in the number of children, if the established customs of the state forbid the exposure of any children who are born, let a limit be set to the number of children a couple may have; and if couples have children in excess, let abortion be procured before sense and life have begun . . ."

[68] Weinfeld, "*Hamitat Ubar*," 139.

[69] See E. R. Goodenough, *The Jurisprudence of the Jewish Courts in Egypt*, Amsterdam, Philo Press, 1968 (reprint of 1929 edition), p. 111, where it is stated that in the Septuagint version of Exodus 21:22–23 "the Greek mistranslates the Hebrew." While this is certainly true, it fails to highlight that what was at work here went beyond just the making of a mistake.

[70] Aptowitzer, "Criminal Law," 88.

figure of Alexandrian Jewry, Philo Judaeus (*c.* 20 BCE – *c.* 50 CE), who undoubtedly used these texts extensively in his erudite philosophic reconciliation of the worlds of Greek and Jewish thought. So thoroughly immersed in the Hellenistic milieu of his day was Philo that his voluminous writings also have been judged by Jewish history to be lacking in Jewish standing. Nevertheless, his profound loyalty to Judaism is unquestioned, and his philosophy clearly represented an attempt to cast Judaism within the mold of Hellenistic ideas, not to step outside the Jewish framework.[71]

In relation to Exodus 21:22–25, Philo took the ideas promulgated by the Septuagint text even further within his *De Specialibus Legibus*:

But if any one has a contest with a woman who is pregnant, and strike her a blow on her belly, and she miscarry, if the child which was conceived within her is still unfashioned and unformed, he shall be punished by a fine, both for the assault which he committed and also because he has prevented nature, who was fashioning and preparing that most excellent of creatures, a human being, from bringing him into existence. But if the child which was conceived had assumed a distinct shape in all its parts, having received all its proper connective and distinctive qualities, he shall die; for such a creature as that is a man, whom he has slain while still in the workshop of nature, who had not thought it as yet a proper time to produce him to the light, but had kept him like a statue lying in a sculptor's workshop, requiring nothing more than to be released and sent out into the world.[72]

Despite the fact that he was aware of the text that would ultimately become part of the Septuagint, in this passage Philo's eloquent prose displays some subtle, though significant, differences from the Septuagint translation.[73] To begin with, Philo seems to depart deliberately from the "two-person paradigm," in preference for that of a sole aggressor

---

[71] Sandmel, *Philo of Alexandria*, pp. 127–134.

[72] *The Works of Philo* (new updated edition, translated by C. D. Yonge), Peabody, Hendrickson Publishers, 1993, *De Specialibus Legibus* III.108–109, p. 605.

[73] Philo actually quotes the Septuagint text in a section of "The Preliminary Studies": "Therefore an indistinct and not clearly manifested conception resembles an embryo which has not yet received any distinct character or similitude within the womb: but that which is clear and distinctly visible, is like one which is completely formed, and which is already fashioned in an artistic manner as to both its inward and its outward parts, and which has already received its suitable character. And with respect to these matters the following law has been enacted with great beauty and propriety: 'If while two men are fighting one should strike a woman who is great with child, and her child should come from her before it is completely formed, he shall be muleted in a fine, according to what the husband of the woman shall impose on him, and he shall pay the fine deservedly. But if the child be fully formed, he shall pay life for life.'" See *The Works of Philo, De Congressu Quaerendae Eruditionis Studies*, 136–137, p. 316.

who is actually engaged in a "contest" with the pregnant woman.[74] This suggests that Philo is referring here to a blow that was purposeful, although the killing of the fetus may not have been the intended outcome.[75] Further, Philo does not make explicit to whom any moneys to be paid would be due, whereas both the Masoretic and Septuagint texts indicate that they would be due to the husband of the victim. The reason for this omission may be that Philo provides two grounds, "the assault" and "preventing nature," upon which one who kills an unformed fetus is fined. This led to speculation that he may be referring to two separate fines that were levied, only one of which was to go to the husband.[76]

But perhaps of greatest moment for the abortion discussion of later centuries, in both Jewish and non-Jewish circles, is Philo's explicit association of "formation" with the point at which the fetus becomes discernibly human in shape and being. Philo makes plain the reasoning that had been implicit within the Septuagint translation by conveying that when this particular juncture is reached, nature has done its essential work of fashioning human life and thereafter is simply incubating the creation until it is ready to emerge. It follows that the intentional killing of the fetus would be tantamount to murder from the moment that formation is achieved, and would be a crime worthy of the penalty of execution. This is consistent with Philo's stated view in the *Hypothetica* that, on pain of death, "no one shall cause the offspring of women to be abortive by means of miscarriage, or by any other contrivance."[77]

There can be little doubt that in arriving at these views Philo leaned heavily towards the Platonic outlook that the fetus was an independent being. This is well illustrated by Philo's understanding of the law of Leviticus 22:28, where the Torah commands that one should not kill an animal together with its young on the same day. Philo subsumes within this provision the instruction that one may not sacrifice a pregnant animal, asserting that Jewish law aims to protect the sensitivities of the animal as well as the vulnerable offspring, both outside and inside the womb.[78] Plainly, this law would hardly be relevant to a pregnant creature,

---

[74] While the Sumerian Laws, the Code of Hammurabi, the Middle Assyrian Laws and the Hittite Laws describe a pregnant woman being struck by a single aggressor, they do not describe it as being in the context of a struggle or "contest."

[75] The fact that the killing of the fetus may have been an accidental result of the "contest" does not appear, in Philo's presentation, to mitigate the consequences.

[76] S. Belkin, *Philo and the Oral Law*, Cambridge, MA, Harvard University Press, 1940, p. 130. Compare how Josephus has been understood to allude to two fines, below, p. 22.

[77] *The Works of Philo, Hypothetica* 7.7, p. 744. Though Philo does not restate here the distinction between a formed and an unformed fetus, he makes his opposition to abortion absolutely plain.

[78] *Ibid., De Virtutibus* 137, p. 653.

unless one held that the "young" fetus had independent standing. From this conclusion, Philo then argues for an extension of the same type of protection to human beings:

And it appears to me that some law-givers, having started from this point, have also promulgated the law about condemned women, which commands that pregnant women, if they have committed any offence worthy of death, shall nevertheless not be executed until they have brought forth, in order that the creature in their womb may not be slain with them when they are put to death.[79]

As will be seen, this position is diametrically opposed to the stance of the Talmud on this matter, which began from the same premise as did the Stoics, namely, that the fetus was a dependent component of its mother.[80]

There are other parts of Philo's writings, however, which appear to be more compatible with this Stoic doctrine of fetal dependence. In the continuation of *De Specialibus Legibus*, Philo opines:

And yet those persons who have investigated the secrets of natural philosophy say that those children which are still within the belly, and while they are still contained within the womb, are a part of their mothers; and the most highly esteemed of physicians . . . agree with them and say the same thing. But when the children are brought forth and are separated from that which is produced with them, and are set free and placed by themselves, they then become real living creatures, deficient in nothing which can contribute to the perfection of human nature, so that then, beyond all question, he who slays an infant is a homicide, and the law shows its indignation at such an action; not being guided by the age but by the species of the creature in whom its ordinances are violated.[81]

Philo, furthermore, describes animal fetuses as "parts of the mothers which have conceived them,"[82] in the context of his commentary on pregnant animals. In both these places, Philo seems to be directly contradicting his previously depicted stance. The offspring appears to remain a part of its mother so long as it is within the womb, and only once it has been born does it become a "real living creature, deficient in nothing."[83] These sources provide the impression that Philo might indeed have concurred that the fetus was not endowed with a fully independent status.

Was Philo "somewhat confused, if not plainly inconsistent"?[84] Was he simply unable to make up his mind as to the nature of the loss that would be sustained if a fetus were killed? It was certainly not indecision that

[79] *Ibid.*, 139, pp. 653–654.   [80] See below, chapter 2, pp. 32–33.
[81] *The Works of Philo, De Specialibus Legibus* III.117–118, p. 606.   [82] *Ibid., De Virtutibus* 138, p. 653.
[83] *Ibid.*   [84] I. Jakobovits, *Jewish Medical Ethics*, New York, Philosophical Library, 1959, p. 179.

characterized Philo's position in this area. In fact, if anything, Philo's apparent equivocation is emblematic of the same complex, blended outlook on the status of the fetus that was discerned in the Septuagint's effective compromise between the Academy's view of fetal independence and the Stoic view of dependence. While this mixed outlook is not evident in the Masoretic text, its echoes in later rabbinic literature[85] led Samuel Belkin to conclude that Philo's writings were not in the least paradoxical: as the unborn child is inherently physically dependent on the mother, while at the same time it has "the legal status of a human being by itself," it follows that "the passage of Philo which says that the unborn child is a part of the mother is not to be considered a contradiction to the passage in which he maintains that the formed foetus is treated like a living creature."[86] It seems correct, then, to assert that Philo's reference to the fetus as being part of its mother is used more as a physical evaluation, imparting the sense of an intertwined destiny of mother and offspring, rather than as a legal description. From an ethical and religious perspective, as well as for purposes of considering the legal consequences of causing the loss of a fetus, Philo can be taken to have been single-minded in viewing the formed fetus as an independent being.

For Philo, then, abortion of this formed, independent fetus would have been an anathema that his reading of the texts would have trenchantly opposed. In this respect he was fully in line with Hellenistic thought. But Philo's outlook diverged markedly from the Hellenistic environment when it came to infanticide. On this subject, Philo had no tolerance for the cavalier attitude of the Hellenistic philosophers and emphasized that infants at birth "become real living creatures, deficient in nothing which can contribute to the perfection of human nature, so that then, beyond all question, he who slays an infant is a homicide, and the law shows its indignation at such an action."[87] It is possible that Philo's rejection of feticide and his determination to frame it as so thoroughly repugnant to Jewish law were components of his strident opposition to the destruction of all early human life. If Jewish law is to take a determined stand against infanticide, the reasoning might have proceeded, then logically it must oppose the taking of life from the moment that "humanness" is recognized.[88] Whatever the reason, the composite nature of Philo's

[85] See below chapter 2, p. 44.   [86] Belkin, *Philo and the Oral Law*, pp. 132–133.
[87] *The Works of Philo, De Specialibus Legibus* III.117–118, p. 606 (as cited above).
[88] Indeed it is precisely this type of argument, pleading for the born creature by analogy to the unborn, that Philo employs in the case of sacrificing an animal with its young on the same day. See *The Works of Philo, De Virtutibus* 137–138, p. 653.

intellectual identity becomes readily apparent here. While in matters of abortion he assumed the classic Hellenistic position, mediated through the Septuagint, when it came to infanticide, he responded with classic Jewish revulsion.[89] Philo's position on abortion, then, although premised upon a clear moral regard for early human life, displays little of the concern for the life of the mother found in the traditional understanding of the Exodus text.[90]

In the concluding decades of the Second Temple period, another significant Jewish commentator addressed the issue of feticide: Josephus Flavius (*c.* 38 CE – *c.* 100 CE). Despite his Jewishness, Josephus' representation of Jewish positions has been treated with a degree of skepticism, because he had, in essence, gone over to the Roman side.[91] Regarding the killing of a fetus, Josephus seems to have taken a somewhat contradictory position on the seriousness of the loss. In *Antiquitates* he wrote: "He that kicks a woman with child so that she miscarries, let him pay a fine in money as the judges shall determine, as having diminished the population by the destruction of what was in her womb, and let money also be given the woman's husband by him."[92] In *Contra Apionem*, however, Josephus describes taking the life of a fetus as murder: "The law orders all offspring to be brought up and forbids women either to cause abortion or make away with the fetus; a woman convicted of this is considered a murderess, because she destroys a living creature, and diminishes the race."[93] The *Antiquitates* extract is reminiscent of Exodus 21:22–25, although it does not address the loss of the woman. But the lines from *Contra Apionem* are more akin to Philo, opposing both abortion and infanticide, albeit without reference to any differentiation between a formed and an unformed fetus. Two types of explanation have been supplied to account for the discrepancy between these two texts. The first considers *Contra Apionem* to be an explanation and an "apologetic" defense of actual, current Jewish practice against non-Jewish attacks on Judaism, and views the *Antiquitates* piece as an informational recounting of Mosaic law.[94] The second, conversely, maintains that *Contra Apionem* is

---

[89] The Jewish tradition has always regarded premeditated infanticide as a heinous transgression. For Jews, unlike for many other peoples, infanticide was "never socially accepted." See L. S. Milner, "A Brief History of Infanticide," at http://www.infanticide.org/history.htm.

[90] See below, chapter 2, p. 30.

[91] R. M. Seltzer, *Jewish People, Jewish Thought: The Jewish Experience in History*, New York, Macmillan Publishing Company Incorporated, 1980, pp. 178–179.

[92] Josephus, *Antiquitates* iv.278.   [93] Josephus, *Contra Apionem* ii.202.

[94] Weyl, *Die juedischen Strafgesetze bei Flavius Josephus*, pp. 50–52; Zipser, *Josephus Flavius Schrift gegen Apion*, pp. 164f.; both cited in Aptowitzer, "Criminal Law," 86–87, n. 117.

not representative of any Jewish practice but is an expression of Josephus' moral evaluation of abortion and should not be considered to be a re-statement of the law, whereas the *Antiquitates* text should be so regarded.[95] Hence, Freund holds that the rationale behind the *Contra Apionem* section is to explain the fine as being "not merely because of the loss of human life, but rather because the decision to terminate any life is one which lies with the state and not with the individual."[96]

Other explanations could be advanced. It is conceivable, for exam-ple, that Josephus was attempting to make a differentiation between the case of an induced miscarriage that is caused by an aggressor, in which the resultant harm could have been unintentional, and the instance of a woman who aborts her own fetus. In the Middle Assyrian Laws, the former case generally resulted in a fine, while the latter was the cause of repugnance and death for the perpetrator; Josephus may be trying to replicate this pattern by articulating a far more stringent standard for the woman who deliberately self-aborts. However, because Josephus de-veloped his ideas within the context of *Eretz Yisrael* (the Land of Israel),[97] although he probably was determined to declare his resistance to the killing of a fetus, particularly at the hands of its mother, in the strongest terms available, he nevertheless held that fining the responsible party was the appropriate penalty for fetal loss.

From the wording of his statement in *Antiquitates*, it seems logical to conclude that Josephus actually envisaged that the assailant would pay two fines, one to the woman's husband, and one "as the judges shall determine." It is quite possible that Josephus based this view on the confusing reading of Exodus 21:22–25 noted above, which called for a fine that was fixed by the husband, yet also required that the protagonist pay according to the order of judges.[98] Whatever its source, it is likely that it was a tradition known to Philo as well, for while nothing in the Septuagint text could be interpreted to call for such a double fine, Philo certainly appears to have been alluding to it in *De Specialibus Legibus*.[99] Belkin holds that this double fine, apparently known to Josephus, Philo, and ultimately the rabbis, was intended to compensate the husband, as head of the family, for the familial loss suffered by the destruction of the fetus, and the wife for the pain and suffering she incurred.[100] Thus,

---

[95] Aptowitzer, "Criminal Law," 86–87, n. 117.
[96] Freund, "Ethics of Abortion," 132. See also Jakobovits, *Jewish Medical Ethics*, p. 180.
[97] For more on the "Land of Israel" (*Eretz Yisrael*) milieu, see below, p. 23.
[98] See above, p. 6.   [99] See above, p. 18.
[100] Belkin, *Philo and the Oral Law*, pp. 136–139.

for Josephus, fetal loss was seen to demand compensation for a double injury, though it was presumably not to be regarded as murder.

In the closing years of the Second Jewish Commonwealth, therefore, it makes sense to speak of a "Palestinian and an Alexandrian point of view"[101] regarding the appropriate punishment for killing a fetus that had reached formation. Indeed, the divergence between the two has been shown to be stark. Answering the question whether the teachers of *Eretz Yisrael*[102] followed "the Alexandrians to their last conclusion, considering the killing of the child in the mother's womb as murder" Aptowitzer emphatically replies, "[t]his question should be negatived with certainty."[103] The Alexandrian point of view, most plainly articulated by Philo, held that the killing, either accidental or intentional, of a formed fetus represented the taking of life in much the same way as did infanticide, and the perpetrator deserved the death penalty. The *Eretz Yisrael* point of view – to which Josephus, particularly through his *Antiquitates* statement, was a witness – would be most explicitly articulated later in the Talmud,[104] and was largely unaffected by Hellenism and the extant Septuagintal texts. Hence, it never deviated far from the plain meaning of the Masoretic text of Exodus 21:22–25, and maintained that, since the fetus was not designated a *nefesh*, the accidental killing of a formed fetus called for no greater punishment than the killing of an unformed fetus; it required compensation through the payment of fines. As to the abortion debate's central interest in intentional fetal destruction, the *Eretz Yisrael* point of view began with indirect data from the *Tanakh*: nowhere was the fetus described as a *nefesh*, and the death penalty, which was mandatory for murder, was only applied to one who intentionally took the life of an individual already born.[105]

With the destruction of the Second Temple by the Romans and the ascendancy of rabbinic Judaism, it would not be long before the Alexandrian point of view would disappear from the operative legal framework of the Jewish people. Vestiges of its ideas would surface in the Talmud,[106] and it would leave traces among the sectarian Samaritans and Karaites.[107] But, for all practical purposes, as the rabbinic period unfolded, the Alexandrian point of view – which was once the outlook

[101] Aptowitzer, "Criminal Law," 89.
[102] The "*Eretz Yisrael*" or "Palestinian" point of view is a shorthand representation. It also would have included the scholars of Babylonia.
[103] Aptowitzer, "Criminal Law," 111. See also Belkin, *Philo and the Oral law*, p. 133.
[104] See below, chapter 2.   [105] Genesis 9:5–6; Exodus 21:12ff.; Numbers 35:31.
[106] See below, chapter 2, p. 34.   [107] Aptowitzer, "Criminal Law," 85–86.

that had been adhered to by the largest Jewish community in the world –
evaporated from Jewish life.

There were two major reasons for the demise of the Alexandrian
approach. The first was that the Philonic-Alexandrian outlook became
the perspective more closely associated with nascent Christianity. Seeing
early Christians embrace the Septuagint as their "Old Testament," made
Jews regard it as less and less suitable for Jewish purposes. Indeed, the
unprecedented religious demands of the Common Era ensured a parting of the ways: "The Jews needed a translation in accord with the
new dominant rabbinic approach to Judaism; the Christians sought one
that would mirror their interpretation of the Hebrew Scriptures."[108]
It comes as no surprise, therefore, that despite the Jewish origins of
both the Septuagint and the works of Philo, the Church would ultimately become the vehicle for the preservation of both sets of texts for
posterity.

In terms of abortion there can be no doubt that the Septuagint would
provide a critical foundation for Christian attitudes on the subject.[109] The
Didache, an early guidebook to Christianity for pagan converts, followed
the Septuagint in regarding the killing of a fetus as murder.[110] Perhaps
even more significantly, major Christian thinkers from the first centuries
of the Common Era, such as Tertullian and Augustine, used the Septuagint as the basis for the view that the killing of a formed fetus was
homicide, deserving of the most severe punishment. Considerable debate ensued among early Christian theologians as to whether formation
should play a central role in determining the punishment for fetal destruction. Some thought that it ought to be completely disregarded, and
there were those, like the fourth-century St. Basil the Great, who seemed
inclined to deem the matter moot,[111] since abortion was generally seen
to be a "serious sin" both before and after formation.[112] The majority,
however, apparently followed Augustine and Gregory in determining
homicide to be a certainty only after formation.[113] It is beyond question, therefore, that the categories at the core of the Septuagint and the

---

[108] L. H. Schiffman, *From Text to Tradition: A History of Second Temple and Rabbinic Judaism*, Hoboken,
Ktav Publishing House Incorporated, 1991, p. 94.
[109] On the influence of the notion of ensoulment on early Christian thought, see below, chapter 2,
pp. 40–41.
[110] Aptowitzer, "Criminal Law," 85, n. 113.
[111] According to St. Basil, "[w]hoever purposely destroys a fetus incurs the penalty of murder. We
do not ask precisely whether it is formed or not formed . . ."; G. Grisez, *Abortion: The Myths, the
Realities and the Arguments*, New York, Corpus Books, 1970, p. 142.
[112] Grisez, *Abortion*, p. 150.   [113] Riddle, *Contraception and Abortion*, pp. 20–21.

Philonic approaches to abortion pervaded and molded initial Christian deliberations on the subject.

The second, and probably more significant, reason for the decline related to the Hellenization of the Philonic and Alexandrian forms of Judaism. As has been shown, there is little doubt that the Septuagintal texts represented an adaptation of the biblical source that diverged far more profoundly from the Hebrew original than did the Masoretic texts used by the rabbis.[114] Since Judaism, at times throughout its history, has substantially accommodated itself to surrounding cultures, this actuality, in and of itself, would not have been fatal to the Alexandrian position. However, the rabbis, who became the predominant force in shaping the Judaism that succeeded the Temple, ordained that the normative Jewish path was the one that grappled with the more original Masoretic texts together with their *Eretz Yisrael* exegesis. Samuel Sandmel, an expert in the period, has written of Philo that "[i]f we ascribe Jewishness to the Rabbis alone, then Philo is essentially not Jewish."[115] This, in essence, would become the fate of the Alexandrian point of view. The rabbis, having taken the Palestinian approach to be the quintessential expression of Jewish thought, left the Alexandrian stance without Jewish status.

The fact, however, that Jewish perspectives on fetal loss became focused increasingly on the *Eretz Yisrael* tradition, founded in the Masoretic text, and distanced themselves both from the Hellenized views of early Christianity and the Hellenistic-Jewish position of Alexandria, was more than just a demarcation of Judaism from other groups. It stood for the repudiation of an attitude that unequivocally held the fetus to be a separate human life and its destruction to be murder. It enunciated the rejection of an outlook that, in large measure, had been formed because of society's utilitarian interests in ensuring fetal survival. Concerned with Divine and moral – rather than in societal – interests,[116] the Jewish approach preserved fundamental characteristics from the time when Exodus first distinguished itself from the other ancient Near Eastern texts. It was a philosophy that was sustained within Judaism principally because it came to be viewed as a more righteous path than the alternatives.

In excess of a thousand years had passed since the Divine revelation perceived by the Jewish people had begun to be transmitted in its carefully structured form. Like many other sections of that unique composition, the verses of Exodus 21:22–25 introduced new ideas that would prove

---

[114] See above, pp. 12–13.   [115] Sandmel, *Philo of Alexandria*, p. 134.
[116] Weinfeld, "*Hamitat Ubar*," 139.

to have profound importance in differentiating the Israelites from their surrounding milieu. Chief among them, and the notion that would later serve as the foundation stone of the abortion viewpoints within Judaism, was the apparent distinction created by Exodus 21:22–25 between the value of a pregnant woman and her fetus. The Torah, oriented towards the value of life as its primary moral concern, placed a premium on the extant life of the pregnant woman that it did not extend to the developing fetus. This distinction, maintained by the teachers of *Eretz Yisrael*, ultimately would become a pivotal Jewish perspective as the early centuries of the Common Era unfolded.

Those first centuries spanned the emergence of rabbinic Judaism and, with it, a period of scholarly elucidation and chronicling of Jewish legal knowledge that was without precedent. This reality would prove to be a significant spur towards articulating a coherent stance on abortion. For though the pre-rabbinic texts had intimated both that the fetus was not a *nefesh*, and that Judaism held the life of the mother to be of elevated status compared to that of her unborn offspring, little detailing of the status of fetal life, or of the permissibility for intentional abortion had been forthcoming. A full discussion of these matters would prove essential to forming Jewish attitudes to abortion; their construal would fall to the rabbis of the Talmudic age and their descendants to specify and make explicit. Among the most significant of the questions to be addressed would be: if the fetus were not a *nefesh*, then what was its standing, and what, if any, implications did this have for the act of bringing its existence to an end?

CHAPTER 2

Evaluating life: rabbinic perspectives on fetal standing

The rabbinic framework pertaining to fetal existence was already largely
shaped by the time the *Mishnah* and *midrashic* texts came to be recorded
in the second and third centuries of the Common Era. In many ways, it
was a structure which served to enlarge and extend the plain meaning of
the Exodus text. The *Tannaïm*, inheritors of the *Eretz Yisrael* approach,[1]
simply continued the legal tradition that regarded the killing of the fetus
as a tort rather than a homicide. They did so, not just in circumstances
such as those depicted in Exodus 21:22–23, but in every context that a
Jew might encounter.

   The *Mishnah* pointedly declares that – among a range of other legal conditions that begin only at birth – one who kills a one-day-old
baby, presumed to be full-term, is criminally liable and deserves the
death penalty; the fetus, however, is not included within this provision.[2]
It is true that there was a *Tannaïtic* view that regarded all fetuses as
being in a state of "doubtful viability." Unless it could be established
that a full nine-month pregnancy had been completed, this condition
continued until the baby came to be regarded as a *bar kayamah*, a viable being, at thirty days after birth.[3] The "doubtful viability" designation must have buttressed the argument against feticide being deemed

---

[1] The age of the *Tannaïm* stretched from the beginning of the Common Era until 220 CE. The age
of the *Amoraïm* followed, lasting from 220 CE until the end of the fourth century CE in the Land
of Israel, and until the end of the fifth century CE in Babylon. See M. Elon (ed.), *The Principles of
Jewish Law*, Jerusalem, Keter Publishing, 1975, pp. 16–17.
[2] *M. Niddah* 5:3. *M. Niddah* 5:1 discusses the fetus in a different context, so it cannot be concluded
that the fetus was simply inadvertently omitted from 5:3. Rather, as the *Gemara* (*Niddah* 44b)
explains it, the definition of homicide is established at one place in the Torah (Leviticus 24:17)
as "if one strikes any *nefesh adam*," meaning if one strikes – and kills – a *nefesh adam* of any age.
Nevertheless, as has been seen, and as the *Rishonim* would repeat (Rashi, *Tosafot* to *Niddah* 44a s.v.
ihu, *Yad Ramah* and *Meïri* to *Sanhedrin* 72b; *Ramban* in *Chiddushim* to *Niddah* 44b), the fetus is not a
nefesh until birth and, hence, its destruction could not be considered homicide.
[3] *Niddah* 44b. The law that one does not mourn a child who has not survived thirty days stems from
this "doubtful viability" provision. See *Sh. Ar. Y. D.* 344:8. See also *Shabbat* 136a.

27

homicide.[4] Nevertheless, the "doubtful viability" doctrine carried with it the risk of the law blurring the distinction between the unborn and the born.[5] Left unqualified, the inference might be gleaned that one who takes the life of a *nefel* (a born child of doubtful viability) commits non-criminal infanticide in the same way that one who takes the life of a fetus commits non-criminal feticide.

Perhaps as a consequence of this risk, the Talmudic discussion coalesces around the absence of the "full person" status of a fetus rather than its lack of viability. Given that the fetus was not designated as a *nefesh* or an *adam*[6] (human) or an *ish*[7] (man), and was, therefore, without any legal standing as a "person," the category of murder was altogether inapplicable. Though the *Tannaïm* never actually provided a reasoned defense of this position, it might be assumed that the Torah's disavowal of feticide as a capital crime must have contained a sufficiently compelling logic that the early rabbis saw no need to question it.

It is predictable, then, that the *Midrash* explicitly reiterates that feticide is a crime that calls for a monetary penalty. The *Mekilta de-Rabbi Ishmael*, a *midrashic* work from the second century CE, provides a rich resource of insights into Exodus 21:22–23 for the *Eretz Yisrael* approach inherited by the *Tannaïm*. Although, in typical *midrashic* fashion, a range of alternative possible explanations are proposed for the difficulties raised by the Exodus verses, the rabbinic conclusions are essentially unequivocal. Thus, the *Tannaïm* reject the suggestion that anybody but the pregnant woman could be the victim of the *ason*.[8] Potential alternative targets are

[4] There are texts that support this view. The *Mekilta*, for example, records: "What then is the purpose of saying: 'And if men strive together?' Because it says: 'And he that smiteth anybody mortally . . . [Leviticus 24:17],' which I might understand to mean even if he kills a child born after only eight months of pregnancy. Therefore, it says: 'And if men strive together,' thereby telling us that one is not guilty of death unless he kills a viable child" (*Mekilta de-Rabbi Ishmael, Masekhet Nezikin*, chapter 8, p. 63). Later scholars would also use "doubtful viability" extensively for somewhat different purposes. See below, chapter 3, pp. 90–91, chapter 4, pp. 97–98. Aptowitzer, "Criminal Law," 111 ff., uses "doubtful viability" together with "not a *nefesh*" to explain the absence of capital culpability for the aggressor.
[5] See *Sanhedrin* 84b and *Shabbat* 135b. At *Sanhedrin* 84b, see particularly the clarification of *Tosafot* at *hakhi garsinan*.
[6] *M. Niddah* 5:3 lists a range of conditions that, while applicable to the *adam*, do not include the fetus. Clear evidence that the fetus is not considered an *adam* is found in the *Gemara, Niddah* 44a, which ruled that "a boy one day old is subject to the uncleanness of leprosy, since it is written, 'When an *adam* shall have in the skin of his flesh (Leviticus 13:2),' implying an *adam* of any age." The Talmud's most extreme example of an "*adam* of any age" is the one-day old, but the fetus is not included. While some independent views can be found which place the fetus within the category of *adam*, the *Netziv, HaEmek Sheëilah*, Jerusalem, 1948–53, volume III, p. 65, 167:17, has shown that the overwhelming majority view is that the fetus is not an *adam*.
[7] *Tosafot* to *Niddah* 43b, s.v. *umetamei be-negaïm*, where the *Tosafists* explain that the term *ish* is used specifically in order to exclude the fetus.
[8] *Mekilta de-Rabbi Ishmael, Masekhet Nezikin*, chapter 8, p. 65.

swiftly dismissed,[9] and the rabbis state definitively, "[W]hen it says 'No harm follows,' it must mean to the woman only; 'He shall surely be fined,' for the children."[10] Hence, they conclude that if no *ason* occurred, then "compensation for causing a miscarriage" is payable to the husband of the pregnant woman, insofar as he is the natural father of the fetus, and the appropriate amount should be reckoned by the judges.[11] If an *ason* does occur, there is at least one *midrashic* opinion that, while conceding that "there is no proof for this," holds that Genesis 42:38 implies that "*ason*" can only be meant to signify the death of the woman,[12] and so "*nefesh tachat nefesh*" is the appropriate outcome.

The *Tannaïm*, furthermore, underscore the accidental nature of the *ason* by determining that the men were actually bent on killing each other, not the pregnant woman. This leads them to confront the question: if the woman is killed, is the existence of the intent of the men to kill each other – although not to kill her – sufficient legal basis to warrant that the attacker should pay with his life for her death?[13] *Sanhedrin* 79a–b provides a most lucid insight into the rabbinic deliberations on this matter:

All is well according to the rabbis, who maintain that if he intended killing one man and killed another, he is liable. For it is written, "If men strive and hurt a woman with child [Exodus 21:22]"; whereupon Eleazar observed: "The verse refers to attempted murder, because it is written, 'And if any *ason* follow, then you shall give life for life [Exodus 21:23].'" But how does Rabbi Simeon interpret "you shall give life for life"? – It refers to monetary compensation, in harmony with Rabbi's [interpretation]. For it has been taught: Rabbi said: "Then you shall give life for life"; this refers to monetary compensation. You say monetary compensation; but perhaps this is not so, life being literally meant? "Giving" [*ve-natatah*] is stated below; and "giving" is also stated above: just as the latter refers to money, so the former too.

Rabbi is clearly of the view, so well explained by Benno Jacob,[14] that the double use of *ve-natatah* must indicate financial compensation for the loss of the woman, just as it does for the fetus.

---

[9] *Ibid*. One suggestion is that the *ason* might have happened to both the woman *and* her offspring. If this were the case, then the Exodus text would convey: "If men fight, and they push a pregnant woman and she miscarries her children, but no injury occurs [to the woman or children], the one responsible shall surely be fined . . ." This led the rabbis to the humorous observation that "If you should interpret it thus – then the husband would even have to pay for the services of a midwife."

[10] *Ibid*., p. 66.

[11] *Ibid*. The rabbis do not propose that a double penalty should be paid, as suggested by Philo and Josephus.

[12] *Ibid*. [13] *Ibid*., pp. 62–63. See also *M. Sanhedrin* 9:2. [14] See above, chapter 1, p. 7.

However, others among the sages plainly thought that, notwithstanding the fact that the woman's death was unintended, the killer, in fact, was guilty of a criminal act and, perhaps, should pay with his life.[15] Further on in the *Mekilta* this same conflicting outlook is again demonstrated; the anonymous view that "it is with life that he must pay for life; he cannot pay for life with money," is almost immediately followed by Rabbi's declaration that *nefesh tachat nefesh* means "monetary compensation."[16] Rashi would later summarize the lack of rabbinic unanimity on this topic:

> Our Rabbis differ on this matter. There are those who say that it actually signifies "life," and there are those who say that it means monetary compensation but not literally life, since he who intends to kill a certain person and instead [inadvertently] kills someone else, is exempt from the death penalty, and has to pay to his heirs his value, as though he were sold in the market.[17]

Those rabbis who thought that the woman's death is worthy of capital punishment arguably read the plain meaning of *nefesh tachat nefesh* differently from the way that Benno Jacob maintains that it always was understood.[18] A possible explanation of why they did so is the one discerned by Greenberg in a similar dilemma within the Toraitic treatment of homicide. As human life is invaluable, it follows that it can never be compensated monetarily; thus, capital punishment is the only appropriate sentence for homicide. But the death penalty involves the further taking of life. Although it is for a legitimate purpose, capital punishment nevertheless challenges the supreme value ascribed to human life. Greenberg concludes: "Yet the paradox must not blind us to the judgment of value that the law sought to embody."[19] Similarly, these rabbis' understanding of Exodus 21 as a call for capital punishment can be seen as a powerful reminder of the supreme legal standing of life. If the woman dies, given that it was not an intentional killing, the paradoxical problem exists that a *nefesh* has been lost; her life cannot be recompensed merely with money. Conversely, the killing is an inadvertent act; it can only be recompensed with money. Effectively, here too the sages focused attention upon the critical "judgment of value that the law sought to embody."

---

[15] Sinclair, "Legal Basis," 110–111. It is worth noting that at this point in Jewish history the death penalty was a theoretical issue, which, in practice, could not be enforced by the rabbis. Nevertheless, the penalty remained an important consideration not just for its powerful symbolic value, but because the potential for its practical revival could not be wholly discounted.

[16] *Mekilta de-Rabbi Ishmael*, p. 67. The notion that *nefesh tachat nefesh* refers to monetary compensation is a singular view, and is always attributed to Rabbi. See *Sanhedrin* 79a and 87b and *Hagigah* 11a.

[17] Rashi to Exodus 21:23 at "*Ve-natatah nefesh tachat nefesh.*"

[18] See above, chapter 1, p. 7.   [19] Greenberg, "Some Postulates," pp. 24–27.

In actuality, however, it seems that the later *halakhah* followed neither the view of the sages nor that of Rabbi, but rather that of *Bei Chizkiyah* as quoted by Rava on *Sanhedrin* 79b:

> Just as in the case of one who kills an animal, you draw no distinction between an unwitting or a deliberate act . . . not acquitting him of it, but imposing monetary liability; so in the case of killing a man you must draw no distinction between an unwitting and a deliberate act . . . not imposing monetary liability, but acquitting him of it . . . But if he is liable for death, surely it is unnecessary to teach that he is not liable to make compensation? Hence it follows that he is liable neither to execution nor to make compensation.

Bei Chizkiyah's approach holds that if the death penalty cannot be applied, monetary compensation is inappropriate in such a case. As one of the foremost Talmudists, Rabbi Adin Steinsaltz, explains:

> The essence of *Chizkiyah*'s system is that when a person commits a crime which contains room for guilt of a capital nature – whether the laws of capital cases are applicable in this instance or whether there is no possibility of applying such laws – since this transgression subsumes an element of the law of death, he is not liable for any compensation in this matter. There are those who say whether the act was deliberate or unintentional he is not liable for any monetary damages caused to others in the course of this serious transgression for which he [in theory] is obligated for his life . . .[20]

Chizkiyah's philosophy, therefore, is that monetary compensation is unthinkable for a capital crime, even in cases where the death penalty cannot be applied because the killer did not intend to kill the woman. Neither penalty is the right solution.[21] Walking in *Chizkiyah*'s footsteps, therefore, the *halakhic* tendency was to join the sages rather than Rabbi insofar as the sages upheld the Torah's plain meaning in demanding something greater than monetary compensation as a suitable recompense for this crime. The dominant view that emerged, then, is that the woman's loss could not be compensated monetarily, in large measure because her death represented the demise of a *nefesh* who was as precious as life itself. The loss of the fetus, by contrast, was regarded as nothing more than a property privation, which, though it deserved financial

---

[20] *Sanhedrin* 79b. *Steinsaltz Talmud*, Jerusalem, 1984, p. 350, see "*shitat Chizkiyah*," in the "*Iyunim*" section.
[21] Later scholars adopt this view: *Hilkhot Rotzeiach* 4:1 exempts the killer who intended to kill someone else from monetary compensation as well as from death. Me'iri *ad loc.* explains it this way as well: as long as an individual commits a capital crime – homicide of the woman – then even though he is exempt from the death penalty, since he did not intend to kill her, he also is exempt from monetary liability.

restitution, was not to be accounted as anything akin to the value of a full human person.

Thus the rabbis affirmed the Torah's powerful distinction between the legal status of a mother and her fetus. The affirmation of this distinction, however, ought not to be construed as a minimization of the fetus' status, much less as any type of warrant for feticide. Indeed, the rabbinic understanding of this unequal status sometimes has been associated incorrectly with the later Talmudic utilization of the principle *ubar yerekh imo*[22] (the fetus is [considered as if it were] a limb of its mother). This occasionally led to the inference that the fetus was a radically subordinated "part," that was totally incomparable in stature to a born human. *Ubar yerekh imo*, though, was never intended to convey diminished fetal status, and the actual instances in which the Talmud uses *ubar yerekh imo* are not life-and-death situations. Rather, the principle is employed, for both animals and humans, in a variety of lesser contexts. It is invoked, for example, to show that the fetus of a purchased animal belongs to the buyer,[23] or to demonstrate that states of ritual impurity are transferred to unborn offspring,[24] or to show that a fetus is considered converted to Judaism as an outgrowth of its mother's conversion.[25] *Ubar yerekh imo* was not, however, a principle that was applied automatically under all conditions, and its use was designed for those situations in which legal changes or decrees that affected the mother were also made applicable to the fetus.[26]

Ubar yerekh imo, then, was not utilized in such a way as to make any definitive statement about the merit or the status of the fetus. Still the idea's prominence led the rabbinic scholar Ephraim Urbach to observe that "[a]mong the *Tannaïm* we do not find anyone who upholds, in the field of *Halakha*, the view that the embryo, while still in its mother's womb, is a separate body, and regards it as a[n independent] living being."[27] It is worth noting that while Urbach narrows his focus to the "field of *Halakha*," there is Talmudic evidence that at least one *Tanna* did espouse the contrary position: "Rabbi Eleazar holds the same view as Rabbi Yochanan...that the embryo is not its mother's thigh."[28] Nevertheless,

---

[22] The Latin counterpart, which was a part of Roman law, was *pars viscerum matris*. See sources in E. Westermarck, *The Origin and Development of the Moral Ideas*, New York, Macmillan Company, volume 1, 1906, p. 415, nn. 8 and 9. *Ubar yerekh imo* does not appear in *Tannaïtic* sources, and is usually an anonymous formula of the Talmud. See Urbach, *The Sages*, p. 794, n. 93.

[23] *Baba Kamma* 78a.   [24] *Nazir* 51a.   [25] *Yevamot* 78a–b.

[26] E. Ellinson, "*HaUbar BaHalakhah*," *Sinai*, volume 66, 1969: 27–29.

[27] Urbach, *The Sages*, p. 243.

[28] *Temurah* 19a. For the *Amoraïc* development of this outlook, see below, p. 44.

there can be little doubt that fetal dependence was the predominant theme among the *Tannaïm*. However, the reality of dependence alone is hardly determinative of any particular attitude to feticide. After all, those who, like Philo, were of the opinion that the formed fetus was to be regarded as a legally independent being considered a deliberate act of feticide as murder. The converse, however, was not true. Those who, like the *Tannaïm*, regarded the fetus as a dependent being, did not necessarily look upon feticide with indifference. Dependence, by itself, revealed nothing about whether or not it was acceptable – under any circumstances – to kill the fetus. All it implied was that, unlike those who were committed to fetal independence from the moment of formation, the *Tannaïm* were open to the possibility that feticide might be condoned in specific situations.

Clues that speak a little more directly to the rabbinic attitude concerning the real value to be accorded to the fetus, and the seriousness with which its loss might be regarded, can be found in the several Talmudic sources that deal with the fetus at different stages during pregnancy. In the Talmudic tractate *Yevamot* the rabbis discuss a case relating to the earliest weeks of fetal existence:

Mishnah: The daughter of a priest who has relations with an Israelite continues to eat *terumah* [the priestly tithe]; if she becomes pregnant, she may no longer eat it.

Gemara: If a priest's daughter were married to an Israelite who died, she may immerse and eat *terumah* the same evening! Rav Hisda said: "She should immerse herself and then eat *terumah* until the fortieth day after conception, for if she was then found not to be pregnant then she never was pregnant, and if she was found to be pregnant, it is considered to be mere water until the fortieth day."[29]

The *Tannaïtic* position, as recorded in the passage from the *Mishnah*, plainly articulates the view that whereas sexual relations with an Israelite did not prevent a priest's daughter from eating *terumah*, pregnancy certainly did. The problem, of course, was that it could not be known for some time whether or not the intercourse had made her pregnant. So long as the matter remained in doubt, was she permitted to eat *terumah*? The *Gemara* answers the question by ruling that if a priest's daughter were married to an Israelite who on their wedding day cohabited with her and then died, she could eat *terumah* on the evening of his death, notwithstanding the fact that she might indeed be pregnant. Rav Hisda

[29] *Yevamot* 69b.

provides the rationale for the decision: until the fortieth day the contents of her womb were considered to be "mere fluid," apparently of insufficient consequence to merit recognition for purposes of considering her truly to be "with child," or to disqualify her from the consumption of *terumah*. Rav Hisda seems to be suggesting, then, that until the fortieth day the developing embryo ought to be considered to possess relatively little legal value.

In the Hellenistic world, of course, day forty had been the most regularly proposed juncture at which formation was said to have taken place. Moreover, day forty was the point at which, according to Aristotle, the male human soul was infused.[30] In this context, it is significant that, immediately after Rav Hisda's observations in the *Gemara*, Abaye is quoted as having said to him: "If so [that before the fortieth day she is not legally to be regarded as pregnant] the final clause [of the *Mishnah*] should be read as: 'If the fetus in her womb is recognizable (*hukar*), she is considered retroactively to have committed an offense [by continuing to eat *terumah*]...' "[31] The rabbinic focus on the fortieth day, combined with Abaye's use of the term *hukar*, cannot help but evoke powerful echoes of the notion of formation, which clearly still had reverberations within the ongoing Jewish tradition.

If anything, the *Tannaïm* made this continuing connection between the fortieth day and the achievement of human form even more explicit within *Mishnah Niddah*:

> If a woman miscarried on the fortieth day, she need not consider it childbirth; but if on the forty-first day, she must continue her periods [of ritual impurity and purity as] for both a male and a female and as for a menstruant. Rabbi Ishmael ruled: "If she [miscarried on] the forty-first day she continues [her periods of ritual impurity and purity as] for a male and as for a menstruant, but if on the eighty-first day she continues [these periods as] for a male and a female and a menstruant; because a male is completely fashioned on the forty-first day and a female on the eighty-first day." The sages, however, maintain that both the creation of the male and the creation of the female are one and the same, each lasting forty-one days.[32]

Close to a millennium after this passage was written, Rashi, commenting on the words "she need not consider it childbirth," would yet make the observation, "for its form is not completed until the conclusion of all forty days."[33] By declaring that the statutory waiting-periods for ritual impurity that applied to childbirth were not operative prior to the conclusion

---

[30] See above, chapter 1, p. 15, n. 64.   [31] *Yevamot* 69b.   [32] *M. Niddah* 3:7.
[33] Rashi to *Niddah* 30a, s.v. *ainah chosheshet le-valad*.

of forty days, the sages confirmed the impression that before this point the fetus was not regarded as possessing the same substantive human-like standing as it would attain thereafter. It is reasonable to assume that the thinking behind this determination was influenced by ideas similar to those that produced the Hellenistic view which determined that the process of creating full human form was brought to fruition at the end of the fortieth day.

The heirs of the *Eretz Yisrael* approach, then, had not been left altogether untouched by the spirit of the Septuagint. Yet, contrary to Philo and to Christianity, the rabbis never chose to elevate the significance of the fortieth day beyond the issues of *terumah* and *tum'ah*. As the attainment of complete human form never inclined the Talmudic authorities toward declaring the fetus a *nefesh* at day forty, fetal standing, from the perspective of criminal sanctions which might be applied for feticide, remained unaffected by the supposed finalizing of the fully human form. Despite the fact that the rabbis maintained that feticide required a financial penalty, both before and after day forty, the *Yevamot* and *Niddah* texts certainly established grounds for perceiving the loss of a fetus younger than forty days to be an event of comparatively minor moment.

After forty days of gestation had passed, however, fetal status was generally seen in a wholly different light. In the *Gemara* to tractate *Niddah*, by way of illustration, fetal existence seems to be depicted as having almost ultimate significance:

Our Rabbis [*Tannaïm*] taught: "During the first three months [of pregnancy], sexual intercourse is injurious to the woman and it is also injurious to the child. During the middle ones it is injurious to the woman and beneficial for the child. During the last ones it is beneficial for the woman and beneficial for the child, for from it the child becomes well formed and of strong vitality." One [*Tanna*] taught: "He who engages in sexual intercourse on the ninetieth day is as though he had shed blood." But how could one know [that it was the ninetieth day]? "Rather," said Abaye, "one proceeds with sexual intercourse, and 'the Lord preserves the simple [Psalms 116:6].' "[34]

Setting aside the medical soundness of the rabbis' observations on sexual relations during pregnancy, it is evident that insofar as injury is deemed possible in these circumstances, one who deliberately engages in intercourse when harm to the fetus is still thought to be possible is seen as behaving in a manner tantamount to a killer. While rabbinic hyperbole is in evidence here – as opposed to any real reference to a capital crime – the

[34] *Niddah* 31a.

implication is nevertheless plain: the fetus, by day ninety and presumably at any point subsequent to day forty, is no longer to be viewed as "mere fluid," but had attained sufficient status that an intentional injury to it could be denounced in terms of spilling blood, the loss of the life force itself. The passage even seems to suggest that day ninety represents some type of qualitative turning point in the pregnancy, a position supported by the notion that it is at this point that movement of the fetus becomes discernible to the mother.[35] Unlike day forty, however, no definitive, practical change in the fetus is described at this juncture. Moreover, once again the rabbis do not seek to formulate any legal conclusions from this apparent enhancement of fetal standing. It is plain, however, that the welfare of this developing being – by the end of the first trimester – had become worthy of their pivotal concern and determined rhetorical calls for protection.

   Though these issues of timing attest to the gravity with which the rabbis might have beheld an act of feticide at a given point during pregnancy, they cannot, of course, be said specifically to have permitted or forbidden feticide. Elsewhere, however, the rabbis were more direct. Within the *halakhic* language of the *Mishnah*, the *Tannaïm* provide two relevant sources. The first text addressing the act of feticide more directly is the classic *Mishnah* text from *Ohalot*, which graphically describes an act of feticide in circumstances in which the mother's life is at stake, in contrast to the accidental miscarriage depicted in Exodus 21:22–25:

If a woman suffers hard labor, the fetus is cut up in her womb, and taken out limb by limb, for her life (*chaiyeiha*) comes before its life (*chaiyav*); if the majority of it has [already] come out, it must not be touched, for the [claim of one] life (*nefesh*) can not supersede [that of another] life (*nefesh*).[36]

Although the *Mishnah*'s use of the term *chaiyav* seems to denote an acknowledgment that the fetus is indeed to be considered a living entity, the *Tannaïm*, consistent with previous Jewish positions, regard it as a living entity whose claim to life is secondary to that of its mother, at least when her life is at stake. Within *Mishnah Ohalot*, however, they go even further: they utilize the assertion of the mother's superior status as a sufficient reason for feticide when the destruction of the fetus is the only way to save the mother's life. Thus, until the moment of birth, when it emerges to the air,[37] the fetus is not only not designated as a *nefesh*, but

35 *Niddah* 8b.   36 *M. Ohalot* 7:6.
37 The *Mishnah* clearly envisages that the moment of birth is when "the majority" of the baby has been born (*yatzah rubo*) – see *Mishnah Niddah* 3:5. Elsewhere, the Talmud makes this moment

feticide is deemed a positive requirement if it is the only way to save an imperiled woman in labor.

The *Tannaïm* further underscore the distance between the treatment of a fetus and that of a full *nefesh* in an altogether different circumstance in *Mishnah Arakhin*: "The execution of a pregnant woman who is condemned to death is not postponed until after she gives birth. But once she is on the birthstool, the execution is postponed until after she gives birth."[38] The *Mishnah*'s view on this matter is obviously diametrically opposed to Philo's position on the same question.[39] While Philo opts to delay any execution until after the birth has taken place, the *Eretz Yisrael* point of view only considers the separate concern of the fetus as a differentiated being when the process of parturition has begun. As the *Gemara* would later explain, once the unborn child has moved from its place in the womb, it is held to be a *gufah acharinah* (separate body),[40] with interests that have to be taken into account independently of the mother. The *Tannaïm* elaborate upon their commitment to execution until the onset of labor within a *midrashic* source:

I might have thought that if she were pregnant they would postpone [the execution] until she gave birth. Therefore, the Bible teaches, "He that smote him shall surely be put to death." I might have thought that if she were three months pregnant, they should not postpone [the execution] until she gives birth; but if she were nine months pregnant, they should postpone [the execution] until she has given birth. Therefore, Scripture teaches: "he shall surely be put to death."[41]

Thus, a woman sentenced to capital punishment was not to have her execution delayed out of consideration for the life of the fetus at any point during pregnancy, even if she had completed nine months of gestation

more precise by declaring birth to be when the head has emerged (*yatzah rosho*) (*Sanhedrin* 72b). This, of course, represents no real contradiction since – in a normal birth – the emergence of the head implies that the majority of the baby has arrived. *Niddah* 29a clarifies that "the majority" was stated particularly for those cases in which the baby came out feet first, in which case it was regarded as born once "the majority" had appeared. The *Yerushalmi* (*Sanhedrin* 8:9) makes the equivalence explicit by stating conjointly that "when the majority and the head" have emerged the baby is considered born.

As far as birth is concerned, then, appearance of "the majority" is representative of the whole. The *Mishnah* (*Niddah* 3:5) further applies this notion to the head, by declaring that if the majority of the head – taken to mean the forehead – has emerged, it represents the whole head, and hence the whole body as well. Maimonides takes this to its logical conclusion by declaring birth to have taken place even if only a majority of the forehead has appeared (*Hilkhot Issurei Biah* 10:6). Effectively, therefore, the baby is considered born when it has reached the end of the vaginal canal and has crowned.

[38] *M. Arakhin* 1:4. [39] See above, chapter 1, pp. 18–19. [40] *Arakhin* 7a.
[41] *Sifrei Zuta* (Horowitz edition) to Numbers 35:22.

but labor had not yet begun.[42] Committed to the general proposition of
fetal dependence, the *Tannäim* were apparently in no doubt that, in this
situation the existence of the fetus required no independent consideration from that of its mother. To the contrary, since fetal life was wholly
dependent on the mother for continuity, if she were subject to the death
penalty then the fetus would share her fate.

Later in *halakhic* history, the *Tosafists* would interpret the *Mishnah*'s
insistence on immediate execution as stemming from a desire to alleviate
the woman's mental anguish concerning her impending demise.[43] If this
view represents the actual thinking behind the *Mishnah*, then the fetus
was plainly subordinate to its mother for causes other than a clear and
present threat to her life. The above *midrash* goes considerably further
in its depiction of the fetus as being sufficiently beneath its mother in
standing that her mental interests – given the prospect of execution –
would be superior to any fetal claim on life.

The *Gemara* to *Masekhet Arakhin* conveys a number of important insights that serve to underscore the elevated status of the condemned
mother in this case. First, the observation is made that were it not for
this *mishnah*'s explicit demand for her death, the mother would in fact
not have been subject to execution, because based on the payment requirement set forth in Exodus 21:22–25, the fetus is the husband's property "of which he should not be deprived."[44] Hence, not only does this
mishnah set the condemned woman's interests over those of her fetus, but

---

[42] It is important to stress that this was a theoretical rather than a practical position. In actuality, as
seen above (n. 15) the carrying out of the death penalty was virtually impossible for the *Tannäim*.
See J. Preuss, *Biblical and Talmudic Medicine*, Northvale, Jason Aronson Incorporated, 1993, p. 421.
Preuss observes that "[I]t is doubtful whether this rule . . . was ever carried out, because, during
the era of Mar Samuel in the second century, the Jews no longer had their own system of criminal
justice. We are thus only dealing with a purely theoretical teaching."

Furthermore, in the case of a woman who was known to be pregnant, her trial would be
postponed until after she had given birth, thereby ensuring that this debate was one of symbolic
rather than substantive significance. See J. D. Bleich, "Abortion in Halakhic Literature" in
Contemporary Halakhic Problems, volume 1, New York, Ktav Publishing House Incorporated, 1977,
p. 365. The noted *halakhic* scholar and ethicist Rabbi David Bleich, citing Rabbi Issar Yehuda
Unterman, states that "[T]he Mishnah in *Erukhin* which provides for the execution of a pregnant
woman is understood by the commentaries as having reference to situations where pregnancy
was not detected until the verdict was announced; when pregnancy was known beforehand, the
trial was delayed until after confinement in order to spare the life of the child."

[43] *Tosafot* to *Arakhin* 7b, s.v. *yashvah*.

[44] *Arakhin* 7a. This Talmudic statement led some later authorities to maintain that – in circumstances
other than those mentioned in the *Mishnah* – the husband's permission would be required before
an abortion could be carried out. See, for example, *Tzitz Eliezer*, volume IX, number 51, below,
chapter 5, p. 163.

over those of her husband, which it is fair to surmise was probably quite a radical notion in the *Tannaïtic* period. Furthermore, in the continuation of the *Gemara*, the rabbis rule as follows: "Said Rabbi Judah in the name of Samuel: 'Before such a woman is executed she is struck across her abdomen, so that the fetus will die prior to the execution, to prevent her dishonor at the time of execution.'"[45] Rashi interprets this "dishonor" to mean that if the fetus did not die, and was expelled from the body after the mother's execution, the bleeding that could result would be a dishonor to the woman.[46] Thus, in addition to the fact that the fate of the fetus was to be given no independent consideration from that of its mother, the law also envisioned that the act of feticide would be carried out separately and deliberately – rather than as a byproduct of the execution – in the interests of the condemned woman's dignity. At no point in the discussion does the *Gemara* demur over the proposed feticide. The *Tannaïtic* ruling goes uncontested: the fetus ought to be killed because the interests of the mother in a swift and "dignified" death far outweigh any consideration due to the unborn.

Aptowitzer makes the case that the *Tannaim* were, in this instance, deeply insightful in enacting these provisions, preferring ethics over politics:

Politics, it is true, would demand the opposite, for it subordinates the welfare of the individual to the interest of the state; ethics, however, protects the individual in the first place. Politics knows subjects of state: taxpayers and soldiers; ethics knows but men. To politics men are members of the state, wheels of a machine; to ethics the state is a union of men. To politics the condemned mother is part of a machine rendered useless, but her expected child is a freshly wrought screw; the former is cast to the heap of old iron, the latter is guarded carefully. To ethics, however, the condemned mother is still a woman having claim to forbearance. Hence, the politically motivated laws of the Egyptians, Greeks, and Romans, refused to admit the execution of a pregnant woman; while the ethically motivated law of the Jews prescribes it.[47]

Aptowitzer certainly deserves credit for a brave defense of Jewish ethics.[48] However, since no matter what happens the woman will die, the case certainly could be made that if "forbearance" for the condemned mother

---

[45] *Arakhin* 7a.   [46] Rashi to *Arakhin* 7a, s.v. *liyedei nivul*.
[47] Aptowitzer, "Criminal Law," 99.
[48] In reality, by deferring the woman's trial, Jews found a way both to show "forbearance" to the woman, and to save the child as well – see D. M. Feldman, *Birth Control in Jewish Law – Marital Relations, Contraception, and Abortion as set forth in the Classic Texts of Jewish Law*, Northvale, Jason Aronson Incorporated, 1998, p. 289.

is the desideratum, then it might be better expressed by allowing her offspring to live, rather than providing her with a speedy death. Still, Aptowitzer surely is correct in emphasizing that the determination to kill the condemned woman without delay is compassionate. It is difficult, however, to support Aptowitzer's view that one approach is dramatically ethically superior to the other. Whether or not Aptowitzer is correct, it is certain that early rabbinic Judaism never unequivocally proscribed feticide, and even came to see it as the "lesser of two evils," at least in these specified circumstances.

The *Tannäim*, then, enshrined within normative Judaism an attitude to fetal standing that was wholly divergent from the Jewish-Hellenistic (Alexandrian) and early Christian views. Never in doubt that the fetus was legally to be regarded as a part of its mother, monetary compensation was the only possible penalty for the loss of a fetus at any stage of development. No objection was raised to the sacrifice of a pregnant animal, in contradistinction to Philo's determined opposition.[49] Decisive contrasts were also to be found in the fact that the death penalty for a pregnant woman was to be carried out immediately, that "formation" was not elevated to a legal turning point, and no law prohibiting abortion was to be found anywhere within *Tannäitic* sources.[50] As a result, by the end of the second century of the Common Era, Judaism and Christianity had embarked upon quite separate paths, which ultimately would result in wholly divergent responses to abortion.

One of the challenges to which these two religious systems reacted with considerable variance concerned the inculcation and fate of the soul. As early as the time of Tertullian in the third century, Christianity had absorbed the Pythagorean Greek view that the soul was infused at the moment of conception. Though this view was confirmed by St. Gregory of Nyssa a century later, it would not be long before it would be rejected by Augustine in favor of the Septuagintal notion that only a formed fetus possessed a human soul. While Augustine speculated whether "animation" might be present prior to formation, he determined that abortion could only be defined as homicide once formation had occurred.[51] Nevertheless, in common with all early Christian thought, Augustine condemned abortion from conception onward. Writing from the Roman Catholic perspective, John Connery observes that:

---

[49] See above, chapter 1, p. 18.   [50] See Weinfeld, "*Hamitat Ubar*," 138.
[51] Grisez, *Abortion*, p. 146.

Abortion was wrong to the early Christians, and this was what concerned them, not what penalty it deserved. They were not interested in comparing one abortion with another for penal purposes. Abortion was wrong whether the fetus was formed or not. One finds in the early Church, then, simple, clear condemnations of abortion without any attempt to distinguish or classify.[52]

During the greater part of Christian history this Augustinian approach was dominant, though there were periods when the earlier view prevailed. In 1869, however, Pope Pius IX affirmed that abortion was murder from the moment of conception, since it was at that moment that the soul entered the body. Pope Pius' stance was the culmination of arguments put by two medical experts, Thomas Fienus and Paolo Zacchia, in the early seventeenth century. Each of them was individually of the view that the soul was infused at or about conception. Over time their outlook came to be accepted, and formed the foundation of Pope Pius' position.[53] It has remained Catholic doctrine ever since.[54] While Christian views can hardly be said to be unanimous either on the moment of ensoulment or on viewing abortion as murder from conception onward, it is reasonable to assert that the early Greek approach to ensoulment at conception not only became a central idea within Christianity, but later came to be widely understood as the definition of life's onset.

It was also during the rabbinic period that Christianity expanded the idea of original sin into the proposition that the soul was in need of cleansing baptism if it were to achieve eternal salvation. Already in Augustine's day it was acknowledged that a fetus that died unbaptized would suffer eternal perdition.[55] An unbaptized fetus, in effect, stood to be subjected to a double wrong: it would not only have its life taken away, but it would also be condemned to an eternity without hope of salvation.[56] Given this stance, it is easy to appreciate why – within traditional Christianity – abortion without baptism came to be regarded as a crime that was actually more heinous than the killing of a born, baptized human person. Unlike the question of ensoulment, however, which determined the timing of Christianity's designation of abortion as murder, the matter of baptism had little practical impact on the

[52] Connery J. R., *Abortion: The Development of the Roman Catholic Perspective*, Loyola University Press, 1977, p. 34.
[53] See Grisez, *Abortion*, pp. 170–177.
[54] L. Lader, *Abortion*, New York, Howard W. Sams and Company Incorporated, 1966, p. 79.
[55] Connery, *Abortion*, p. 56. [56] See Connery, *ibid*., p. 310.

Christian response to abortion. It only served to stiffen Christianity's already firm anti-abortion resolve.[57]

The Jewish attitude to these matters of the disposition of the soul was altogether different from that of nascent Christianity. The essential distinctions, however, were not so much to be found in matters of actual substance as in approach. Where Christianity, grounded in the Septuagint, began from a stance of determined opposition to abortion, rabbinic Judaism did not. Consequently, discussions over the inculcation and fate of the soul developed within the context of each system's primary orientation. While the rabbis gave credence to the idea that the soul entered the body at conception, and were concerned with the life of the soul in the "world to come," their thinking on these issues seems to have remained largely a speculative pursuit. Unconcerned with securing a particular position in relation to fetal status, the rabbis appear to have given little, if any, consideration to translating philosophical reflection about the soul's nature into definitive *halakhic* outcomes, and, as a result, such translation never took place.

Thus, the Talmud records this famous dialogue between the Roman Emperor Antoninus and Rabbi:

Antoninus said to Rabbi: "From when is the soul endowed in man, from the time of conception or from the time of formation?" Rabbi replied: "From the time of formation." The emperor demurred: "Can meat remain three days without salt and not putrefy? You must concede that the soul enters at conception." Rabbi [later] said, "Antoninus taught me this, and Scripture supports him, as it is said: 'and Your visitation has preserved my spirit (Job 10:12).' "[58]

---

[57] John Connery (*ibid.*, p. 315, note 1 to chapter 1) depicts the Catholic view in these terms: "The claim is frequently made that the concern of the Catholic Church for the fetus was related chiefly to the question of baptism, that is, the eternal welfare of the fetus. History certainly testifies to the concern of the Church for the spiritual welfare of the fetus, but it testifies with equal clarity that the prior concern was with the taking of fetal life. It was because abortion constituted the taking of fetal life that it was condemned. If the one responsible for the abortion was also to blame for allowing the child to die without baptism, this was an additional fault. But even if the fetus could have been baptized after the abortion, the Church would not have condoned it . . ." These representations of the Church's understanding of baptism certainly appear to represent Christian ideas faithfully. Thus, contrary to the perspectives of Rabbi Immanuel Jakobovits (Jakobovits, *Jewish Medical Ethics*, p. 175) and Rabbi David Feldman (Feldman, *Birth Control.*, p. 269), baptism was not a "crucial factor determining the [Christian] attitude to abortion;" rather, it was a fundamental concern which reinforced Christianity's primary aversion to abortion.

[58] *Sanhedrin* 91b. A variant reading of this text appears in the *Midrash* (*Genesis Rabbah* 34:10). In the *midrashic* version Rabbi's initial response to Antoninus – before Antoninus encourages reconsideration – places ensoulment at birth: "Antoninus said to Rabbi: 'From when is the soul endowed in man, from the time he leaves his mother's womb or from before that time?' Rabbi replied: From the time he leaves his mother's womb."

Rabbi is depicted in this source as being persuaded of the view that conception and ensoulment indeed do coincide. There is, moreover, a range of *aggadic* (rabbinic lore) insights which similarly appear to dictate an early time of ensoulment if they are to make sense: Jacob and Esau are said to have begun their struggles while yet in Rebecca's womb,[59] and fetuses in general are envisaged taking part in *shirat Mosheh* (the song of Moses),[60] accepting the Divine law,[61] cursing hypocritical individuals,[62] denouncing teachers who withheld *halakhic* instruction,[63] and studying the entire Torah in preparation for a righteous life.[64] None of these depictions of "life" in the womb would have been conceivable without the presence of a soul.[65] However, although these texts strongly suggest that the rabbis perceived the fetus to be endowed with some type of "life" which was independently animated, no fully developed theory of the timing or nature of ensoulment ever crystallized. Without such a coherent theory, there arose no barrier to academic notions of early ensoulment continuing to coexist side-by-side with legal positions that did not seek to criminalize feticide. For example, the *Yad Ramah*, a Talmudic commentary of the thirteenth-century Rabbi Meir Abulafia, cannot be more plain in interpreting Rabbi's position to mean that the soul is infused at conception. Yet Abulafia concomitantly continued to accept feticide under limited conditions, on the basis that the fetus was not considered a *nefesh* until birth.[66]

Similarly clouded was rabbinic thought regarding when a developing human becomes "fit to enter the world to come."[67] This inquiry received no fewer than five different Talmudic answers: at conception, at birth, at *brit milah*, at the onset of speech, and along with the ability to respond "Amen."[68] In rabbinic Judaism, however, the soul is regarded as pure and untainted from the outset,[69] and is consequently in no need of any baptismal act, so its return to the Divine reservoir of being is assured, no matter which of these five answers was seen to be the most conducive. Put another way, even should the developing human being die prior to

---

[59] *Genesis Rabbah* 63:6.   [60] *Berakhot* 50a; *Ketubot* 7b; *M. Sotah* 6:4; *Mekilta* to Exodus 15:1.
[61] *Midrash Shoher Tov*, Warsaw, 1893, to Psalm 8:3.   [62] *Sotah* 41b.   [63] *Sanhedrin* 91b.
[64] *Niddah* 30b.
[65] Nevertheless, the fact that Rabbi and Antoninus end up concurring, as their conversation continues, that the *yetzer ha-rah* (the evil inclination) is only imbued at birth, in all probability implies that the rabbinic acceptance of some notion of early ensoulment did not correspond to the fullness of the term "soul" as it is generally understood.
[66] *Yad Ramah*, Sloniki, 1798, reprinted Jerusalem, 1971, to *Sanhedrin* 91b, 72b.
[67] *Sanhedrin* 110b; *Yerushalmi Shvi'it* 4:8.   [68] *Ibid*.
[69] See, for example, *Berakhot* 60b.

attaining "the world to come," Judaism foresaw no deprivation or suffering that would result. The rabbis, therefore, felt no particular urgency to arrive at a resolution of the matter, and consequently left this issue, too, within the realm of surmise.

From a Talmudic perspective, then, it emerges that while the questions of the inculcation of the soul and its fate were intellectually tantalizing, they had no connection to the legal status of the fetus.[70] As Rabbi David Feldman, a leading authority on abortion in Judaism, succinctly put it, "The conclusion is inescapable that these Aggadic or theological reflections...have no bearing on the abortion question."[71] A subject that would come to have undeniable influence upon Christian attitudes to abortion thereby was rendered essentially non-germane as a Jewish issue by the rabbis' inconclusive approach to matters they treated as largely conjectural. It was not, of course, that the rabbis regarded such matters as being unimportant. It was just that, as these issues did not impinge upon the realities of the world of deed and action, there was no cause for them to influence the realm of *halakhic* thinking.

It is important to note that, as the *Amoraïc* replaced the *Tannaïtic* period, a number of these *aggadic* reflections expressed a subtle shift in the dominant *Tannaïtic* commitment to the concept of fetal dependence. The Talmud records an alteration in *halakhic* attitudes in the name of the third-century *Amora* Rabbi Yochanan, who plainly maintains the view that *ubar lav yerekh imo*, the fetus was not to be considered a limb of its mother.[72] The various *aggadic* descriptions of conscious, independent fetal response, set out above, reveal that the position recorded in Rabbi Yochanan's name had become more than the stance of just one individual. Indeed, while it is even possible that an occasional *Tanna* may have held the same outlook,[73] by the time of the *Amoraïm* "indications are to be discerned in the Talmudic discussions that a change of view had taken place."[74] However, this "change of view," from a position that formulated *halakhic* provisions based on a presumption of fetal dependence to one that also gave acknowledgment to the possibility of fetal independence, occasioned no discernible new legal restrictions for Jews in the area of feticide. Yet again the rabbis appear to have taken substantive philosophical strides while not making any correlating legal adjustments.

Nevertheless, the *Amoraïc* period did yield three significant perspectives on the nature of the fetus, each of which, in its own way, would come

[70] Jakobovits, *Jewish Medical Ethics*, pp. 182–183.   [71] Feldman, *Birth Control*, pp. 274–275.
[72] *Temurah* 25a.   [73] See above, p. 43.   [74] Urbach, *The Sages*, p. 245.

to have a profound influence on later Jewish thinking about abortion. The first, a statement found in the continuation of the *Gemara* in *Masekhet Arakhin*, dealt with what should be done to assist a "trapped" fetus on *Shabbat*. It is worth recalling that the *Mishnah*, in *Masekhet Shabbat*, had already provided unambiguous permission for transgressing the *Shabbat* to assist a pregnant woman in difficulty, given that the very fact of her pregnancy was seen to place her in a category associated with an element of risk to life. This permission, however, was provided with the primary intent of preserving *her* life, not that of the fetus.[75] Elsewhere, in the famous passage in *Masekhet Yoma*, in which a pregnant woman is allowed to eat pork on *Yom Kippur* (the Day of Atonement) if it becomes necessary to satisfy her cravings, Rashi presents the reasoning behind the ruling as the alleviation of potential danger to both mother and fetus if she does not eat.[76] In both cases, however, the holy day is to be overridden when the life of a full *nefesh* is potentially at stake. Indeed, the rabbis explicitly predicate the duty to contravene the *Shabbat* or *Yom Kippur* on their interpretation of Leviticus 18:5, "which, if a man performs them [the commandments], he shall live by them." While the *Amoraïm* understood this to convey that "he shall live by them and not die because of them,"[77] it was the "man" who was the focus of this statement, and the fetus, of course, was not considered to be a "man."[78] The question, then, remained, should one contravene the *Shabbat* in order to save a fetus?

In *Masekhet Arakhin*, the issue of *Shabbat* violation arises within a context that efficiently eliminated all maternal interest from the picture:

Rav Nachman said in the name of Shmuel: "If a woman who has been sitting on the birthstool died on a *Shabbat*, one may bring a knife and cut her womb open to take out the child." But is this not self-evident? What is he doing? He's only cutting flesh.[79] Rabbah said: "It is necessary [to allow for] the fetching of the knife by way of a public thoroughfare." And what is he informing us? That in a case of doubt one may desecrate the *Shabbat*. But we have already been taught: "If debris falls on one and there is doubt whether he is there or not, whether he is alive or dead, whether he is a Canaanite or an Israelite, one may remove the debris from him." You might have said: "There [permission was given] because

---

[75] *M. Shabbat* 8:3.   [76] Rashi to *Yoma* 82a, s.v. *ubarah sheherichah*.

[77] *Yoma* 85b. In other words, one must take all measures to ensure that one does not sacrifice life through the observance of *mitzvot*.

[78] See above, p. 28.

[79] There is only a prohibition on the cutting of the living – other than for life-saving purposes – on *Shabbat*. If the woman were dead, then cutting her flesh would be no more prohibited than cutting meat on *Shabbat*.

[the person] had presumption of being alive, but here where it [the fetus] did not have such original presumption of life, one might say no [desecration of the *Shabbat* shall be permitted]." Therefore we are informed [that it is].[80]

The discussion depicts a woman who dies in labor, though the *Gemara* does not indicate whether the pregnancy is full-term or if the fetus is to be considered viable. Indeed the *Gemara*'s comment that "here the fetus did not have such original presumption of life" possibly could indicate that, unlike one buried in debris, the normal assumption in rabbinic times was that any fetus in this condition would not be found alive. Regardless, the Talmud directly calls for the overriding of *Shabbat* so that a knife can be brought, and so that the fetus, whose "presumption of life" is wholly questionable, can be extracted. On the surface, the text seems to communicate that even at stages of pregnancy short of full-term – and even if the fetus is not yet viable – if labor has commenced, then the "life" represented by the fetus is not just some academic construction, but is of enough weight and reality that it deserves the breaching of commandments on its behalf, even if saving it is no more than a doubtful proposition.

Indeed, it is the issue of doubt that seems to be at the forefront of Shmuel's consideration in this text. The rabbinic rule of *mechalelin al hasafek* (transgressing the law in a case of doubt), which was applied in order to override *Yom Kippur* for the sake of the pregnant woman[81] – even though the threat to life was remote – is also central here: "in a case of doubt one may desecrate the *Shabbat*." The analogy offered by the Talmud to the instance of a person buried in debris highlights the very same feature: even though his life is in doubt, nevertheless *mechalelin al hasafek* applies. Clearly, Shmuel is of the view that just as *mechalelin al hasafek* is appropriate in the case of a *nefesh*, so too it is appropriate in the case of a fetus.

Given, however, that such exertions on behalf of a fetus might suggest that it has a standing akin to that of a *nefesh*, later scholars sought to explain the apparent contradiction between Shmuel's permission to override the *Shabbat* and the status of the fetus, by understanding the text in a different way. Earlier in the *Arakhin Gemara*, the fetus had been perceived as making the transition from being part of the mother's body to being "another body" at the onset of labor.[82] Hence, the woman's death on the birthstool could be regarded as the effective entrapment

---

[80] *Arakhin* 7a–b.
[81] *M. Yoma* 8:6–7, *Yoma* 83a–85b, *Shulchan Arukh Orach Chayim* 329 and 330:5.   [82] *Arakhin* 7a.

of a newly independent baby, trapped within the mother's dead tissue. Nachmanides, in his *Torat Ha'Adam* commentary would succinctly summarize this outlook:

> But there are those who assert that one should not desecrate the *Shabbat* to save a fetus ... but when she dies on the birth-stool the fetus is considered to be born already, no longer her limb and not dependent on her, but alive and prevented from emerging, as the door is closed before him. Thus, because it lacks only prior status as living, and we are lenient when it comes to saving lives [we can desecrate the *Shabbat* to save it].[83]

This nascent child, as it were, is essentially locked in, without means to actualize its independence through the birth process. It is, as the *Tosafot* would later depict it, "like something enclosed in a package."[84] Viewed in this manner, this trapped being could be said to have been "born," after a fashion, at least in terms of having been irrevocably separated from the life-creating and sustaining nurturing of its mother. Indeed, the *Tosafists*, who were major proponents of this approach to *Arakhin*, took the position that one stranded by the death of its mother in this way is like an encased newborn, and, hence, if it were to be killed, the perpetrator ought to be considered a murderer.[85] If this is indeed the correct understanding of the Talmud's intent, then the reason for transgressing the *Shabbat* by bringing the knife becomes obvious: the rescuing of a child considered to have been born is a clear-cut case of *pikuach nefesh* (saving a life). It follows, given this understanding of the passage, that the *Arakhin* text need not, in fact, be perceived as presenting any particular exception to the general rules about saving life, or as providing any new information about the standing of a fetus. Seen in this light, the purpose of the text is simply to instruct that, in the exceptional case of the mother's demise – and only in such circumstances – although the child has not yet "emerged," it ought to be treated as if it had.

However, in the ninth century, the *Halakhot Gedolot* adopted an altogether different approach to the *Arakhin Gemara*. The author emphasized that the rabbis had intended to maintain an unmistakable differentiation between the born and the unborn, and that the reason for violating the *Shabbat* in this case arose not from considerations of the fetus as a present human life, but from an altogether different motivation:

> As the *Mishnah* states regarding a one-day-old infant, that capital punishment is prescribed for murdering it, for a one-day-old infant but not a

---

[83] Nachmanides, *Torat Ha'Adam, Kitvei HaRamban*, Jerusalem, 1963, volume II, p. 29.
[84] *Tosafot* to *Niddah* 44a–b, s.v. *miyat be-reisha*.   [85] *Ibid.*

fetus . . . nevertheless with regard to keeping the laws (i.e. the *Shabbat*) we set them aside for it . . . since the Torah declared "set aside one *Shabbat* that he might keep many *Shabbatot*."[86]

The *Halakhot Gedolot*, unwilling to accept any conflation between a *nefesh adam* and a fetus – even if labor had begun – held that it was appropriate to break the *Shabbat* and to save the fetus, not out of consideration of its current status, but because of its future potential as a full life. It is fitting, according to this reasoning, to override one *Shabbat* even when life itself is not at stake, in the interests of possibly assuring a life that may come to be. There is, however, no logical rationale why such a principle should be limited to a fetus whose mother has died in labor. The *Gemara* imposes no condition on fetal viability in order to make *Shabbat* contravention appropriate. If, then, it was actually future considerations that represented the truly pivotal issue, this ought to imply that one should override the *Shabbat* in order to save any fetus that is *in extremis*. Nachmanides would later understand the *Halakhot Gedolot* as wanting to convey just this message:

> According to the *Baʾal Halakhot Gedolot* the reason for bringing the knife is that according to the Torah one desecrates one *Shabbat* so that one will be able to fulfill many *Shabbatot*. Therefore the opinion of the *Halakhot Gedolot* is that the *Shabbat* is desecrated even to save a fetus that is less than forty days in the womb, and which has no life at all.[87]

Nachmanides clearly comprehends the *Halakhot Gedolot* to be saying that the future life which any fetus portends is sufficiently compelling that it makes the act of trying to save the threatened fetus worthwhile, despite the *Shabbat* desecration involved. This, Nachmanides maintains, remains true even for a fetus that could not live, such as one that was less than forty days old. If the reason for saving the fetus was its future potential life, then, given that future life is dubious for all fetuses, all ought to be treated alike: praying for the miraculous, one should override the *Shabbat* in the hope that future life will be granted. Nachmanides' understanding notwithstanding, this approach of the *Halakhot Gedolot* certainly circumvented the difficulty of regarding a potentially non-viable fetus as possessing, on the basis of its current condition, a claim to similar extreme life-saving measures as one already born. At the same time, the notion of "future potential" allowed for the retaining of the *Gemara*'s sense that the welfare of the fetus was important enough to overtake the *Shabbat*, if necessary.

---

[86] *Halakhot Gedolot, Hilkhot Yom HaKippurim* 26.   [87] Nachmanides, *Torat HaʾAdam*, p. 29.

The actual import of the *Arakhin* text has remained obscure. Some later scholars came to regard the whole discussion of *Shabbat* violation on behalf of the fetus as a theoretical rather than a practical matter, since they beheld any threat to the fetus as *ipso facto* a threat to the mother, and there was no doubt that it was appropriate to override the *Shabbat* for her.[88] However, this view notwithstanding, it is difficult to escape the impression, from the vantage point of the *Amoraïc* framing of the text, that the rabbis wanted to convey a sense that the fetus, if not "a born human life," nevertheless represented a nascent life form of great significance. Though this perspective was never framed within a legal context, the suggestion that the *Shabbat* should be infringed upon to rescue a fetus that "did not have original presumption of life" certainly seemed to imply that fetal existence was not to be treated lightly, and that the saving of the fetus was a high priority.

The second critical *Amoraïc* observation concerning the fetus, which would have profound implications for abortion deliberations within Judaism, focused on the fetus as a potential *rodef*. A *rodef* is one who pursues another with intent to kill, and ought, if possible, to be killed before innocent blood is shed.[89] While debating the parameters of the *rodef* regulations, the rabbis raise the question whether a child might be killed as a *rodef*. In response, they rule that, since the aim of the law is to save the innocent person being pursued, and since there is no requirement that the *rodef* be able to comprehend any sort of forewarning before it is killed, it does not matter whether the pursuer is old or young; behaving as a *rodef* deserves death, without regard to the age of the *rodef*.[90]

Reflecting upon this decision, Rav Hisda raised the following difficulty, based on *Mishnah Ohalot*: " 'Once the head[91] has emerged it may not be harmed.' Why [should this be so]? Is it not a *rodef*? The answer is that it is considered to be from heaven that she is pursued."[92] Rav Hisda seems to have reasoned as follows: if, indeed, one can be deemed a *rodef* at any age, then why does *Mishnah Ohalot* advocate that one should not harm

---

[88] For example, *Rosh* to *Yoma* 8:13 who avers: "I do not know what is the need for all these particulars, since it does not occur that there is a danger to the fetus without a danger to the woman, and there is no danger to the woman without danger to the fetus." Presumably in a case of the mother's death, such as that described in *Arakhin*, those of this view would either intervene on the *Shabbat* on the basis that it is no longer a fetus, but rather a "newborn" that is at issue, or would argue for no intervention.

[89] *M. Sanhedrin* 8:7.   [90] *Sanhedrin* 72b.

[91] *Mishnah Ohalot* 7:6 refers, of course, to "the majority," rather than "the head." See above, p. 36, n. 37.

[92] *Sanhedrin* 72b.

a baby that has just emerged in circumstances in which the mother's life is endangered? After all, is not the baby threatening her life, and is it not, therefore, behaving as a *rodef*, pursuing its mother to kill her? Consequently, ought it not to be killed forthwith, in accordance with the Talmud's approach to the *rodef*? The anonymous answer provided by the *Gemara* is unambiguous: the newborn was not to be considered a *rodef*, but rather it was heaven itself – an elusive *rodef* to impede – that was pursuing the mother. Since the *Gemara* did not explain its logic, this ruling naturally evoked the question why a young child should be regarded as a *rodef*, but a newborn not?

Though the Talmud offers no answer to this inquiry, later scholars would.[93] Steinsaltz, in his elucidation of this part of the *Gemara*, evokes their rationale: "The baby does not act in this way through any reasoning of its own, and the matter is not determined by its will and, therefore, we do not subordinate its life to the life of its mother."[94] This argument posits that even though a young child's reasoning and will might be immature, these capabilities are still functional to an extent that makes the child's behavior less than innocent; the same, however, cannot be said of the newborn. If the view that the newborn could not be a *rodef* because it did not yet possess the abilities to behave as a *rodef* is indeed the correct explanation of the Talmud's logic, then it could reasonably be held that the fetus certainly could not be deemed a *rodef*, for it was even further from attaining the requisite qualifications that would make *rodef* status possible. From the text of *Sanhedrin* 72b, though, this line of thinking cannot be considered to be more than supposition, since the Talmud does not reveal whether or not the rabbis regarded the fetus as a *rodef*. All that can be stated with certainty is that the *Sanhedrin Gemara* did not consider the newborn to be a *rodef*.

The issue of whether the fetus might be considered a *rodef* is made more complicated by three texts in the *Talmud Yerushalmi* that all put forward a different view from that of the *Talmud Bavli*.[95] In the case of a baby whose head already has emerged, the *Yerushalmi* maintains that it is impossible to determine whether it is the baby killing its mother or the mother killing her baby. The scholar, Elyakim Ellinson, points out that the *Yerushalmi* text itself does not actually invoke the *rodef* argument,

---

93 See, for example, the approach of Israel Lipschutz, below, chapter 4, p. 97.
94 *Sanhedrin* 72b. *Steinsaltz Talmud*, Jerusalem, Israel Institute for Talmudic Publications, 1984, p. 321, s.v. *de-mishmaya ka radfi la*.
95 *Yerushalmi, Avodah Zarah* 2:2. Also to be found with slight variations at *Yerushalmi, Shabbat* 14:4 and *Yerushalmi, Sanhedrin* 8:9.

but regards this as a case of *pikuach nefesh*. He clarifies that since there is no basis within Jewish law for preferring one *nefesh* over another, and since "the situation in the birth process is so shrouded in uncertainty that it cannot be assumed that there is a simple choice between the life of the mother and the life of the newborn" if an intervention were to take place, the *rodef* argument cannot be operative here. *Shev ve-ʿal taʿaseh* (take no intervening action) is the appropriate response.[96] The commentators[97] explain that it would be inappropriate to kill the baby as a *rodef*. In the case of the fetus, the *Yerushalmi* never states that the fetus ought to be regarded as a *rodef*. Nevertheless, since the *Yerushalmi*'s principal argument for rejecting *rodef* status for the emerging baby is that one cannot tell who is killing whom, it could be held that this problem is of far less significance when considering the fetus. After all, in *Mishnah Ohalot*, it is the stated threat to the life of the mother that is the paramount concern, and there seems to be no confusion over who is being pursued. One could, then, hold that the *Yerushalmi* leaves open the possibility that the fetus might be considered to be a *rodef*, even while rejecting the notion that the newborn could be.[98] This is, however, an argument from silence, for the *Yerushalmi* never asserts that this is so.

The Talmud, therefore, never declares the fetus a *rodef*. Of course, the fact that the Talmud did not take this approach merely implies that, in circumstances in which the mother's life is at stake, there would be no obligation to kill the fetus because of it being a *rodef*. Nevertheless, the provision that requires the death of the fetus because "her life takes precedence over its life,"[99] remains in force, so that, from a practical standpoint, even if the fetus is not eligible to be a *rodef* it makes no difference: the fetus is to be killed to save the life of the mother. However, as noted above, even though the Talmud never states it, the reality that "her life takes precedence over its life" might also form the basis of a position that the fetus is behaving as a *rodef* after her life.

This source, then, might well have been considered to be little more than an intellectual curiosity within the developing foundations of the abortion framework. Indeed the *Amoraïm* probably did not regard *Sanhedrin* 72b as being at all critical in defining the parameters of permissible feticide. Centuries later, however, this text would provide inspiration

---

[96] Ellinson, "*HaUbar BaHalakhah*," 42.
[97] *Penei Moshe* to Avodah Zarah, Korban HaʾEidah to Shabbat, Marei Panim to Sanhedrin.
[98] There are logical problems inherent in this argument – see below chapter 3, pp. 60–61 – but they do not make the argument unthinkable.
[99] *M. Ohalot* 7:6.

for a decisive legal reformulation, which would come to shape abortion
deliberations in new and unexpected ways.[100] From the *Amoraïc* viewpoint, though, since the fetus was not described as a *rodef*, the permissibility of killing it could not be extrapolated from any "pursuer" status.

The third important *Amoraïc* perspective[101] constitutes the only explicit Talmudic limitation on abortion, and is addressed specifically to
Noahides (non-Jews). According to Jewish law, non-Jews are obligated by
seven laws derived by the rabbis from the instructions given to the sons
of Noah in Genesis 9. In full, Genesis 9:6 – one of the verses from which
the Noahide laws are derived – is usually translated "Whoever sheds the
blood of man, by man shall his blood be shed; for in His image did God
make man." The rabbis extend this verse as follows:

> In the name of Rabbi Yishmael they said: "[A Noahide receives capital
> punishment] even for [destroying] a fetus." What is the reason of Rabbi
> Yishmael? It is the verse "he who sheds the blood of man, in man (*adam
> ba'adam*) shall his blood be shed" (Genesis 9:6). What is the meaning of "man in
> man?" This can be said to refer to a fetus in its mother's womb.[102]

As pointed out above, the rabbis never regarded the fetus as being included in the term *adam*. Clearly, however, this did not prevent the rabbis,
within the context of this *midrash halakhah*, from seeing the expression *adam
ba'adam* as being a suitable synonym for the fetus. The Hebrew, *adam
ba'adam*, allows for the interpretation "man in man," and it is from this
variant reading that the rabbis determined that capital punishment becomes appropriate for the Noahide who has killed a fetus. The linguistic
link, established by the translator of the Septuagint, between this idea
and Exodus 21:22–23, together with its implicit connection between
homicide and feticide, probably also appealed to the rabbis and further
motivated them to outlaw abortions for non-Jews.[103] This rabbinic legal
innovation was not only exceptional in that it specified the first broad
prohibition on abortion to have been created within the tradition, but
also for the fact that it transcended the theoretical realm, and became
part of the accepted *halakhah*.[104]

Scholars have hypothesized about the core intent of this text. One view
contends that the position attributed to Rabbi Yishmael was an attempt

---

[100] See below, chapter 3, pp. 59ff.
[101] The timing of this material is uncertain but it is most probably *Amoraïc*. Even though Rabbi
Yishmael was an early second-century *Tanna*, the law was explicitly stated in the names of the
Amoraïm, Rabbi Ya'akov bar Acha (*Sanhedrin* 57b) and Rabbi Chanina (*Bereishit Rabbah* 34:19).
Despite the attribution to Rabbi Yishmael, Ellinson contends that no source exists for it in
Tannaïtic literature. See Ellinson, "*HaUbar BaHalakhah*," 31.
[102] *Sanhedrin* 57b.   [103] See above, chapter 1, p. 14.   [104] See below, chapter 3, p. 62.

to battle the prevalent culture of abortion within Roman society.[105] Aptowitzer declares this approach to be temporally impossible – "a good joke" – and holds instead that the passage was formulated for internal rather than external consumption, as "an interpretation of the Noahide law important to the Jewish court."[106] This perspective maintains that the outlook ascribed to Rabbi Yishmael comprised a more stringent legal stance on abortion within rabbinic thinking, which, though it would come to be the dominant view within developing Christianity, was ultimately jettisoned by the rabbis.[107] While this position is conceivable, it must be noted that the absence of further evidence for such a stricter attitude to abortion among the rabbis means that it is difficult to accept that this theory is anything stronger than a possibility. It cannot, therefore, be stated with certainty exactly what goal this source was intended to achieve.

The impact of this source is, however, far easier to trace: even though Jews are required to observe commandments, and are not specifically subject to the Noahide laws, the strong stance of this source inevitably raised the question whether it was truly tenable that abortion could so definitively be deemed a crime worthy of capital punishment for the non-Jew, and yet not even be prohibited to the Jew? But this inquiry would only arise in a later period of *halakhic* history.[108] In Talmudic times, these words from *Sanhedrin* suggested that feticide, as carried out by non-Jews, was sufficiently odious to the rabbis that they did not hesitate to use their tools of exegesis in order to outlaw the practice. While the rabbis, for the most part, had no jurisdiction over non-Jews, this source plainly gave voice to their opposition to forms of unbridled abortion that were beyond rabbinic regulation.

It is apparent then, that, by the time the Talmud came to a close, the rabbis had included in their great compendium only one text that enacted definitive restrictions on feticide – its constraints not being incumbent upon Jews – and but a small number of passages relevant to feticide and to the status of the fetus in life and death matters. One final source from the rabbinic period holds significance for the history of abortion, insofar as it speaks of direct evidence of approved abortions being carried out by Jews:

---

[105] I. H. Weiss, *Zur Geschichte der Jüdische Tradition*, volume II, p. 23, as cited in Aptowitzer, "Criminal Law," 114, n. 187.

[106] Aptowitzer, "Criminal Law," 114, n. 187.

[107] See Geiger A., *HaMikrah VeTirgumav*, Jerusalem, 1948, p. 280, and Alon G., *Mechkarim BeToldot Yisrael*, Tel Aviv, 1967, volume I, p. 280.

[108] See below, chapter 3, p. 62.

If a qualified physician who is engaged in healing under the authority of the court causes injury, he is not liable if [the injury is] inadvertent; if [the injury is] intentional, he is liable – in order to promote the public welfare.

If one cuts up a fetus in its mother's womb, under the authority of the court, and causes injury [to the mother], if [the injury is] inadvertent, he is not liable; if [the injury is] intentional, he is liable – in order to promote the public welfare.[109]

These provisions, established in order to indemnify the physician and to ensure that he would not abstain from healing,[110] suggest that the rabbis approved, at least in theory, of giving doctors license from the court to practice medicine and to perform authorized abortions.[111] There is, however, no reason to believe that the authorized abortions under discussion would have included any circumstances other than a direct threat to the life of the mother, as described in *Mishnah Ohalot*.[112]

What is striking about the rabbinic material, besides the paucity of relevant texts, is the absence of any reference to unauthorized abortions. The rabbis were, generally speaking, not reticent in their attempts to eliminate practices which they deemed to be unbecoming of Jews.[113] Had they regarded unapproved abortion as a problem of serious dimensions, it might well have been expected that rabbinic literature would contain sources railing against the phenomenon. There are, however, no such passages. While arguments from silence can be no more than tentative, this conspicuous lack of response suggests one of two possible conclusions. One explanation is that the rabbis had no particular qualms about abortions carried out for reasons other than a threat to the life of the mother, but did not say so explicitly. This is highly unlikely, given both the comprehensive nature of rabbinic deliberations and the rabbis' unambiguous opposition to abortion for Noahides. Had there been any systematic consideration of Jewish abortions in situations less than a direct threat to the mother's life, it is reasonable to expect that there would be textual evidence of this thinking.

The other, far more credible, explanation is that little unauthorized abortion took place among Jews during rabbinic times. Children and

[109] *Tosefta Gittin* (Lieberman edition), 3:8–9.
[110] S. Duran, *Tashbatz*, Amsterdam, 1739, volume III, number 82.
[111] M. Elon, *Jewish Law: History, Sources, Principles*, Jerusalem, The Jewish Publication Society, 1994, volume II, p. 604, n. 249.
[112] Duran, *Tashbatz*, volume III, number 82.
[113] One example – of many that could be cited – is pre-marital sexual relations. As for feticide, there is no explicit Toraitic prohibition on such relations, yet the rabbis established numerous "fences" to restrict the practice. It is reasonable to assume that, in so doing, they were responding to what they perceived to be deplorable behavior that called forth a decisive response.

large families were seen as a blessing,[114] and, as in the biblical period, pregnancy was depicted as an event touched by the miraculous.[115] Child rearing was a central occupation of women, as women were largely occupied with domestic duties, and effective contraception was unavailable. Perhaps as a result, pregnancy was more apt to be welcomed than regarded as an inconvenience. With this background, it is not difficult to imagine that an abortion, for reasons other than a direct threat to the life of the mother, was simply not part of the cultural landscape of the Jews. If this theory is correct, then the rabbis' lack of attention to this area could provide testimony that unauthorized abortions were sufficiently rare that they did not provoke a legal or social controversy thought to be worthy of requiring a rabbinic response.

What, then, can be said of the overall rabbinic attitude to the permissibility of taking the life of the fetus? Since circumstances apparently did not press the rabbis to refine a definitive, coherent answer to this fundamental question, it is hardly remarkable that a careful comparison of the relevant sources displays some sizable inconsistencies between critical texts. Despite these disparities, it is possible to arrive at a number of conclusions that appear to have received rabbinic accord. First, while feticide was considered a capital crime for the non-Jew, the rabbis, rhetoric notwithstanding, showed no inclination to raise feticide above the legal level of a tort for Jews. Second, the rabbis specifically legislated that a fetus ought to be aborted if its continued existence directly threatened the life of its mother, or in the near impossible event that its mother faced impending death for a capital crime. Third, the rabbis conveyed that if a fetus were to be lost, then that loss would be of least significance during the first forty days of pregnancy, but of far greater moment thereafter, with the onset of labor denoting an initial measure of legal independence, and birth the transition to becoming a *nefesh*.

Finally, the rabbis left the impression that they had no argument with the fetus being regarded as some type of "life" from conception onward. To be sure, the nature of this "life" was thought to undergo crucial transformations – both during pregnancy and upon birth – but its status as nascent human life seems to have been generally accepted. Like Aristotle, who thought that a vegetative soul, an animal soul, and finally a human soul enter the fetus at different stages, so the rabbis seem to convey that life progressively developed in significance.[116] Nevertheless,

---

[114] *M. Yevamot* 6:6, *Yevamot* 63b.   [115] See above, chapter 1, pp. 2–3.
[116] See above, chapter 1, p. 15, n. 64.

at each stage the fetus was regarded as "life." Rav Hisda's view that until day forty the fetus was to be considered "mere fluid" seems to have been the exception to this rule, since it could be seen as equating "life" with formation. If, though, Rav Hisda saw no "life" before forty days, it is nonetheless possible that he held the developing entity to be "potential life." If he literally meant "mere fluid," then he apparently did not represent the majority opinion. Apart from Rav Hisda's *Yevamot* declaration, those texts which suggested that the fetus possessed a lesser standing did so not as a rejection of the fetus' standing as "life," but by way of indicating its subordinate status to its mother. Indeed, the combined evidence of *Mishnah Ohalot*'s statement that "her life takes precedence over *its life*," along with the evident rabbinic acceptance of the concept of ensoulment at conception, *Masekhet Arakhin*'s call to override the *Shabbat* in order to save a fetus whose age and viability were indeterminate, and the sentence of capital punishment for a Noahide who killed any fetus, powerfully indicates that the dominant rabbinic view saw the fetus as "life." This "life" was not considered the equivalent of the life that inhered in a *nefesh*, but to use a lesser term would be to discount the essence of the rabbinic approach to the nature of fetal existence.

Thus, while the rabbis, from a legal perspective, continued to regard the fetus as "property" in the same way as Exodus had done, a clarification of attitude had been made during the Talmudic period. Notwithstanding the fact that the penalty for causing the improper death of a fetus remained one appropriate to property loss, the rabbis suggested that the fetus be seen as representing some form of life. The rabbis, then, effectively echoed the dialectic that had earlier been discerned within Josephus' *Antiquitates* and *Contra Apionem*. While in the eyes of the law unjustified feticide was essentially a property crime, its moral significance was far more weighty.[117]

By the time that rabbinic and *Geonic* Judaism yielded the historical stage to the *Rishonim*, the foundations for a *halakhic* response to abortion had been established. Though the rabbis had left the matter of abortion itself largely untouched, they had provided an approach to the question of the significance of the fetus and the seriousness of its loss that would inform and shape all subsequent Jewish attitudes to abortion. As has been seen, the sages left a somewhat ambiguous legacy, which, while regarding feticide as a capital crime for non-Jews, continued to view the act as a tort for Jews – albeit a tort of undeniable seriousness given that

[117] See above, chapter 1, p. 22.

"life" was at stake. Centuries later, prominent scholars would subject this dichotomy between Jew and non-Jew to rigorous challenge. But even before such a reevaluation would occupy *halakhic* thought, two of history's greatest rabbis, Rashi and Maimonides, would formulate divergent perspectives on the permissible rabbinic limits to taking the life of the fetus. These insights would be made possible by the wisdom of the rabbis, who, through generations of scholarship, had distilled the essential elements critical to the future developments to come.

CHAPTER 3

Divining a prohibition: the positions of the Rishonim *and* Acharonim

Five hundred years had passed since the close of the Talmud. The locus of Jewish legal thought had shifted from *Eretz Yisrael*, Sura, and Pumbedita to the lands of Europe. The period of the *Geonim* (heads of the Babylonian academies) had faded into history. Yet, in a manner characteristic of Jewish legal authorities, Rashi (1040–1105), the Talmud's preeminent commentator, wrote as if the passage of time and the changing cultural geography had all meant nothing.[1] In large measure, Rashi's position re-iterated the rabbinic view of fetal status, albeit with one significant elaboration. In the case of a woman undergoing treacherous labor, Rashi's prescription and rationale could hardly have been clearer or more reminiscent:

It is removed limb by limb, for, as long as the being did not come out into the world, it is not a *nefesh* and it is permitted to kill it and to save its mother. But, if the head has emerged, it may not be harmed, because it is considered as fully born, and one may not take the life of one *nefesh* in favor of another.[2]

Just as his rabbinic forebears were, Rashi was plainly in no doubt that when the woman's life was threatened, the interests of the unborn were subordinate to those of its mother. Rashi's rendering, however, takes the *Mishnah* one fundamental step beyond what had previously been

---

[1] Rashi lived at the beginning of the period of the *Rishonim*, "early" scholars. While the era of the *Rishonim* is not precisely fixed, it is generally held to extend from the decline of the Babylonian academies in the middle of the eleventh century to the renewal of ordination in the middle of the fifteenth century. The era of the *Acharonim*, the "later" scholars, followed that of the *Rishonim* and concluded with the emancipation of European Jewry at the end of the eighteenth century. See Elon (ed.), *Principles of Jewish Law*, pp. 17–18.

[2] Rashi to *Sanhedrin* 72b, s.v. *yatzah rosho*. As *Sanhedrin* 72b makes clear, this ruling is based entirely on *M. Ohalot* 7:6. It is worth noting that almost all later authorities concur that the *Mishnah* does not just allow, but, in such circumstances, requires that the fetus be sacrificed for the sake of its mother. One exception to this general agreement is Shlomoh ha-Kohen of Vilna, who is of the view that while the *Mishnah* makes it possible to save the mother by killing the fetus, it does not make it a requirement. See *Yedei Mosheh* 4:8.

articulated. Where *Mishnah Ohalot* simply states that the fetus ought to be removed forthwith "for her life (*chaiyeiha*) takes precedence over its life (*chaiyav*)," Rashi chooses to explain the mother's precedence by reasoning that the fetus "is not a *nefesh* and it is permitted to kill it and to save its mother." According to Rashi, then, the mother's priority was not to be perceived as some arbitrary determination, but stemmed from a subservience of the fetus which could be understood logically: lacking *nefesh* status, it was subject to being killed in the name of the predominant need of a full *nefesh*.

Rashi's explanation, of course, is formulated under the circumstances of a woman in a life-threatening situation. Nevertheless, his interpretation allows for the question of whether there might be conditions under which other, less extreme, physical or emotional traumas to the mother might also countenance abortion of the fetus. After all, if the mother's standing as a "full" *nefesh* meant that her claim to life superseded that of the non-*nefesh* fetus, could not her superior position as a *nefesh* also imply that her claim to health and well-being might overwhelm any claim to life on the part of a non-*nefesh*? Rashi's position makes this a possibility.

It would not be long, however, before Moses Maimonides (known as Rambam, 1135–1204), the intellectual giant of Jewish legal codification and philosophy, would offer an entirely unexpected and decidedly challenging perspective on the subject matter under discussion in *Sanhedrin* 72b:

This too is a negative commandment: not to have compassion[3] on the life of the pursuer (*rodef*). Therefore, the sages ruled that when a woman has difficulty in labor it is permitted to dismember the fetus within her, either by drugs or by surgery, because the fetus is like a *rodef* pursuing her to kill her. But once the head has emerged, the fetus may not be harmed, for we do not set aside one life for another. This is the natural course of the world.[4]

This position, which would later be echoed by other Codes,[5] is surprising from several points of view. Maimonides, in keeping with the tradition,

---

[3] As *Ravad* discerns, *ad loc.*, Maimonides here follows the *Sifrei* to Deuteronomy 25:12 in understanding the requirement to subdue the *rodef* as being based in the Torah's *mitzvah*, "*lo tachos einekhah*," "you shall show no pity" (Deuteronomy 25:12). Coincidentally, this Toraitic injunction is also set in the midst of a struggle between two men. On this occasion, the wife of one of them is punished for her intervention.

The Talmud, however (*Sanhedrin* 73a) holds that the correct source for opposing the *rodef* is "*lo ta'amod al dam rei'ekhah*," "you shall not stand idle while your neighbor bleeds" (Leviticus 19:25). Maimonides' choice of sources here will later be interpreted to be both deliberate and significant. See below, p. 83, and chapter 4, p. 104.

[4] *Hilkhot Rotzeiach* 1:9.   [5] *Sefer HaChinukh*, number 600, *Shulchan Arukh, Choshen Mishpat* 425:2.

cleaves to the ruling of the *Mishnah* in *Ohalot* that a fetus that has not yet
emerged may be killed in order to save the life of its mother. If it has
emerged, however, it may not be sacrificed. The logic of Maimonides'
supporting argument, however, is unprecedented. Despite the fact that
the *Yerushalmi* offers no contradiction to Maimonides' position,[6] *Sanhedrin*
72b rejects the *rodef* categorization even for a newborn, and the Talmud
never sought to apply it to the fetus.[7] Yet, Maimonides maintains that
the reason the fetus may be dismembered in the womb and the mother's
life preserved is not because it is a "non-*nefesh*," but rather because it is
a *rodef* "pursuing her to kill her."

Without doubt, this hitherto unexpressed insight had dramatic potential ramifications for the parameters of permissible abortion. For
Maimonides could reasonably be understood to be proposing that the
fetus was only subject to destruction insofar as it was behaving "like a
rodef" and presenting a credible threat to its mother's existence. Were it
not behaving in this manner, Maimonides could be – and indeed was –
comprehended as implying that one who kills it is guilty of murder.[8] If
this were the correct discernment of the Maimonidean position, a subject that would be debated by later scholars, it presumably would imply
the preclusion of any abortions performed for reasons other than the
mother's life being in imminent peril.

But identifying the fetus as a *rodef* under these conditions was unanticipated in an even more perplexing way. Maimonides follows the *Mishnah*
in declaring the emerging newborn to be a *nefesh* that may not be harmed.
This is consistent with the approach of *Sanhedrin* 72b which declares that,
unlike a child or an adult, the emerging newborn is not considered a *rodef*
and there is, consequently, no duty to kill it in order to save the mother.
However, Maimonides' decision to deem the fetus a *rodef*, and then –
seemingly arbitrarily – not to apply the *rodef* classification to the emerging
newborn, appears to defy logic. While it might be argued that birth is
an occasion for status change, and that the fetus could cease to be a *rodef*
as it becomes a *nefesh*, this is problematic. After all, unlike becoming a
"*nefesh*," the "*rodef*" appellation does not attach to a given stage, but to
a type of behavior, and if the fetus is regarded as an aggressor prior to
birth, because of the threat it poses to its mother, then there is no coherent
reason why this should change at the moment of crowning, particularly if
the threat to the mother is ongoing. Since Maimonides himself provides

---

[6] See above, chapter 2, pp. 50–51.   [7] See above, chapter 2, pp. 49ff.
[8] See, for example, the views of Unterman, below, chapter 5, pp. 138ff.

no explanation for his assignation of the *rodef* principle to the fetus, or why it should not apply to the newborn, subsequent generations were left to grapple with his reasoning, as well as with the restrictive nature of his insight.[9]

Maimonides, then, seems to establish an altogether different legal approach to the fetus whose mother is at risk, from the view promulgated by the Talmud and Rashi, which sees the fetus as simply possessing a lesser status.[10] Whereas Rashi's understanding appears to leave open the potential for lenient rulings in cases of abortions when the mother's life is not at stake, Maimonides' use of the *rodef* designation as the reason for fetal destruction seems to rule out any contemplation of such matters as far as he is concerned. Both positions had their supporters. Thus, two great scholars of the thirteenth century reiterate Rashi's viewpoint: Rabbi Meir Abulafia writing, "So long as he [the fetus] is inside [the womb], it is not a *nefesh*, and the Torah has no pity upon it,"[11] and Rabbi Menachem Mèiri affirming, "It is permitted to dismember the fetus in the womb…since it is not designated as a *nefesh* so long as it has not emerged."[12] Conversely, one of the greatest Codes of the *Acharonim*, the *Shulchan Arukh*, incorporates Maimonides' language verbatim.[13] Since it was not immediately obvious how the positions of these two pivotal *Rishonim* could be reconciled, an interpretative interchange began in an attempt to harmonize their approaches. Through the course of a millennium, it remained a conundrum that would continue to evade definitive resolution.

Later generations, however, would not just have the divergent perceptions of Rashi and Maimonides with which to contend. For in the centuries concurrent with and following Maimonides, the *Tosafot*,[14] in their commentary to the Talmud, would provide the first explicit prohibition of abortion to be applied to Jews. They based this prohibition on

[9] According to Sinclair, there is yet another unexpected and unexplained outcome of Maimonides' rendition, namely that Maimonides greatly strengthens the case that the fetus ought to be considered a life: "by invoking the aggressor principle to justify the ruling in *Mishnah Ohaloth*, Maimonides implies that the foetus is a life, for why else would he have recourse to a justificatory principle normally applied to the killing of a fully viable human being?"; Sinclair, "Legal Basis," 121.

[10] It is not possible to say more than that he "seems" to do this, since there would be those who would assert that the views of Rashi and Maimonides were actually quite close to each other. See, for example, the outlook of Bacharach, below pp. 75ff.

[11] *Yad Ramah* to *Sanhedrin* 72b.

[12] *Beit HaBechirah*, Avraham Sofer Edition, Jerusalem, 1965, to *Sanhedrin* 72b.

[13] *Shulchan Arukh, Choshen Mishpat* 425:2.

[14] The *Tosafot*, a grouping of rabbinic scholars, began with the generations after Rashi, and are generally considered to span the twelfth to the fourteenth centuries.

the Talmudic interpretation of Rabbi Yishmael, who held that abortion was a capital offense for Noahides.[15] Maimonides had codified this interpretation in his *Mishneh Torah*, along with a statement that revealed his view of the serious societal consequences of feticide: "A Noahide who kills a *nefesh*, [or] even a fetus in its mother's womb, is killed because of it... The Jewish court must provide judges for these resident aliens to judge for them in accordance with these laws [of the Sons of Noah] so that society not corrupt itself..."[16] The *Tosafot* connect this Noahide restriction to the principle which is mentioned just once in the Talmud,[17] "there is nothing which is permitted to a Jew but prohibited to a non-Jew:"

A gentile (*oved kokhavim*) is culpable for the death of a fetus, while a Jew is forbidden to cause its death but is not culpable. Even though [a Jew] is not culpable, nevertheless it is not permitted. What of their statement that when a woman in labor is having difficulty, if its head emerges one does not touch it for one *nefesh* is not set aside for another, but prior to the head emerging one dismembers the embryo within her to save her life, even though this is forbidden to a gentile? There are those who say that here likewise a Jew is commanded to save her, and it is possible that a gentile is also permitted to save her.[18]

In the *Tosafot* to *Masekhet Chullin* the same position is enunciated even more explicitly: "Even though a gentile (*ben Noach*) is given capital punishment for aborting a fetus, as it is stated in *Sanhedrin* 58b – while a Jew is not killed – despite the fact that [a Jew] is not liable for capital punishment, nonetheless [aborting a fetus] is still not permissible for a Jew."[19] Two important positions emerge from these *Tosafot* writings: First, the *Tosafot* hold that because a Jew is not bound by the Noahide laws, and since the fetus is a non-*nefesh*, the Jew is not subject to capital punishment for an act of feticide. Still, the *Tosafot* state that such an act is not permissible for a Jew. Second, the *Tosafot* tentatively relax the prohibition on the non-Jew in the case of a therapeutic abortion and permit the non-Jew to abort a fetus in circumstances where a Jew would be commanded to do so.

All of this would be clear enough were it not for the fact that another *Tosafot* in *Niddah* reads: "And there are those who say that in any case because of *pikuach nefesh* we transgress the *Shabbat* for [the fetus'] sake, even though it is permitted to kill it, as in the case of a *goses be-yedei adam*[20]

---

[15] *Sanhedrin* 57b. See above, chapter 2, p. 52.   [16] *Hilkhot Melakhim* 9:4, 10:11.
[17] *Sanhedrin* 59a.   [18] *Tosafot* to *Sanhedrin* 59a, s.v. *lica*.   [19] *Tosafot* to *Chullin* 33a, s.v. *echad*.
[20] A *goses* is usually defined as a person who has been inflicted with a mortal wound and whose death is expected within seventy-two hours. There are, however, problems with this definition. Rabbi Faitel Levin (*Halacha, Medical Science and Technology*, New York, Maznaim Publishing Corporation, 1987, p. 57, n. 28) makes this observation: "A definition of the *goses* state has been discussed by,

where one who kills him is not liable…"[21] What exactly the *Tosafot* intend
here by "it is permitted to kill it" is the subject of some disagreement.
Is this text in fact contradicting the other two *Tosafot* selections that
prohibit feticide for the Jew, or can it be harmonized with them? Tzvi
Hirsch Chajes (known as Maharitz, 1805–55), in his Gloss to *Masekhet
Niddah*, regards the texts as being inconsistent because the *Tosafot* in
Chullin instruct the Jew that it is "*a priori* forbidden to kill a fetus, whereas
the words of *Tosafot* here [*Niddah*] convey that it is *a priori* permitted."[22]
But the *Acharon* Rabbi Jacob Emden (known as Yaʿavetz, 1697–1776)[23]
is of the view that the language of the *Tosafot* in *Niddah* "is not precise,
for who would permit the killing of a fetus without reason even if the
death penalty would not be incurred?"[24] Those who, like Yaʿavetz, find
the phraseology of the *Tosafot* in *Niddah* to be deceptive, point to the
context of this *Tosafot* and note that the situation under consideration is
what to do about the "trapped" fetus whose mother has already died.[25]
In such a circumstance, they deduce, there could not possibly be any
thought of granting permission to kill the fetus. Rather, they suggest that
the *Tosafot* use the words "it is permitted to kill it" to communicate that
although one might consider the fetus to be a quasi-independent being
in this situation, whose destruction might be thought to warrant death
for the perpetrator, this is not the appropriate punishment. The *Tosafists'*
decision to invoke the *goses* is significant in this context because, while

and in the main has evaded, contemporary Halachists. However, many concur on the opinion
that this is a state no more than three days prior to death. However, today when the classical
symptoms of the *goses* state are reversible, and the need arises to redefine the essential criterion of
this state, various possibilities exist. Three days prior to death is one. A person definitely moving
towards death may be another. (And yet other possibilities exist.) Hence, one might suggest that
even before three days prior to death, if death is certain, all the laws of *goses* will be applicable.
There has been some discussion of differences between different types of *goses* and a person
who is *tereifah*. However, as Steinberg points out, from a Jewish ethical standpoint there exists no
differences between any individuals; the distinctions are only legal (with regard to punishment
for murder etc.)." These legal distinctions are, however, of some significance to the abortion
discussion. Thus, three different states may be discerned (see *Sanhedrin* 78a and *Hilkhot Rotzeiach*
2:7–9):
    The *tereifah* – one who is suffering from an injury, for which there is no cure or hope of
recovery. One who kills him is not liable for the death penalty (though he may be subject to
Divine punishment).
    The *goses be-yedei shamayim* – one whose death is imminent and is dying from a terminal illness
brought on by heaven. One who kills him is liable for the death penalty.
    The *goses be-yedei adam* – one whose death is imminent and is dying from some primary injury
brought about by human hands. Though there is a Talmudic debate concerning the appropriate
fate of one who kills him, the consensus follows the Sages and Rava in declaring him not liable
for the death penalty.

[21] *Tosafot* to *Niddah* 44b, s.v. *ihu.*   [22] *Hagahot Maharitz* to *Niddah* 44b.   [23] See below, pp. 78ff.
[24] *Hagahot Yaʿavetz* to *Niddah* 44b.   [25] See above, chapter 2, pp. 45ff.

the *Shabbat* may be violated to save a *goses*, nevertheless one who murders him is not liable for death.[26] Plainly, if indeed this argument is correct and the *Tosafot* are actually referring to the absence of capital punishment, as opposed to any permission to kill the fetus, no disparity would exist between the *Tosafot* texts.

Bleich holds strongly to this position. In an extensive treatment of the subject, Bleich first dismisses Chajes' argument: "A close examination of the line of reasoning employed by *Tosafot* shows that the conclusion reached by *Mahariz Hajes* cannot be supported..." He then goes on to make the case for the other side, which he summarizes as follows: "The conclusion, then, is that there is no evidence that the destruction of a fetus whose mother had preceded it in death carries a statutory punishment. That the taking of a life of a fetus is forbidden does not at all come into question according to this understanding of *Tosafot*." But Bleich goes even further. He maintains that the *goses* analogy employed by the *Tosafot* is unhelpful: "According to any interpretation, the comparison by *Tosafot* of a fetus to a *goses be-yedei Adam* defies comprehension..." The failure of the analogy, Bleich contends, leaves open the possibility that overriding the *Shabbat* to save the fetus "establishes that it is therefore a human life whose destruction is punishable."[27]

It is possible, then, that the outlook of Chajes may point to a thread in the tradition that questioned the solidity of the prohibition enunciated by the *Tosafot*. It seems more likely, however, given the widespread post-*Tosafot* acknowledgment that some form of ban was extant,[28] that the Ya'avetz view of a coherent prohibition – other than in life-saving circumstances – was dominant during the time of the *Rishonim* and *Acharonim*.

Nevertheless, the basis of the *Tosafists'* extension of the prohibition to Jews is not at all plain. For, although the principle "there is nothing that is permitted to a Jew but prohibited to a non-Jew," might provide a pretext for a prohibition being plausible, it offers no logically compelling argument. Indeed, the *Tosafists'* reasoning in this matter has been described as "circular,"[29] since they use their formulated prohibition on feticide as evidence of the Talmudic principle's validity. From their declaration that "despite the fact that [a Jew] is not liable for capital punishment, nonetheless [aborting a fetus] is still not permissible," the *Tosafot* make plain that no firmly grounded legal interdiction of the Jewish conduct of

[26] *Yoma* 84b.
[27] Bleich, "Abortion in Halakhic Literature," pp. 328–330, n. 4.   [28] See below, generally.
[29] Sinclair, "Legal Basis," 115.

abortion was to be found in the received *halakhic* heritage, upon which they could stake their claim. It is not, after all, an unreasonable assumption to hold that had a stronger objection to feticide been available to the *Tosafot* they most surely would have mentioned it.

Indeed, Sinclair goes so far as to posit that the prohibition discerned by the *Tosafot* derived more from a process of eisegesis on their part than one of exegesis:

> Moreover, it is quite consistent with their style that the Tosafot would seek to derive a legal prohibition on abortion, however vague and indefinite, and irrespective of the historical texts used, in order to provide support for a generally accepted notion. In this they were very possibly influenced by the methods applied in the analysis of Roman and Canon Law by the Medieval French jurists, who tended to disregard the original historical sense of the text under analysis in order to reach the desired end.[30]

Sinclair hardly could be clearer. The *Tosafot*, in his view, had produced a prohibition in order better to address the societal reality in which they found themselves, notwithstanding the fact that this may not have done justice to the true contextual sense of the sources.[31]

The "vague and indefinite" standing of the prohibition, moreover, was little alleviated by its explicit enunciation on the part of the *Tosafot*. Pivotal questions remained unresolved: was the prohibition to be seen as biblical in nature, conveying that the Torah, by analogy to the Noahide, forbade the Jew from taking fetal life as a form of murder? Alternatively, was it a rabbinic edict, allowing for much greater flexibility in its application? There is cogent evidence that the great Spanish *Rishon*, Rabbeinu Nissim (*c.* 1310 – *c.* 1375) took the latter view. In his commentary on Alfasi,[32] Rabbeinu Nissim provides an unexpected reason for the *Arakhin* text's call for the speedy execution of a pregnant woman condemned to death. Rabbeinu Nissim rejects the *ubar yerekh imo* argument – which would imply that the fetus was condemned to the same fate as its mother because it was a dependent part of her – choosing instead to

---

[30] *Ibid.*, 120.
[31] Indeed, there is further evidence from a famous non-legal text, the kabbalistic *Zohar*, released to the Jewish world in the thirteenth century, that Jews had assumed a decidedly negative attitude to fetal destruction. While it is possible that this negative response arose from the Jewish textual heritage already in place, it seems likely that outside influences may well have added to its strength: "There are three who drive away the *Shekhinah* from the world, making it impossible for the Holy One, blessed be God, to fix God's abode in the universe, and causing prayer to be unanswered ... [The third is] the one who causes the fetus to be destroyed in the womb, for such a one destroys the artifice of the Holy One, blessed be God, and God's workmanship ... For these abominations the Spirit of Holiness weeps ..." (*Zohar, Shemot* 3b).
[32] At *Chullin* 58a.

favor the *ubar lav yerekh imo* position. Hence, Rabbeinu Nissim postulates that "in the case of a woman about to be executed, we do not wait until she gives birth, not for reasons of *ubar yerekh imo*, but rather because, given that she is condemned to death, we do not delay her sentence; and, as concerns the fetus, since it has not emerged into the world, it does not call forth our consideration."[33] It is, of course, not plausible that Rabbeinu Nissim would permit an unjustifiable destruction of the fetus. Consequently, Rabbeinu Nissim has been understood here as conveying that the prohibition against fetal destruction is lifted by the rabbis out of sensitivity to the plight of the condemned woman.[34] Plainly, if the ban were biblical in nature, the rabbis would have no such power, and it would be difficult indeed to make sense of Rabbeinu Nissim's reasoning.[35] While Rabbeinu Nissim's position is not entirely certain, it seems apparent that, even at a time close to the ban's articulation, its standing was by no means settled.[36]

It is small wonder then, given the contributions made to the abortion landscape by Rashi, Maimonides, and the *Tosafot*, that the *Acharonim* would be confronted with an extensive task of textual reconciliation and explication. Several problems would continue to be matters of pressing interest for later generations. There was the subject of how to comprehend the Maimonidean use of the *rodef* classification, and how to correlate it with Rashi's position. There was the issue of the nature of the prohibition articulated by the *Tosafot*. Did it imply that, as for the Noahide, abortion was to be considered a capital offense for the Jew? Or was there another rationale that made the prohibition applicable to Jews? Was the origin of the prohibition biblical or rabbinic? Was the prohibition in force through all stages of pregnancy? And did the prohibition apply to all circumstances except a direct threat to the mother's life?

The first among the *Acharonim* to deal tangentially with some of these issues was Rabbi David ibn Zimra (1479–1573). Zimra, who was born in Spain, left Spain in 1492 because of the Spanish expulsion of the Jews and died in *Eretz Yisrael*. Like many other scholars, his path from Spain

---

[33] Ran, Commentary to *Chullin* 58a, *Perek Shlishi*, s.v. "*ule-inyan*."
[34] See *Sheëilot UTeshuvot Achiezer* (Rabbi Chaim Ozer Grodzinsky), New York, 1946, volume III, number 65, section 14.
[35] It is always possible, of course, that Nissim might have determined that there were other biblical proof-texts that buttressed the prohibition – as would a number of the later *Acharonim* – but if so, murder would not be their concern.
[36] For a more detailed exposition of Nissim's position that *ubar lav yerekh imo* see below, chapter 4, p. 106.

took him to Safed, which had become an important center of Jewish life. In 1513 Zimra went to Cairo, where he became head of the local Jewish community, chief rabbi, and head of the rabbinic court. Zimra is particularly remembered for his commentary on Maimonides' *Mishneh Torah* and for his responsa, of which there are more than ten thousand in existence.[37] Zimra's thoughts relevant to the above questions appear in two separate *teshuvot* (responsa). In the first, Zimra is asked about the regular phenomenon in Egypt of women dying in childbirth: given that some women had taken to beating their bellies in order to hasten the death of the fetus, was this to be considered a form of murder (*netilat neshamah*), and, if it occurred on the *Shabbat*, was it to be considered a transgression of *Shabbat*?[38] While condemning such behavior, Zimra unambiguously states that so long as the fetus has not emerged, and so long as it has not attained status as a viable being, one who kills it is not guilty of murder. Even if the fetus is moving, it is not considered a living being.[39] The fetus is not like a *goses*, who does have standing as a viable being. Hence, while all steps should be taken to prevent such conduct, killing the fetus would not be considered murder, and nor would there be any transgression of *Shabbat*.

In his second *teshuvah*, Zimra is asked whether a *kohen* who deliberately struck a pregnant woman and caused her to miscarry becomes ineligible to perform priestly rites.[40] Consistent with his other *teshuvah*, Zimra rules that, notwithstanding the fact that Maimonides stated that even a *kohen* who spilled blood inadvertently becomes ineligible, this *kohen* does not lose his eligibility because he did not kill a *nefesh* that had standing as a viable being. Significantly, Zimra uses this opportunity to place his ruling in the context of his understanding of *Mishnah Ohalot*. Zimra maintains that, in fact, the "true reason" that the *Mishnah* held that the fetus might be killed to save the mother is because the fetus is not a *nefesh*, not because it is a *rodef*. Furthermore, there is, says Zimra, irrefutable proof for his position on the *kohen*'s eligibility in Exodus 21:22–23. The assailant, who, in the Torah passage, was guilty of causing a miscarriage, was required to pay a financial penalty to the husband as compensation for the loss

---

[37] "Rabbi David Ibn Zimra" in "Biography," in *The Responsa Project*, a *ShuT* CD-Rom, Bar-Ilan University, Version 6.0, 1972–98.

[38] References and quotations concerning this Zimra *teshuvah* are from *ShuT HaRadbaz*, volume II, number 695.

[39] While the fetus certainly is alive and is considered "life," it is not a living being in the sense of being of viable standing.

[40] References and quotations concerning this Zimra *teshuvah* are from *ShuT HaRadbaz, Orach Chayim*, volume VIII, number 22.

of the fetus. So, too, in the case of the *kohen*. He likewise is obligated to pay a financial penalty. Making him ineligible for priestly rites would go beyond what is required. Zimra, then, takes an unequivocal stance; favoring Rashi's view over that of Maimonides, he offers little comfort for the *rodef* approach, holding instead that feticide cannot be regarded as murder because the fetus is not a *nefesh*.

A very similar view of the divergent positions of Rashi and Maimonides was expressed by the renowned Polish scholar, Rabbi Joshua Falk (1555–1614), in his *Sefer Meïrat Einayim* commentary on the *Shulchan Arukh*. Despite the fact that the *Shulchan Arukh* had recorded Maimonides' position precisely, Falk was of the view that those who based "their halakhic decisions on the Shulchan Arukh alone without investigating sources, remained ignorant of the sources and rationale of the law and rendered incoherent halakhic decisions."[41] Thus, the *Shulchan Arukh* notwithstanding, Falk had no compunction in deeming the *rodef* argument to be of little relevance. What is significant is that the fetus is not a *nefesh*. Though the fetus is surely alive, its non-*nefesh* status is "evidenced by the fact that the person who strikes a pregnant woman is only required to pay compensation, and is not called a murderer, nor is he liable to the death penalty."[42] Like Zimra, Falk certainly offers support for Rashi's perspective.

While Zimra and Falk provide early perspectives on the differing approaches of Rashi and Maimonides, the first *Acharon* to grapple substantially with the prohibition on fetal destruction was the *Sefaradi halakhist* Rabbi Yosef Trani (known as Maharit, 1568–1639). Maharit, who was chief rabbi of Turkey and head of a large *yeshivah* in Constantinople, authored two *teshuvot* pertinent to abortion.[43] When read together, these two *teshuvot* present a confusing and seemingly dichotomous approach to the subject, which, although amenable to harmonization, is open to variant interpretations.[44] How these *teshuvot* ought to be comprehended has been the subject of much debate. David Feldman states that "[t]hese two Responsa must be taken together; probably a printer's confusion separated and disarranged them."[45] Rabbi Eliezer Waldenberg also holds

---

[41] S. Eidelberg, "Falk, Joshua ben Alexander Ha-Kohen," in *Encyclopaedia Judaica*, Jerusalem, Keter Publishing House, volume VI, pp. 1158–1159.
[42] *Sefer Meïrat Einayim, Choshen Mishpat* 425:8.
[43] Y. Trani, *Maharit*, Lemberg, 1861, volume I, numbers 97 and 99.
[44] Compare, for example, the understanding of Al-Chakam (see below, chapter 4, pp. 113–114) with that of Feinstein (see below, chapter 5, pp. 174–175).
[45] Feldman, *Birth Control*, p. 256, n. 30.

firmly to this view, maintaining that sections that belong to one responsum actually somehow became mixed into the other, thereby muddling the correct understanding.[46] Sinclair writes that "the resolution of the two apparently contradictory responsa of Trani has exercised a number of authorities and it is by no means clear that the two responsa are dealing with the same issue; it is very likely that they are not…"[47] All three essentially maintain, therefore, that both *teshuvot* contain the authentic views of Maharit, albeit on two somewhat different matters that have become awkwardly tangled together.[48] It seems most cogent, however, to see the *teshuvot* as somehow linked, given that they deal with the same general subject matter.

These two *teshuvot*, therefore, might be understood best as follows. In *teshuvah* number 99, Maharit was asked whether or not it was permitted for a Jew, presumably a doctor or midwife, to assist a non-Jew by performing an abortion for her, and whether such an action would constitute murder. The inquiry was probably prompted by the vast difference in proposed penalties for Jews and non-Jews: if the abortion were performed by a gentile, the act would be worthy of capital punishment; whereas, while the procedure would be forbidden to a Jew, a Jew would go unpunished. In his answer, Maharit vigorously denies any possibility that murder was involved as far as a Jew is concerned. He points to *Mishnah Arakhin*, which calls for the speedy execution of a pregnant woman condemned to death, thereby subordinating the interests of the fetus to those of its mother.[49] Maharit echoes the Talmudic view that it is appropriate – at least in theory – to bring forward fetal death out of consideration for the "dishonor" and the delay which the mother otherwise might suffer. Maharit, however, focuses most particularly upon the reaction of the *Gemara* to *Mishnah Arakhin*'s ruling: "*Peshita!*," the *Gemara* proclaims; "It is self-evident!" that she would be executed forthwith as the fetus is seen to be a part of her body. If it is entirely self-evident, however, why is there any need to state that the woman should be killed forthwith? Maharit replies that without this instruction one might have thought to delay her execution on account of the mandate in Exodus 21:22 that one who brings about a miscarriage is penalized by being required to pay compensation to the husband. Hence, the Talmud is attempting to convey

[46] E. Waldenberg, *Tzitz Eliezer*, Jerusalem, 1963 and on, volume IX, number 51; see below, chapter 5, p. 161.
[47] D. B. Sinclair, unpublished chapter: "The Interplay of Legal Doctrine and Moral Principle in the Halakhah of Abortion," p. 27, n. 113.
[48] On this question, see also the views of Feinstein below, chapter 5, pp. 174–175.
[49] See above, chapter 2, p. 37.

that, the husband's interests notwithstanding, one nevertheless proceeds with the capital punishment. From the *"Peshita"* response of the *Gemara*, Maharit concludes that there is not the faintest suggestion that murder is involved when a Jew takes the life of the fetus: "if, out of concern for the disgrace of the mother, we kill the fetus without concern over murder (*ibud nefashot*), it follows that – where Jews are concerned – for the 'need' (*tzorekh*) of the mother it is permitted to cause her to abort since it is for the mother's healing."[50] In this *teshuvah*, then, Maharit displays a rather lenient approach to abortion for Jews. While he does not define what would constitute an appropriate "need," his connection of this "need" to the "dishonor" mentioned in *Arakhin* certainly implies that Maharit foresees abortions for Jews in circumstances that are less serious than a threat to the mother's life.

Turning his attention to non-Jews, Maharit, in discussing the appropriateness of rendering any type of medical help to a gentile, recounts a *teshuvah* of Rabbi Solomon ben Abraham Adret (known as Rashba, 1235–1310), a renowned rabbinic scholar from Barcelona. Rashba had written about the manner in which Nachmanides had rendered assistance, in return for payment, to a non-Jew by helping her to conceive. Maharit's decision to report about this *teshuvah*, it appears, was designed to demonstrate that there was nothing improper about providing such assistance to non-Jews. Immediately after this example of Jewish aid given to a non-Jew, Maharit proceeds to aver that not only is abortion not to be considered as murder for a Jew, it is not to be considered as murder for a gentile either.[51] Given that one is permitted to offer medical treatment to a non-Jew, this lenient approach is a logical outgrowth of Maharit's position on fetal standing for Jews. In *teshuvah* number 99, then, Maharit's discussion essentially revolves around the question of "ought there to be a ban on feticide as a form of murder?" Concluding that no

---

[50] As Bleich puts it: "An act of murder certainly would not be condoned simply in order to spare the condemned [woman] undue agony or to prevent dishonor to a corpse"; "Abortion in Halakhic Literature," p. 336. See also Bleich's n. 23 on p. 336 where he lists those authorities who reject this line of argument since they contend that the fetus – as part of its mother – is subject to the same sentence, and it is for this reason that the *Gemara* would find the *Mishnah*'s ruling to be obvious.

[51] It is important to note that there is no small measure of confusion as to how this section of Maharit's *teshuvah* ought to be understood. There is at least one prominent twentieth-century figure who understood Maharit quite differently. According to Unterman, the reference to abortion is connected, in fact, to the *teshuvah* about Nachmanides, such that Nachmanides ought to be seen as helping the non-Jew to conceive, and subsequently to abort (see the views of Unterman below, chapter 5, pp. 137ff.). For reasons that will shortly become clear, if this were the correct reading, Nachmanides' behavior would be problematic indeed and would require explanation.

murder is involved, Maharit does not see murder as the reason for an abortion ban for either Jews or non-Jews. If murder were Maharit's only concern, therefore, *teshuvah* number 99 would bar a Jew neither from abortion, nor from assisting a non-Jew to abort.

Murder, however, was not Maharit's only concern. For, in *teshuvah* number 97, Maharit displays no doubt whatsoever about the existence of a prohibition on abortion: "The *Tosafot* wrote that a non-Jew is liable [for punishment] for fetal death, while a Jew is not liable. [But] even though a Jew is not liable, it is not permitted [to kill the fetus], and hence [it follows] that there is a prohibition in this matter."[52] If, however, murder was not at stake, then what, in Maharit's view, was the fundamental reason for this prohibition of the *Tosafot*? What crime was committed if a Jew sought an abortion with non-therapeutic motivations? According to Maharit, the crime was that of *chabbalah*, wounding the body. The proof-text for the ban on unlawful wounding is Deuteronomy 25:3. *Baba Kamma* 90b records in the name of Akiva that "he who injures himself, even though it is not permitted, is exempt from punishment, whereas others who injure him are liable."[53] Maimonides, in *Hilkhot Rotzeiach* 1:4, explains that the *halakhah* regards the body as God's possession, which no human being has the right to damage. Hence abortion, in Maharit's view, represented a prohibited act of *chabbalah*. Indeed, the provision of *Masekhet Arakhin*, which called for sacrificing the fetus of the woman about to be executed, fitted logically into Maharit's explanation, since worries over unlawful *chabbalah* are inapposite to one about to be lawfully executed. Moreover, because wounding for the purposes of healing is permitted within the law, the *chabbalah* explanation helps to clarify why abortion in therapeutic circumstances would be acceptable.[54]

In response to Maharit, some sources took the view that the *chabbalah* provision did not prevent wounding part of one's own body.[55] Hence, the *chabbalah* reasoning – as a later respondent would point out – may imply no censure at all if a woman decided voluntarily to self-abort.[56] The *chabbalah* explanation certainly has not been enthusiastically endorsed as the most cogent justification of the prohibition on feticide. Feldman declares *chabbalah* to be "a weak answer" to the question of the nature of the crime that prompted the ban.[57] *Chabbalah* nevertheless has proved to

[52] *Teshuvot Maharit*, volume 1, number 97.
[53] This law is codified in *Hilkhot Chovel UMazzik* 5:1 and *Sh. Ar. Ch. M.* 420:6.
[54] See *Sanhedrin* 84b.
[55] *Yad Ramah* to *Baba Kamma* 90b and *Tur Ch. M.* 420:6 convey that self-wounding is not forbidden.
[56] See *Seriedei Eish*, 349.   [57] Feldman, *Birth Control*, p. 256.

be sufficiently compelling and enduring that later scholars have utilized it in their discussion of the abortion prohibition.[58]

A Jew, then, according to *teshuvah* number 97, could not perform a non-therapeutic abortion on a Jew because of the *chabbalah* prohibition. Was it permissible, though, to assist a non-Jew, as was asked in *teshuvah* number 99? Notwithstanding the fact that murder is not involved, Maharit reminds his readers, the non-Jew is specifically enjoined not to abort by the "man in man" provision of the Talmud. Hence, in Maharit's view, as the non-Jew is banned from abortion on pain of death, for a Jew to carry out such an abortion would transgress the biblical principle of "do not place a stumbling-block before the blind."[59] Maharit cites the Talmudic examples of the use of this verse in forbidding someone to place a cup of wine in front of a *nazir*, one who has forsworn the consumption of alcohol, or to offer a limb torn from a wild animal to a gentile,[60] for whom consumption of such a limb is explicitly prohibited by the Noahide laws.[61] These examples seem to indicate that Maharit perceived such an assisted abortion as an insinuation to the non-Jew that transgression was acceptable, when, in fact, for the non-Jew, the consequences would be dire indeed. In *teshuvah* number 97, then, Maharit rules that a non-Jew should not be assisted in the performance of a non-therapeutic abortion.

It is worth emphasizing that Maharit never refers to Maimonides' *rodef* argument. He never suggests that an abortion is only acceptable if the mother is being pursued or if her life is threatened.[62] Maharit simply concludes that abortion without sufficient reason is prohibited by the *chabbalah* ban for Jews and by the "man in man" prohibition for non-Jews.[63] If, then, these two *teshuvot* are designed to be consistent one with the other, it can be posited that Maharit intended to convey that, although there is an extant *chabbalah* prohibition in place, in instances of maternal "need," for purposes of "healing," this ban could be overridden. Consequently, Maharit could be identified with the "Rashi school"

---

[58] See below, chapter 5, pp. 145, 151.   [59] Leviticus 19:14.
[60] Maharit cites these examples in *Teshuvot Maharit*, volume 1, number 97.
[61] The Talmudic reference for these examples is *Pesachim* 22b.
[62] Some, however, did understand Maharit as only allowing abortions when the mother's life was in danger. See D. Meislich, *Binyan David*, Ohel, 1935, number 60.
[63] It is important to record that Maharit was not alone in the Turkish rabbinate in holding negative views about assisting non-Jews to procure an abortion. His student, the famous Rabbi Chaim Benveniste (1603–1673), rabbi of Smyrna, and "one of the greatest of the Jewish codifiers," was the author of *Knesset Ha-Gedolah*, a work hailed by *Ashkenazim* as well as *Sefaradim*. In it, he too adjured Jews not to help gentiles in this way, for such behavior would represent a "stumbling block," causing others to transgress. See *Knesset Ha-Gedolah*, *Yoreh De'ah* 154:6.

of thought since he does not exclude the possibility of abortions in situations other than imminent maternal jeopardy.[64]

Maharit, then, had provided the first cogent, if not wholly convincing, explanation of the abortion prohibition. It would not be long, however, before a second reason would be advanced, this time from within the *Ashkenazi* milieu. It came from the renowned Talmudic scholar Rabbi Yaïr Chayim Bacharach (1638–1702), who was born in Germany in the year before Maharit's death. Three years before his own demise, when he was already deaf and sick, Bacharach published *Chavvot Yaïr*, his great collection of *teshuvot*. *Chavvot Yaïr* was a *tour de force*, which displayed Bacharach's prodigious comprehension both of rabbinic texts and of the science and culture of his time.[65] Within *Chavvot Yaïr*, Bacharach responds to the question of whether a woman, who is in the early stages of pregnancy, who has conceived in the context of an adulterous relationship, and who is now profoundly remorseful and in deep sorrow for what she has done, may abort.

Bacharach begins his answer by asserting that there is absolutely no difference between a *mamzer* (a bastard) and a legitimate child, with the exception of the ban on "entering the community[66] and serving on the Sanhedrin."[67] Logically, therefore, Bacharach proceeds to analyze the abortion issue broadly, only returning to reply to the original inquiry at the end. Bacharach first reformulates the question: "I glean that the essence of your question generally is whether the sin of murder [would be involved] after she became pregnant, were the fetus to be damaged, killed and aborted." Bacharach then points out that various stages of pregnancy are sometimes invoked in such a discussion, such as the passage of forty days signifying that the fetus is more than "mere water,"[68] or the completion of three months when the fetus is sensed, or later on

[64] See M. Washofsky, "Abortion and the Halakhic Conversation," in W. Jacob and M. Zemer (eds.), *The Fetus and Fertility in Jewish Law*, Pittsburgh, Rodef Shalom Press, 1995, pp. 45–46. Washofsky's allying of Maharit's views with those of Rashi appears appropriate.
[65] J. Haberman, "Bacharach, Jair Hayyim ben Moses Samson," in *Encyclopaedia Judaica*, Jerusalem, Keter Publishing House, volume IV, pp. 46–48. Haberman describes the immense richness of *Chavvot Yaïr*: "This epoch-making work, which has gone through many editions, demonstrates not only Bacharach's exhaustive knowledge of all branches of rabbinic learning, but also the whole extent of his knowledge of the general sciences, such as mathematics, astronomy, and music, and shows also his opposition to the distorted type of *pilpul* [theoretical discussion on Jewish law] current in his day . . ."
[66] This is a Toraitic ban that came to imply that a *mamzer* was forbidden from marrying anybody except another *mamzer*.
[67] Unless otherwise specified, all Bacharach references and quotations are from Y. Bacharach, *Chavvot Yaïr*, Lemberg, 1896, number 31.
[68] See above, chapter 2, pp. 33–34.

when fetal movement is detected. However, Bacharach declares, he intends to rule not "from mental inclination and the logic of the belly," but "according to the law of Torah." Clearly, Bacharach is signaling his determination to prefer a textual approach to decide the appropriateness of such an abortion, undifferentiated by distinctions based on physical developments.

In his analysis, Bacharach, like Maharit, rejects the notion that abortion should be considered murder. He quotes the Talmudic sources which demonstrate that while the killer of a one-day-old baby would be guilty of murder, this is not so in the case of the fetus. In fact, were it not for the reality that there is a prohibition in place, Bacharach implies, there would be nothing to prevent a Jew from killing a fetus up to the onset of labor.[69] If, though, the fetus becomes a *nefesh* at birth, why does Bacharach stop at the onset of labor, as opposed to birth itself? Bacharach argues that *Mishnah Ohalot* might lead one to contend that since the fetus is not a *nefesh* until birth, one could kill it with impunity up to the moment before it emerged. However, given that in *Ohalot* the mother was in life-threatening difficulty, there is an implication that the permission to kill only applies when the mother is endangered. If this were the case, then such an authority to kill with impunity – in circumstances in which the mother is imperiled – obviously would extend throughout the pregnancy until the moment of birth. It is for that reason, Bacharach maintains, that the *Gemara* in *Sanhedrin* 72b refers to the mother as being pursued: it conveys that only in circumstances where her life is being pursued may one kill the fetus without punishment at any point during gestation. To understand what happens in other circumstances, when the mother's life is not being pursued, Bacharach – as did Maharit before him – relies heavily on *Masekhet Arakhin*. From the *Mishnah*'s instruction that execution ought to be delayed for a woman who has gone into labor, Bacharach concludes that this is because the fetus is now a "separate body" that may not be touched after the commencement of labor. Conversely, the rabbis propose in the *Arakhin* text that before the onset of labor the fetus may be sacrificed out of concern for the possible "dishonor" of the mother. Bacharach derives from this that if a fetus may be killed out of consideration for the "dishonor" of a condemned woman, then these Talmudic passages certainly would not regard the killing of a fetus, before the onset of labor, as a criminal act, even if the mother were not at risk.

---

[69] When the fetus, having moved from its place, becomes a *gufah acharinah*. See above, chapter 2, p. 46.

Moreover, as Bacharach explains it, when the *Arakhin Gemara* allows for the transgression of *Shabbat* in order to save a fetus, this is completely consistent with his point of view. After all, Bacharach points out, the *Gemara* speaks of a woman who dies while "on the birthstool." Clearly, if she is on the birthstool, then the fetus has already become a "separate body." As a separate body from its mother, but not yet a *nefesh*, it would be – following the *Tosafot* – in much the same *halakhic* position as the *goses*: although killing it would be forbidden, such killing would not be considered a capital crime, and the *Shabbat* certainly could be violated on behalf of the fetus. According to Bacharach's view, however, none of this would apply prior to the onset of labor for "certainly if it is permitted to kill [the fetus], it is impossible to state that we would transgress the *Shabbat* on its behalf."

Bacharach further maintains that it is a general principle that, before the beginning of labor, the laws of the Torah can only be overridden out of concern for the welfare of the mother, but not for the fetus. Thus, when a pregnant woman is permitted to eat pork on *Yom Kippur*,[70] there must be a concern for her that is at stake – not just the fetus – because "for danger to the fetus alone we certainly would not transgress *Shabbat*, nor would we feed its mother."[71] Hence, from Bacharach's perspective, not only is it not murder to abort a fetus, but until labor is underway, saving the life of the fetus is a sufficiently low legal priority that it would not warrant disturbing the *Shabbat*.

But if it is "not murder" to abort a fetus when the mother's life is not threatened, then, while this might be consistent with Rashi, it would seem to be at odds with Maimonides.[72] Undeterred by such ostensible difficulties, Bacharach claims that the seemingly varying approaches of Rashi and Maimonides are actually not in conflict: Maimonides probably would concur with Rashi that the fetus is not a *nefesh*, and that the nature of its existence cannot be equated to that of a born human being. However, as Bacharach sees it, Maimonides' ruling is limited to the circumstances of *Mishnah Ohalot* in which the mother's life is at risk. If, however, Maimonides would agree that the fetus is not a *nefesh*, presumably there should be no problem with killing it in order to save its mother. Given that this is so, why would Maimonides have any need to invoke the *rodef* categorization? According to Bacharach's explanation, Maimonides needed the *rodef* designation in order to deal with the

---

[70] *Yoma* 82a. See above, chapter 2, p. 45.
[71] For similar outlooks, see above, chapter 2, p. 45.   [72] See above, pp. 58–61.

extant prohibition upon a Jew killing a fetus.[73] It is true, as the *Tosafot* made clear, that in an instance of danger to the mother, the prohibition is lifted and "a Jew is commanded to save her."[74] Maimonides, however, requires some sort of justification that can explain in *halakhic* terms why an otherwise operational prohibition ought to be set aside in order to save the life of the mother. In Bacharach's view, Maimonides' utilization of the *rodef* argument is his answer to this technical *halakhic* conundrum.

Bacharach derives this explanation from a careful examination of Maimonides' use of language. Maimonides stipulates that when the mother's life is threatened, "it is permitted to dismember the fetus... because the fetus is like a *rodef*," whereas *Mishnah Ohalot* had simply stated that "the fetus is dismembered." The permission, then, to dismember the fetus, the prohibition notwithstanding, stems from the fact that the fetus is behaving as a *rodef*. Were it not conducting itself as a *rodef*, there could be no basis for overturning the prohibition, even if the mother were dying. Thus, Bacharach submits that Maimonides would concur that the fetus is not a *nefesh*, that killing the fetus is not murder, that it is nevertheless forbidden to kill the fetus, and that this prohibition can only be lifted insofar as the fetus acts like a *rodef*.

While Maimonides, as Bacharach perceives it, has an effective explanation for the rationale behind the lifting of the prohibition when the mother is at risk, what is still lacking is an overall reason for the prohibition itself. Bacharach, like those before him, is concerned to answer the question: if murder is not the root problem behind the prohibition, then what is? Bacharach discerns an entirely different *halakhic* reason for the ban from the *chabbalah* justification proffered by Maharit. The real issue, in Bacharach's view, is the wanton spilling of male seed (*hotzaʾat zerah levatalah*). Spilling of male seed, of course, can be a form of contraception: semen that is emitted but not deposited in the womb, either through masturbation or *coitus interruptus*, frustrates reproduction, and is seen to

---

[73] For Bacharach's explanation to be sustainable, it would seem necessary to hold that Maimonides was aware of the ban on feticide for Jews that was first recorded by the *Tosafot*. Despite the geographic separation, this is credible, given that Maimonides was contemporaneous with the early *Tosafot*. Even had they not overlapped in time, the fact that the *Tosafot* were the first to document the prohibition, does not preclude the possibility that the tradition was actually older, and may have been independently known to Maimonides. No matter the historic realities involved, it is clear that Bacharach assumes that Maimonides would have known of the Tosafists' position.

[74] *Tosafot* to *Sanhedrin* 59a, s.v. *lica*, see above, p. 62.

be an affront to the *mitzvah* to be fruitful and multiply.[75] Implicit in Bacharach's thinking, then, is the notion that if it is unacceptable to block child-bearing via the destruction of male seed before conception, then it should be improper after conception as well. Hence, Bacharach holds that the prohibition on feticide is subsumed within the tradition's strenuous objection to the wanton spilling of male seed:

As Yochanan stated: "Whoever emits semen in vain deserves death, as it says, 'What he did was evil in the sight of the Lord, and [God] took his life also' (Genesis 38:10)." Rabbi Yitzhak and Rabbi Ammi said: "It is as though he shed blood, as it says, 'You who inflame yourselves among the terebinths, under every verdant tree; who slaughter children in the valleys, among the clefts of the rocks' (Isaiah 57:5)."[76]

Bacharach understands Isaiah's reference to slaughtering "children in the valleys" to connote feticide, and reasons that one is prohibited from killing the fetus because of the destructive spilling of male seed that would thereby be involved.

There are two noteworthy features of Bacharach's rationale. First, although this prohibition against wasting male seed is understood to apply to men, Bacharach, basing his position in prior declarations of the *Rishonim*, states that women are also included in the ban. He is careful to ensure that nobody draws the conclusion that his "destruction of seed" reasoning could exempt women from the abortion prohibition.[77] The second significant aspect of Bacharach's explanation is that it makes his insistence upon paying no heed to the physical stages of pregnancy, and only ruling according to the words of Torah, all the more comprehensible.[78] After all, if the reason for the ban were indeed the spilling of male seed, then the ban would apply equally at every moment of pregnancy, without differentiation. The traversing of various physical stages becomes, consequently, immaterial to Bacharach's perspective.

---

[75] It is, according to tradition, forbidden to destroy male seed, or to spill it without procreative intent. This is referred to as the ban on onanism after the biblical figure Onan (Genesis 38:7–10). There is a strong line of thought to the effect that such behavior is biblically prohibited. See *Tosafot* to *Sanhedrin* 59b, s.v. *ve-ha*, where the *Tosafot* conclude that "[O]ne who is commanded concerning 'be fruitful and multiply' is commanded [implicitly] not to destroy seed."

[76] *Niddah* 13a.

[77] Bacharach quotes the *Tosafot* to *Yevamot* 12b, s.v. *shalosh*, which expresses the view that women are also prohibited from such destruction. He also refers to the *Tosafot* to *Gittin* 41b, s.v. *lo*, which conveys that despite the fact that women are not specifically included in the commandment to "be fruitful and multiply," women are still an indispensable and responsible part of the Divine design to populate the world.

[78] See above, pp. 73–74.

Just as they had done to Maharit, later scholars would criticize
Bacharach's justification for the abortion prohibition, and would find
inconsistencies and loopholes within it.[79] Nevertheless, by the time that
Bacharach finally provided the questioner with a conclusion to the original inquiry, the great *Acharon* had contributed significantly to the abortion
rulings of the Middle Ages. In the end, Bacharach's answer to the inquiry before him is in the negative: "Therefore, according to what we
have shown, the law of the Torah would permit what you ask, were it
not for the widespread practice among us, and among them, to seek to
establish a fence to curb the immoral... Whoever assists [in such an
abortion] gives a hand to transgressors." In theory, then, according to
Bacharach, but for the prohibition, the law might not have had a specific objection to such an abortion before the onset of labor. In reality,
however, the prohibition against destruction of male seed argued against
such an abortion, even if the pregnancy were begun in adultery and the
fetus thereby was destined to be a *mamzer*.

Clearly Bacharach, then, unlike Maharit, can be said to be closer
to the "Maimonidean school" insofar as he regarded it as significant
not only to grapple with Maimonides' approach, but to make the *rodef*
principle fit into his own understanding. Bacharach's notion that the
prohibition could only be lifted if the fetus behaved as a *rodef* is, after
all, entirely absent from Maharit's writings. This rather stark difference
led the *halakhic* scholar Rabbi Mark Washofsky, Professor of Rabbinics
at the Hebrew Union College – Jewish Institute of Religion, to this
observation:

In the seventeenth century, it was not at all obvious that the fetus could be
aborted *only* when it threatened the mother's life. It was not at all obvious that
Rambam's interpretation of the Talmudic material was correct. Nor, as Trani's
responsum shows, did it seem obligatory to take his position into account in
reaching an *halakhic* conclusion. Jewish law was hardly univocal on the subject
of the warrant for abortion.[80]

This multi-vocal stream, moreover, was not about to narrow any time
soon. In 1697, five years before Bacharach's death, Rabbi Jacob Emden
(Ya'avetz) was born, also in Germany. Like Bacharach, Ya'avetz was well
versed in the secular sciences, but he was unusual in the sense that he
possessed a good knowledge of non-*halakhic* Jewish literature as well.
Apart from a brief five-year period as rabbi of Emden, Ya'avetz never

[79] See, by way of example, the view of Ouziel, below, chapter 4, p. 126.
[80] Washofsky, "Abortion and the Halakhic Conversation," p. 47.

held a communal position, which made it possible for him to be critical of the practices he saw around him, and thereby ensured that he became a figure of controversy. One scholar wrote of him, "[t]he independence, originality, and stormy temperament of Emden are noticeable in his halakhic works. In certain subjects he takes up an extreme view against the majority opinion, and in others he is outstandingly lenient…"[81] It was this lenient side of Yaʿavetz that came to the fore within his *teshuvah* on abortion. Coincidentally, Yaʿavetz's *teshuvah* on the subject responded to a question almost identical to that put to Bacharach a century earlier: is there "a prohibition on the destruction of a fetus in the belly of a mother who had committed adultery," and does it make a difference "if she is single[82] or a married woman"?[83]

Yaʿavetz opens his answer by reviewing Bacharach's previous reply to the matter. Bacharach had begun by contending that, when it comes to feticide, it makes absolutely no difference if the fetus was a developing *mamzer* or was without taint. Yaʿavetz, however, strenuously disagrees with this view. In the case of a married woman who has committed adultery, he points out, the Torah provides for capital punishment for her crime. In Yaʿavetz's day, of course, the rabbis could not administer the death penalty. "In any case," though, writes Yaʿavetz, "she deserves death according to the law of heaven." Theoretically, were the intent of the law fulfillable, the execution of such an adulteress would be carried out without regard to her pregnancy.[84] Indeed, Yaʿavetz notes, the *Arakhin Mishnah* called for just such an outcome, and that was when the pregnancy was presumed to have been independent of whatever crime the condemned woman had committed. Here, where the pregnancy was a direct result of the transgression, how much more would the *Arakhin* text suggest that one not hesitate to execute her forthwith. "It is obvious," avers Yaʿavetz that

[81] M. S. Samet, "Emden, Jacob," in *Encyclopaedia Judaica*, Jerusalem, Keter Publishing House, volume VI, pp. 721–724.

[82] In which case adultery would not be involved. As Jewish law – at least theoretically – allowed for polygamy until the *cherem* (ban) of Rabbeinu Gershom was applied in the *Ashkenazi* world, no single woman could ever be guilty of adultery because she could be taken to be an additional wife. While polygamy has disappeared, present day *halakhah* continues to omit the single woman from those who potentially might be classified as adulteresses.

[83] Unless otherwise specified, all Yaʿavetz references and quotations are from J. Emden, *Sheʿilat Yaʿavetz*, Altona, 1739, number 43.

[84] In the course of his discussion, Yaʿavetz refers to the requirement for *hatraʾh*, forewarning. If capital punishment were applicable, the rabbis required that the witnesses be able to testify that *hatraʾh* was heard by the alleged criminal, warning him/her that the act about to be undertaken was a crime, which would result in a capital penalty. Without *hatraʾh* there would be no capital punishment, and Yaʿavetz seems to regard it as a requirement in these circumstances as well. On *hatraʾh*, see *Hilkhot Sanhedrin* 12:2.

in such an instance there would be no delay out of "concern for [the fetus], and it would be killed [on account of] its mother."

Ya'avetz's implication is clear: the life of such a woman can effectively be regarded as forfeit, even though he certainly did not advocate that any practical ramifications should follow from this assertion. However, in his subsequent statements in the *teshuvah* – which have been described as "rather astonishing,"[85] and are deeply controversial given the general tenor of *halakhah* – Ya'avetz does articulate some potential consequences for such a woman. He suggests that even though the death penalty is no longer practicable, still, as the woman's life is "forfeit," there would be no punishment – presumably from heaven – if she were to commit suicide. Indeed, Ya'avetz cites the suicide of King Saul – deemed an appropriate act by the rabbis – and opines that, given the circumstances of the case before him, such an act might even be regarded as meritorious for the adulteress. While it is unlikely, of course, that any woman would readily avail herself of the opportunity to attain such merit, what is significant is the inference which Ya'avetz goes on to draw. If an adulteress may, with impunity, destroy her very being in this way, one logically can deduce that she certainly may destroy a part of her body. It follows, therefore, that in such a case, there would be no legal barrier to the killing of the fetus. Since, from a legal perspective, this fetus would have been killed in the process of its mother's execution, no prohibition could now stand in the way of its destruction. Despite the fact, then, that Bacharach and Ya'avetz had been asked to respond to essentially the same inquiry, their conclusions hardly could be more divergent. Where Bacharach forbids the abortion of a fetus destined to be a *mamzer*, seeing it to be just as protected by the abortion prohibition as any other fetus, Ya'avetz permits such an act on the basis of the exceptional legal provisions to which he perceives this fetus to be subject. Indeed, Ya'avetz is so sure of the appropriateness of fetal subordination in this instance that he is prepared to advocate "commandment" language:

I have stated my clear opinion that [in this case] it is permissible [to perform an abortion], and perhaps performing an abortion under such circumstances is close to earning the merit of a *mitzvah* (commandment)... We make no distinction whether the father of the fetus is a Jew or a non-Jew... As a married woman, the mother is liable to the death penalty, and the rights of the fetus [to life] certainly do not exceed those of the mother.

[85] Bleich, "Abortion in Halakhic Literature," p. 364.

Yaʿavetz, then, is unquestionably of the view that there are circumstances other than a direct threat to the mother's physical existence[86] that would come close to compelling abortion.

Disparities between Yaʿavetz and Bacharach, however, arise not only within their conclusions, but also within the reasons they provide for the prohibition. Where Bacharach maintains that the prohibition is grounded in the absolute injunction against the "wanton spilling of male seed," Yaʿavetz is of the view that the emission of semen is only forbidden if it were truly *levatalah* – purposeless. Citing the Talmudic example of the three types of women permitted to use a *mokh*,[87] Yaʿavetz maintains that there can be no objection to the non-procreative emission of semen if it is for a worthy end: "we learn from this that this serious prohibition [the wanton spilling of male seed] [becomes] absolutely permitted when there is a need [to fulfill] a mitzvah." It follows that while "spilling seed on the ground" might be thoroughly objectionable, it is an altogether different matter to emit seed into the womb with procreative intent. The latter act cannot be defined retroactively as "the wanton spilling of male seed." If, then, Bacharach's reasoning for the prohibition is the most cogent available, Yaʿavetz would have to be understood to hold that the fundamental problem which the prohibition had been enacted to address was not problematic under all circumstances. While this does not necessitate a questioning of the prohibition itself, it suggests that the prohibition appeared to Yaʿavetz as an arbitrary construction, rather than a coherently grounded restriction.

Yaʿavetz does not attempt to provide an alternative understanding of the prohibition. His approach, therefore, is one that is respectful of the prohibition, while at the same time refusing to embrace the reasoning put forward to support it. Not surprisingly, then, when Yaʿavetz briefly digresses from the case at hand to address abortion generally, his response is consistent with this philosophy:

---

[86] Of course, one legitimately might contend that being condemned to death is "a direct threat to the mother's physical existence," and that this is not, therefore, an exceptional case. However, a closer examination reveals that this argument is unsatisfactory. In all "normal" instances of a "direct threat" to the mother, fetal destruction is called for as an act of *pikuach nefesh* in order *to save the mother's life*. Here, fetal destruction, while dictated by the mother's fate, is disconnected from her fate. If saving the mother were the aim, the court could alter its sentence, and feticide would become unnecessary.

[87] A *mokh* is an absorbent material designed to frustrate conception. It could be used either during coitus or as a post-coital absorbent. It was permitted for use by three categories of women for whom conceiving could present some type of danger. See *Yevamot* 12b and 100b; *Ketubot* 39a; *Niddah* 45a; *Nedarim* 35b.

And even with a legitimate fetus, there is reason to be permissive (*lehakel*) where there is "great need" (*tzorekh gadol*), so long as it [the fetus] has not uprooted itself [i.e., labor has not yet begun]. [This is so] even if it were not to save the life of the mother, but to save her from the adverse consequences which "great pain" would cause her. The matter requires further consideration.

There can be no doubt that, as Rashi portended, Ya'avetz is explicitly advocating that there are circumstances less severe than a threat to the life of the mother – situations in which one would want to relieve the mother of the serious outcome of some unspecified "great pain" which was liable to befall her – that would warrant an abortion.

To be sure, Ya'avetz is not advocating any generalized leniency. He remains of the view that there is an extant prohibition on fetal destruction. Nevertheless, the prohibition is clearly one that, from Ya'avetz's perspective, may be transcended in those rare cases in which a "great need" dictates such an action. While Ya'avetz does not specify the parameters of this "great need," it would become an important term for those wishing to take a more lenient approach to abortion.[88] The fact of its use, however, led Sinclair to comment, "[T]he criterion of 'great need' ... is a direct result of the non-homicidal nature of foeticide and the absence of any clear legal prohibition on abortion."[89] It is difficult to argue that Sinclair is incorrect: Ya'avetz's legacy in this area seems to affirm that the prohibition still lacked legal clarity, and that if feticide could be acceptable for interests less important than saving the mother's life, then the act of destroying the fetus assuredly could not be considered murder.

Further evidence for the prohibition's persistent dearth of legal clarity may be adduced from the ongoing uncertainty about whether the ban was to be considered as biblical or rabbinic in nature. Rabbi Jacob Schorr, a seventeenth-century *Acharon*, whose *teshuvah* on the subject is to be found in the eighteenth-century collection *Teshuvot Geonim Batrai*, suggests that the answer may be dependent on the proposed method of fetal destruction.[90] Schorr, in attempting to resolve the differences between the views of Rashi and Maimonides, notes that Maimonides did not write that the fetus is an actual *rodef*, but rather is *ke-rodef*, "like a *rodef*." The reason for Maimonides writing in this fashion, according to Schorr, is that otherwise one might conclude that it is permissible to kill

---

[88] See, for example the use made of "great need" by Weinberg, below, chapter 5, pp. 152–153, and Waldenberg, below, chapter 5, p. 166.

[89] Sinclair, "Legal Basis," 124.

[90] Unless otherwise specified, all Jacob Schorr references and quotations are from Y. Schorr, in *Geonim Batrai*, Turka, 1764, number 45.

the fetus by use of drugs, but not by surgical means.[91] Maimonides' use of the term *ke-rodef* implies that *lo tachos einekhah* (one should have no pity) on the fetus in a situation that is life-threatening for the mother, just as one would have no pity on a *rodef*. No concerns over a *mitah yafah* (an easy death[92]) should impede the destruction of the fetus, and one should use whatever measures are necessary in order to eliminate the threat that the fetus poses. Schorr conveys that Maimonides' employment of the term *ke-rodef* is only intended to show that the treatment of the fetus shares this particular similarity with that of the *rodef*. In the course of making this point Schorr also implies that but for Maimonides' instruction in this regard, a differentiation might otherwise be made between the permissibility of destroying the fetus by less direct, chemical means – which might be more easily allowed – and by direct, physical means – which might be considerably more problematic.

Although Schorr uses the potentially divergent standings of the two methods of fetal destruction for explanatory purposes, a succeeding *Acharon*, Rabbi Yehudah Ayash (died 1760), utilizes them for an actual *halakhic* viewpoint. Ayash was a scholar of renown from the revered Ayash family of Algiers, who eventually made *aliyah* to Jerusalem. In his responsa collection, *Beit Yehudah*, Ayash is asked generally about women who become pregnant while still nursing a child, and where there is fear that continued pregnancy may cause danger to the suckling infant. Ayash is asked to rule on whether it would be forbidden to use a medication to induce abortion.[93]

Ayash's ruling sets forth an analogy between the case before him and the Talmudic discussion of castration.[94] Since a woman is not commanded concerning procreation,[95] she is biblically permitted to consume a potion that would result in her own sterilization. By analogy, Ayash maintains, although the rabbis would prohibit it, there would be no biblical obstacle to her consumption of an abortifacient drug: "In the case of the drinking of a drug that aborts, since it is permitted there [in the case of sterilization] to drink a 'cup of roots,' as it does not touch

---

[91] Those who accepted such a distinction were of the view that the use of drugs was merely rabbinically proscribed, whereas surgery was barred by a biblical prohibition. For a fuller explanation, see the logic of Yehudah Ayash, below.

[92] *Sanhedrin* 45a quotes Nachman, in the name of Rabbah b. Abbahu, as interpreting "Love your neighbor as yourself" (Leviticus 19:18) to mean "choose an easy death for him." Rashi comments that an easy death implies a quick death.

[93] Unless otherwise specified, all Yehudah Ayash references and quotations are from Y. Ayash, *Beit Yehudah*, Leghorn, 1746, *Even HàEzer*, number 14.

[94] *Shabbat* 111a.   [95] The commandment to procreate is addressed to males.

the limbs of the seed, here too it is permitted…" Hence, Ayash states, "in [the case of] one who drinks a medication to abort, the prohibition, whatever it may be, is rabbinic." Ayash, however, is of the view that the same is not true vis-à-vis the physical destruction of the fetus, which certainly constitutes "touching the limbs of the seed," and, like castration, would be biblically proscribed.[96] Consequently, Ayash concludes that while physical destruction of the fetus would be unacceptable, the mother in this instance should be permitted to contravene the rabbinic prohibition on taking a drug to abort, because of the danger to the nursing child. Plainly, from Ayash's analysis, whether the prohibition on abortion was biblical or rabbinic was in large measure dependent on the intended operational procedure. A significant aspect of this *teshuvah* lies in the fact that Ayash plainly considers the needs of an individual other than the mother in weighing the abortion decision. While this fetus might indeed be regarded as a *rodef*, it is clear that its mother is not the one in any imminent danger.

Like Ayash, his northern contemporary, Rabbi Isaac Schorr of Galicia (died 1776) was also confronted with a question about abortion in circumstances of danger. Schorr, who was the author of a collection of responsa under the title *"Koach Shorr,"* gave extensive consideration to a number of the abortion issues that had concerned the other *Acharonim*. Schorr was asked whether a surgeon is permitted to abort the fetus of a woman who is suffering from a dangerous, potentially life-threatening illness, given that the fetus is not the cause of her difficulties.[97] Schorr is in no doubt that if the fetus is the direct cause of the malady, then it certainly may be killed, and the surgery unquestionably should proceed. If, however, the fetus is not the direct cause of her disease, or if the cause is uncertain, then – if Maimonides is read literally – the matter becomes much more complex.

It is quite possible, of course, that the abortion may be indicated even if the fetus is not the cause of the mother's problem, as the presence of the fetus may be exacerbating her condition or impeding her recovery. From a *halakhic* perspective, however, Schorr suggests that this may be

---

[96] The difference between the two methods is that physical destruction is considered to be direct, whereas a drug is regarded as indirect causation (*geramah*). Ayash cites another example of such indirect causation, found in *Moed Katan* 18a, in which one who carelessly discards fingernail clippings is regarded as an evil person, because of the possibility that a pregnant woman might get such a fright from walking upon the nails that it could result in a miscarriage. Such discarding, therefore, is prohibited by the rabbis.

[97] Unless otherwise specified, all Isaac Schorr references and quotations are from I. Schorr, *Koach Shorr*, Kolomea, 1888, volume 1, number 20.

troubling. In his discussion of Maimonides' use of the *rodef* principle, Schorr maintains that, strictly speaking, a pursuer can only come under the *halakhic* category of being a *rodef* if the direct commission of a homicide is anticipated. For example, one who imprisons another such that the victim dies of starvation cannot be considered a *rodef* as the cause of death is hunger, and not the direct action of the aggressor. Schorr opines that "the case in which Torah permits the saving of the life of the pursued and the killing of the *rodef* is only if he [the *rodef*] pursued after him to kill him with his own hands," and death would be the immediate result of inaction. "We have not heard," writes Schorr, "that it would be permitted to save the pursued by taking the life of one who wants to prevent a benefit necessary for the life of his fellowman." Consequently, the fetus whose presence is an obstacle to effective medical treatment cannot be considered a *rodef*.

In this context it is worth noting the observation of an Italian contemporary of Schorr, Rabbi Isaac Lampronti (1679–1756). Lampronti's credentials were not only as a rabbi, responsa-writer, and author of the monumental *halakhic* encyclopedia *Pachad Yitzchak*, but as a physician as well. Lampronti is definite in his view that when the threat to the mother stems from a source other than the fetus, the fetus is clearly not a *rodef*, and abortion is not warranted: "It follows that we may not induce an abortion... to save her from a disease deriving from... other 'fevers'... in the sixth month of her pregnancy... for only a pursuer may be killed in self defense or for defense of another... but this fetus is no pursuer... We must save her by other treatments."[98] Feldman suggests that "[i]f 'other treatments' are not an effective alternative, the author would presumably rule otherwise."[99] Lampronti, though, does not indicate definitively that this is so.

In Schorr's *teshuvah*, however, the matter does not end with the denial of *rodef* status for the fetus. Schorr goes on to compare the situation with which he is confronted to two well-known Talmudic passages. The first concerns a group of Jews who, when traveling along a road, met up with gentiles. The gentiles said, "Give us one of you and we will kill him, or if not we are going to kill all of you." The *Yerushalmi* instructs: "Even if all of them are [certain to be] killed they must not turn over one Jew."[100] The second passage relates the instance of two people, traveling far from

---

[98] *Pachad Yitzchak, Erekh Nefalim* 79b.   [99] Feldman, *Birth Control*, p. 282.
[100] *Yerushalmi, Terumot* 8:4. Both the *Yerushalmi* and Schorr go on to discuss special circumstances like that of Sheva ben Bikhri (see below, chapter 4, pp. 96–97), but Schorr's insight is based on this core statement.

habitation, one of whom has a flask of water in hand. If both of them drink the water, both will die from insufficient hydration; if one of them drinks, he will be able to reach settlement. The *halakhic* solution, which follows Rabbi Akiva's reasoning, is that the one who has the water should drink and live.[101] Schorr avers that, although these two sources reach quite different practical conclusions, the common thread between the two texts is that neither requires an active (*kum ve-áseh*[102]) intervention that would lead to the death of another. In other words, both passages prefer to maintain the *status quo*[103] rather than have a Jew take an action that would be a contributing cause of a death, beyond whatever deaths the circumstances might already dictate. Extrapolating from this insight to the case before him, Schorr observes that as the fates of mother and fetus are similarly intertwined, these Talmudic texts convey that a *kum ve-áseh* intervention might be inappropriate. If, then, the fetus is not the direct cause of its mother's illness, it follows – on the basis of the arguments presented by Schorr – that the fetus may neither be killed as a *rodef*, nor may its life be taken in the interests of saving one life in a case where both might be lost. According to Schorr's explanation, moreover, this *halakhic* logic would hold true even if there were an element of doubt about whether or not the fetus was the cause of the mother's disease. Unless it could be ascertained beyond question that the fetus was the origin of the mother's problem, it would seem to be forbidden – even on the basis of a strong supposition – to sacrifice the fetus in order to save the mother.

However, Schorr's *teshuvah*[104] changes direction when he calls attention to the fact that all of the foregoing can only be accepted if one is prepared to read Maimonides on nothing more than the straightforward (*peshat*) level, and if scant heed is paid to Rashi's interpretation of *Sanhedrin* 72b. From Schorr's perspective, this is untenable. After all, if Rashi's position is given its deserved credence, then the logic behind taking the life of the fetus stems from the reality that the mother is endangered, and the fetus is subordinate to her because it is not a *nefesh*. Given that it is not a *nefesh*, Schorr inquires, if the mother is at risk, what practical

---

[101] *Baba Metzia* 62a. Ben Petora's view, that both should drink and both die, though recorded in the Talmud, was rejected by the tradition in favor of Akiva's position.

[102] A *halakhic* concept literally meaning, "get up and do." Adin Steinsaltz describes it as "[a] mitzvah or positive act whose fulfillment requires a specific deed." See A. Steinsaltz, *The Talmud: The Steinsaltz Edition – A Reference Guide*, New York, Random House, 1989, p. 251.

[103] Even though the *status quo*, in the *Yerushalmi*'s case, may result in a higher number of deaths.

[104] The *teshuvah* contains considerably more *halakhic* arguments than those enumerated here. Those discussed here attempt to provide an overall sense of Schorr's position.

difference would it make if the fetus were the cause of her difficulties or not?

In fact, Schorr contends, Rashi and Maimonides do not actually hold contradictory positions at all. Maimonides surely would agree with Rashi that the fetus is not a *nefesh*. Maimonides' application of the *rodef* designation was never intended to restrict abortions solely to those cases in which every single aspect of the *rodef* classification was fulfilled, such as the mother's life being "pursued" with the fetus being the direct cause of her jeopardy. Like Jacob Schorr, Isaac Schorr points to the fact that Maimonides, who was very precise about the use of language, does not write that the fetus can only be sacrificed when it is a *rodef*, but rather when it is *ke-rodef* – "like a *rodef*." On those occasions when it shares certain, although not all, characteristics in common with the *rodef*, it becomes permissible to kill it. But which characteristics of the *rodef* laws does Maimonides have in mind when he makes this connection between the *rodef* and the fetus? According to Schorr, Maimonides is particularly concerned to highlight the ruling that one who kills a *rodef* when it is possible to save the pursued by incapacitating the *rodef* is not to be held liable for the killing.[105] It is for this reason, maintains Schorr, that Maimonides adds the words "either by drugs or by surgery" in the *Mishneh Torah*. The *Mishnah*'s instruction to remove the fetus "limb by limb" might lead to the conclusion that one should perform a procedure to disable but – insofar as was possible – not to kill the fetus. Hence, the "either by drugs or by surgery" statement is important in order to teach that one should speedily take whatever steps are necessary to avert the danger posed by the presence of the fetus, without regard to liability issues. Thus, Isaac Schorr suggests, echoing the standpoint of Jacob Schorr, that from a practical point of view, Maimonides implies that one should first use abortifacient drugs in order to remove the threat posed by the fetus, followed by surgery if the drugs do not have the desired effect. There can be no doubt, then, that Schorr, like Bacharach before him, was persuaded that Rashi and Maimonides were united in the view that the fetus is not a *nefesh* and that it can be killed in circumstances not limited to a direct fetal threat to the mother's life because it lacks *nefesh* status. Schorr concludes that in a situation in which the danger to the mother stems from a source other than the fetus, such as the instance described in the *she'eilah*, an abortion is warranted.

---

[105] *Hilkhot Rotzeiach* 1:7. Schorr notes that Maimonides is more lenient in this regard than was Yonatan ben Shaul (*Sanhedrin* 74a), who rules that where disabling the *rodef* is possible, one who kills him is liable for his death.

Two further significant points arise from Schorr's discussion. First, Schorr clarifies that the Torah did not in fact intend that the fetus would have a different legal standing depending on whether a gentile or a Jew is being addressed:

> It would be a matter far distant from logic if the Torah did not consider the fetus to be a *nefesh* for us, but considered it a *nefesh* for them... Rather, one would have to say that, in reality, the fetus is also not a *nefesh* for them, just as it is not for us; but the Torah took a more stringent approach for gentiles, making them liable for the murder of a fetus – even though the fetus is not considered a *nefesh*... Hence, for them as well it [the fetus] is not a *nefesh*, and they are therefore permitted to make it subordinate to the *nefesh* of its mother... (One ought to reject the consideration that the matter depends on calling [the fetus] "*nefesh*...").

According to Schorr, the fetus is not a *nefesh* for Jew or gentile, and hence the killing of a fetus is not murder for either. The gentile, however, is enjoined by a special regulation that carries a capital penalty for an abortion performed when the life of the mother – the *nefesh* – is not at risk.[106] Consistent with this approach, Schorr determines that, concerning the question of whether a gentile is permitted to save a woman's life by performing an abortion, a gentile doctor may carry out the operation if a Jewish doctor is not present.[107] Like Maharit, Schorr reasons that, ordinarily, asking a gentile physician to do this would be a transgression of the commandment "you shall not place a stumbling-block before the blind."[108] However, this *mitzvah*, as with all but three of the negative *mitzvot*[109] – may be disregarded in the name of saving life. Moreover, recalls Schorr, Rabbi Moses Isserles rules[110] that in order to save a life this *mitzvah* might be overridden even if the resulting "stumbling block" is the enactment of one of the three "cardinal sins."[111] Hence, within this context, murder would not be a consideration for the non-Jew, and the non-Jew would be permitted to perform an abortion if the mother's life were at risk.

---

[106] Feldman, *Birth Control*, p. 261, observes, "[p]resumably other justifications... would likewise be admissible."

[107] The *Tosafot*, of course, instruct that a Jew is commanded to save her, but leave the matter in doubt as regards the non-Jew. See above, p. 62.

[108] See above, p. 72. This *halakhic* insight, although mentioned by Maharit and Schorr, presumably was widely accepted.

[109] Sexual transgressions (usually understood as adultery and incest), murder, and idolatry are the three transgressions to be avoided even if life must be sacrificed. See Maimonides, *Hilkhot Yesodei HaTorah* 5:2.

[110] *Yoreh De'ah* 157:1.

[111] See above, n. 109. This is the term used by Bleich, "Abortion in Halakhic Literature," p. 370.

The second additional point arising from Schorr's *teshuvah* is that he does not accept Maharit's view that concern over *chabbalah* is the essential issue behind the *Tosafists'* prohibition on Jews carrying out non-therapeutic abortions. Schorr points out that Deuteronomy 25:3, upon which the *chabbalah* interdiction is based,[112] depicts a form of wounding imposed by sentence of a court (*Beit Din*). Schorr infers from this that the prevention of *chabbalah* cannot be applicable even to minors, much less to fetuses, because they would never have been subject to this form of judicial punishment.[113] Schorr does not advance an alternative explanation for the prohibition. While he certainly upholds the prohibition, his *teshuvah* nevertheless serves to broaden the boundaries of permissible therapeutic abortion that would not be subsumed under the ban.

At the same time that Schorr was dealing with many of the central issues that were already part of the abortion discussion, a contemporary responded to a question that previously had not been considered directly. Rabbi Meir of Eisenstadt (died 1744), in his responsa collection *Panim Mëirot*, was asked about a case in which both a woman and her baby were in life-threatening difficulty in the midst of the birth process, and the majority of the baby had already emerged.[114] Would it be permissible in such an instance to sacrifice the baby in order to save the mother, or should there be strict adherence to the *Mishnah*'s injunction not to set aside one *nefesh* for the sake of another? Notwithstanding the literal reading of the *Mishnah*, Meir tentatively concludes that, if the alternative is the death of both, the mother should rather be saved. Meir states, however, that this type of situation requires further reflection beyond his preliminary reaction. While not a case of abortion *per se*, later rabbinic authorities would use this precedent in addressing similar pre-birth cases.[115]

The writings of Meir and Schorr were produced entirely in a period before the dramatic revolutions that would open the door to modernity. The same, however, cannot be said of "one of the most famous rabbis of the close of the classical *Ashkenazi* rabbinic era,"[116] Rabbi Ezekiel Landau (1713–93). Landau began his career in Poland, and eventually served in

---

[112] See above, p. 71.
[113] Aryeh Lifshutz, in *Aryeh Devei Ilai*, Vishnitz, 1850, *Yoreh Dèah*, number 6, employs the same logic to suggest that Maharit is really concerned with prohibiting abortion as *chabbalah* done to the mother.
[114] M. Ashkenazi, *Panim Mëirot*, Sulzbach, 1738, volume III, number 8.
[115] See, for example, the approach of Lipschutz, below, chapter 4, pp. 95–98.
[116] M. S. Samet, "Landau, Ezekiel ben Judah," in *Encyclopaedia Judaica*, Jerusalem, Keter Publishing House, volume x, pp. 1388–1391.

the prestigious position of rabbi of Prague. His commanding intellect
and prodigious output are seen clearly in his great *halakhic* work, *Noda
bi-Yehudah*. For most of Landau's life, the Jewish people accepted rabbinic authority over Jewish communal life without question. Ultimately,
however, in his later years, Landau would be among the first who would
have to respond to the stirrings of "the new situation arising from the
opening of the gates of the ghetto and the consequent entry of the Jews
into general non-Jewish society."[17]

It was in 1781, just as this unprecedented set of circumstances was about
to unfold, that Landau, in the context of correspondence with Rabbi
Isaiah (Pick) Berlin of Breslau,[18] addressed some of the latter's disquiet
in relation to feticide.[19] It is clear from Landau's *teshuvah* that Berlin
harbored some concern over whether killing a fetus really only ought
to be considered an offence worthy of a monetary penalty; perhaps it
should be regarded as a capital crime? Landau replies that as one cannot
be certain of viability before birth,[20] one who kills a fetus is not guilty of
a capital offence. Landau further writes that the fetus is not within the
category of being an *ish*, which would imply capital punishment for its
killer. Any suggestion, moreover, that the fetus might be a *nefesh* ought to
be rejected as well, as Rashi taught. Nevertheless, just as one may not
take the life of a *tereifah*, even though such an act would not carry capital
liability, so one may not take the life of the fetus. Landau sees no possible
justification for sacrificing the life of a *tereifah*, even in the name of saving
an unafflicted individual. By analogy, therefore, no justification would
exist for saving the life of the mother by killing her fetus, "were it not
considered as something of a *rodef*."[21] Maimonides' depiction of the fetus
as *rodef* is necessary to Landau's analysis, then, because without it, one
would have no permission to intervene in order to save the mother's life.
It is a logical corollary of Landau's position that abortion would not be
countenanced unless the mother is in fact in a life-threatening situation, a
situation directly caused by the fetus behaving as a *rodef*. Landau further
illuminates Maimonides' use of the *rodef* characterization in the case of
the fetus by quoting those sources that convey that one is not permitted

---

[17] *Ibid.*

[18] Berlin (1725–99) regularly corresponded on *halakhic* matters with the great authorities of the
day. In fact, he was in communication with Tzvi Hirsch of Brody on this very same subject.
Brody's response, like that of Landau, sought to reassure Berlin in this area.

[19] Unless otherwise specified, all Landau references and quotations are from E. Landau, *Nodah
Bi-Yehudah*, Vilna, 1904, *Choshen Mishpat*, number 59.

[20] The principle that we "follow the majority" in considering whether infants are viable is rejected
in the case of fetuses within the discussion between Landau and Berlin.

[21] This is a controversial matter. For a different point of view, see the position of Lipschutz, chapter
4, pp. 95–98.

to kill a *rodef* if it is possible to neutralize its impact by disabling it. Only if one cannot save the life of the pursued by impairing the *rodef* is it acceptable to take its life. Landau's understanding of Maimonides in this regard, is altogether different from that of Isaac Schorr.[122] Near the end of his *teshuvah*, Landau admits that it is unclear to him why Maimonides uses the *rodef* classification before the fetus is born, but is unwilling to apply it after birth. What is plain, however, is that as far as Landau is concerned, the lack of assured fetal viability, combined with the *rodef* designation, is what allows for abortion to proceed, but only under very limited circumstances.

A younger contemporary of Landau, Rabbi Joseph Teomim (1727–92), famous for his *Peri Megadim*, a super-commentary to the *Shulchan Arukh*, arrives at a resolution of the divergence between Rashi and Maimonides different from that of Landau. The *Peri Megadim*[123] joins several predecessors in commenting that Maimonides' view is that the fetus is like a *rodef*, but is not an actual *rodef*.[124] The mother is essentially "being pursued from heaven."[125] Further on, the *Peri Megadim* provides an illustration of how the fetus is "like a *rodef*," noting that should the mother miscarry, one would fear danger to her, and, therefore, would violate the *Shabbat* on her behalf. The *Peri Megadim* observes that in the case of a *rodef*, too, one should be saved from the *rodef* even if it requires that the *Shabbat* be overridden. Quoting Rashi's position, the *Peri Megadim* holds: "And it should be said that so long as the fetus has not emerged, its viability is in doubt, and an [instance of] doubt does not overwhelm an [instance of] certainty . . ." It seems that the *Peri Megadim* connects Rashi's stance that the fetus is a non-*nefesh* to the issue of the questionable viability of the fetus.[126] Unlike Landau, then, the *Peri Megadim* cleaves closer to Rashi's outlook, maintaining that there are circumstances in which

---

[122] See above, p. 85.

[123] Unless otherwise specified, all Teomim references and quotations are from *Peri Megadim* (*Mishbetzot Zahav*) to *Shulchan Arukh*, *Orach Chayim* 328:1.

[124] Beyond those mentioned above, there are others who make the same point. One of the best known names is Yonatan Eybeschuetz (1690–1764) of Altona, in his *Urim VeTumim*, Karlsruhe, 1755, number 30:103.

[125] *Sanhedrin* 72b uses this language when the mother is in danger after birth. See above, chapter 2, pp. 49–50.

[126] In this context, however, the following sentence from the *Peri Megadim* contains somewhat curious wording. Referring to *Mishnah Ohalot*, the *Peri Megadim* states that the mother represents a "more important *nefesh*, since one who kills her deserves death, something which is not true for the *nefesh* of the fetus [*nefesh haúbar*], and this requires further investigation . . ." The *nefesh haúbar* construction is strange here, given the *Peri Megadim*'s apparent acquiescence with Rashi's emphasis on the fact that the fetus is not to be considered a *nefesh*. It is possible that the *Peri Megadim* is uncomfortable leaving the fetus without any type of *nefesh* status, but this is wholly speculative.

the fetus may be killed because of its lesser status, and limiting the *rodef* definition.

Teomim died just three years after the French Revolution. The age of Enlightenment and Emancipation had arrived. The sociological nature of Jewish life together with the entire intellectual landscape that Jews encountered, was about to undergo dramatic convulsions in the years ahead. The result would be a Jewish milieu that was vastly different from anything that the *Rishonim* and *Acharonim* had ever known.

The *Rishonim* and *Acharonim* bequeathed a varied legacy to this new era. Three points can be enumerated with some certainty. First, none of the *Rishonim* or *Acharonim* took the position that abortion – no matter what the motivating factor – constituted murder for a Jew, and there was strong opinion that this was true for the non-Jew as well. Second, the predominant outlook of the *Rishonim* and *Acharonim* seems to have regarded abortion in order to save the life of the mother as required for a Jew and permitted for a non-Jew. Third, non-therapeutic abortion conversely was seen to be the subject of a specific prohibition, notwithstanding the fact that murder was not involved. The *Rishonim* and *Acharonim* were of the view that a non-Jew ought to be condemned to death for performing such an act in contravention of the Noahide Laws, whereas a Jew was to go unpunished.

Beyond these three matters of general agreement, other issues remained unresolved during this epoch. Although the prohibition, which was first articulated in this period, was explained in a variety of different ways, none of the proposed reasons attained widespread support. Whether the prohibition was biblical or rabbinic – or, perhaps, partook of both – also remained a subject of contention. The extent of the prohibition was another inconclusive discussion. Those who held to a straightforward (*peshat*) reading of Maimonides forbade abortion in any circumstance other than a direct threat to the mother's life, while those who were inclined to read the *Mishnah* through Rashi's lens contended that other conditions – for example, a fetus conceived in adultery – could overcome the prohibition. Those who wrote about the discrepancies between Rashi's and Maimonides' positions usually tried their hardest to resolve the apparent contradictions between the two.

Despite the lack of resolution in these matters, it is nevertheless possible to discern some overall trends. These trends appear likely to have enjoyed the assent of a plurality of the *Rishonim* and *Acharonim*. The first such trend was that abortion usually became a consideration for the *Rishonim* and *Acharonim* only when concerns arose for the mother, not for the fetus or anyone else. This tendency was, of course, a continuation of the preeminent position accorded to the mother that stretched all the way back to Exodus 21:22–23. While it is clear that Ayash's ruling permitting an abortion in order to save an existing child was anomalous in this regard, it was the exception that proved the rule. Generally it was the life or health of the mother alone that dictated whether or not extreme measures could be taken.

A second trend that emerged arose from the discussion on the differences between what a non-Jew and a Jew could do. It is true that the *Tosafot* essentially had built an "unequal parallel" between Jew and non-Jew by structuring the prohibition for Jews around the perceived Noahide ban on abortion for the non-Jew. As time went on, however, the parallel seems to have become increasingly equal, as more rabbis advocated shrinking the practical distinctions between the two groups. Thus, while there was an opinion that a Jew ought not to assist a non-Jew in procuring an abortion, this coexisted with the view that abortion, in truth, was not to be considered as murder for a non-Jew. From this latter position, some gave permission to non-Jewish physicians to perform an abortion to save the mother if a Jewish doctor were unavailable. As this type of procedure represented the preponderance of real abortion cases, the actual – as opposed to the theoretical – divergence between Jew and non-Jew appeared to decrease.

A third discernible trend can be found in the fact that few of the scholars of these centuries were inclined to restrict themselves to a strict interpretation of Maimonides. A greater number sought to moderate and limit the understanding of "like a *rodef*" so that it better comported with Rashi's stance that the fetus, at times, could be sacrificed on the basis that it was not a *nefesh*. While Yaʿavetz probably went the furthest of all in proposing abortions in situations in which the mother was not herself at risk, few seemed inclined to rule in a way that completely precluded such possibilities.

To be sure, insofar as the questions which came before the *Rishonim* and *Acharonim* were indicative of the social realities of their times – and whether or not these *sheʾelot* were representative is wholly uncertain – there seemed little pressure to address abortions short of the most extreme circumstances. Hence, even had the *Rishonim* and *Acharonim* been inclined to be conservative where the risks to the woman were less dire, there was little call to state such positions decisively.[127] Indeed, it is worth observing that it was Landau, the *Acharon* of note who lived closest in

---

[127] It is quite possible that the *Rishonim* and *Acharonim* saw no need to state an opposition to abortion in less severe circumstances because it was regarded as obvious. The Jewish physicians of the period who recorded their views on abortion provide evidence that such opposition may well

time to the nineteenth century, who gave voice to what was probably the most explicitly restrictive position among the *Acharonim*. Perhaps he sensed something in the winds of change that suggested that a more rigorous approach was appropriate, or maybe it was simply his reading of the sources that took him in this direction. We can only speculate. In general, though, the *Rishonim* and *Acharonim* were in no hurry to deny all abortions contemplated for reasons other than saving the life of the mother.

By the end of the era of the *Rishonim* and *Acharonim*, it made sense to speak of a range of responses to abortion within Jewish law. Judging from the number of *teshuvot* written on the subject during the course of these generations, abortion was no more than a peripheral area of the *halakhah*. Nevertheless, by the close of the eighteenth century the parameters of abortion discourse had been established within a framework that the rabbis of the Talmudic period had never made explicit. When looked at collectively, it can be said that the *Rishonim* and *Acharonim* had navigated a centrist course: they had put in place a hitherto unspecified prohibition on Jewish abortion, but they had also provided extensive opposition to the notion that abortion was murder, they had preserved abortion to save the mother's life, and – within the contours of the Rashi-Maimonidean dialectic – they had kept open the potential for, and at times had even permitted abortion in non-life-saving circumstances. Their prohibition, then, can be regarded as neither absolute nor inflexible.

For many decades to come, this template, formed by the *Rishonim* and *Acharonim*, would continue to be utilized in fashioning Jewish responses on abortion-related matters. Although the nineteenth century, in many ways, would be revolutionary for Jews, the approach of the *Rishonim* and *Acharonim* to abortion issues would continue to exert its influence. Under the surface, however, the seeds of modification were about to be planted. Modernity was at hand.

---

have been regarded as a societal "given." Thus, Amatus Lusitanus of the sixteenth century in "The Oath of Amatus" proudly records that "[N]o woman has ever brought about an abortion with my aid," and Jacob Zahalon of Rome in a seventeenth-century piece called "The Physician's Prayer" made oblique reference to his aversion by entreating, "[m]y God, deliver me from the hand of the wicked, from the palm of the perverter and oppressor and place me not in his hand even for one moment lest he entice me to practice wantonness (God forbid!) to administer a poison or drug to injure some man or some pregnant woman . . ." See H. Friedenwald, *The Jews and Medicine*, New York, Ktav Publishing House Incorporated, 1967, volume 1, pp. 277, 369.

CHAPTER 4

No clear consensus: the sages of a rising modernity

The *halakhic* statements relevant to abortion that were written during the greater part of the nineteenth century displayed no evidence whatsoever that a watershed in Jewish history was being traversed. Yet, in almost every significant area of Jewish life, that was precisely what was happening. Monumental transitions were underway. Citizenship, economic mobility, the disintegration of autonomous community, the rise of secular law, the challenge of reason to revealed religion, the development of scientific thought and of a critical study of the past – among many other factors – were all having profound and irrevocable effects upon Jews and Judaism.[1] Eventually the impact of these unprecedented phenomena would be seen clearly in the abortion area, but the early rabbis of modernity were decidedly more engaged in the deliberations of the *Acharonim* than in responding to their own *Zeitgeist*. Despite its avowed revolutionary nature, when it came to *halakhic* matters that were less than pressing, modernity, it seems, called forth a slow process of percolation that eventually would culminate in altered perspectives, rather than immediate effects.

Thus it was that Rabbi Israel Lipschutz (1782–1860), who was born during the early stages of the Enlightenment and lived through the first decades of modernity, accepted the inheritance of the *Rishonim* and *Acharonim*, without displaying any apparent influences from the events of the outside world.[2] When Lipschutz in his famous commentary to the *Mishnah*, *Tiferet Yisrael*, dealt with *Ohalot* 7:6, he immediately entered one of the central discussions of the *Acharonim* concerning Maimonides' use

---

[1] A great deal has been written on the nature of the impact of modernity on the Jewish people. See, for example, "The Modern Period," in Seltzer, *Jewish People, Jewish Thought*, pp. 507 ff.

[2] It should be remembered that Lipschutz lived in Germany, where Emancipation was relatively late in arriving. Nevertheless, Germany was an important center for the early reforms in Judaism undertaken by some Jews as a response to modernity. Lipschutz hardly can have been unaware of the profound changes that were stirring.

of the *rodef*. He did so while considering the very difficult question of "late-term abortion": is it permitted to abort one in the process of being born, and, if so, until what point?

Lipschutz begins, "[W]e do not judge it like a *rodef*," thereby concurring with the Talmudic view of this matter.[3] Lipschutz then advances a reason for this contention: while the infant is being born it possesses no intention to kill its mother. In making this assertion, Lipschutz seems to imply that one cannot be a *rodef* without an intention to kill. If this were indeed the case, it would have profound ramifications for the position taken by Maimonides. Lipschutz proceeds to demonstrate that it is not even proper to treat such a baby as though it shared characteristics with a *rodef*. He does so by responding indirectly to an issue that had first been dealt with by Rabbi Meir of Eisenstadt a century before.[4] Meir had been asked whether it is appropriate to intervene to save one life when both mother and child are at risk during the birth process and the majority of the child has already emerged. The *Mishnah* declares that once the "majority" has come out, one life is not to be set aside in favor of another.

While Rabbi Meir had offered scant reason for his conclusions, Lipschutz is far more expansive.[5] Lipschutz first provides several *halakhic* examples of cases in which an individual unintentionally places others in a situation in which they could die. Sheva ben Bikhri, for example, is one of Lipschutz's citations.[6] As related in 2 Samuel 20:4–22, Sheva ben Bikhri, a rebel against the leadership of King David, took refuge in the town of Avel while being pursued by King David's troops. King David's commander, Yoav, made it abundantly clear to the townsfolk that he was going to destroy Avel together with all its inhabitants, unless Sheva ben Bikhri was handed over to him.[7] Thus, Sheva ben Bikhri inadvertently put the citizens of Avel face-to-face with death. By analogy, Lipschutz contends, a baby in the process of being born, which poses a threat to its mother, does precisely the same thing. It, too, unintentionally confronts its mother with the real possibility of imminent demise. One important difference, however, between the baby and Sheva ben Bikhri is that once Sheva ben Bikhri entered Avel he was marked for certain death, at the hands of either Yoav or the townspeople. The only question at Avel was

---

[3] *Sanhedrin* 72b. See above, chapter 2, p. 49.   [4] See above chapter 3, p. 89.
[5] All Lipschutz references and quotations are from *Tiferet Yisrael – Boaz* to *Mishnah Ohalot* 7:6.
[6] Lipschutz here expands upon an argument already made by Rashi about the connection between the *rodef* and Sheva ben Bikhri. See Sanhedrin 72b, s.v. *yatzah rosho*.
[7] The account concludes with a wise woman persuading her fellow citizens that they should kill Sheva ben Bikhri themselves and provide Yoav with his severed head.

whether the townspeople would be saved. However, in the matter before Lipschutz, it is perfectly possible that the mother could die and the baby, the "cause" of her mortal danger, could be saved. Hence, while Sheva ben Bikhri was destined for death at Avel, how can one decide, asks Lipschutz, which one must die – the baby or the mother – in the circumstance before him?

There is a further disparity between the likes of Sheva ben Bikhri and the baby which makes the case before Lipschutz more difficult. Sheva ben Bikhri, according to Lipschutz, cannot be considered a *rodef* to the people of Avel, as he had no intention to pursue them and kill them.[8] Nevertheless, since he willfully placed them in mortal danger[9] while contravening the law, it is appropriate to treat him "like a *rodef*."[10] The same is not true, however, for the emerging baby. The baby is subject to the forces of nature and is neither willfully placing its mother in danger, nor acting against the law. As the *Gemara* holds, therefore, when the majority of the baby has emerged it cannot be considered a *rodef*[11] and, hence, no differentiation between mother and baby can be made on this basis. In Lipschutz's view, then, such an infant, is neither a *rodef* nor "like a *rodef*," and, therefore, should not be treated in the same manner that one would treat a *rodef*. It is difficult to see how Lipschutz, having denied *rodef* standing to the baby being born, might apply it to the fetus, especially given that fetal intent must be considered to be at least as low as that of the emerging baby, if not less. Plainly, Lipschutz's stance in this regard is one that raises a serious challenge for the Maimonidean outlook.

Rather than using the *rodef* designation, then, Lipschutz attempts to respond to this problematic case in another way. Obviously troubled by the notion that doing nothing would result in the death of both mother and baby, Lipschutz suggests appealing to the "doubtful viability" argument,[12] namely, that the child's standing is uncertain until it reaches

---

[8] Lipschutz is by no means alone among later scholars in insisting that the *rodef* classification requires demonstrable intent on the part of the perpetrator. Clearly, unless one maintains that different rules pertain prior to birth – which, while possible, seems arbitrary – this makes Maimonides' designation of the fetus as a *rodef* all the more difficult to understand. For an alternative approach to the issue of intent, see the views of Zalman, below, pp. 104–105.

[9] Even though he may never have intended that the citizens of Avel should die, he could have avoided placing them in any danger simply by not entering the town.

[10] Jews are instructed, of course, to kill a *rodef* if it is at all feasible. Lipschutz hereby justifies the actions of the people of Avel.

[11] *Sanhedrin* 72b.

[12] This argument had been used before, most recently by Landau. See above, chapter 3, p. 90.

thirty days of life. This strategy provides an impartial reason to extend
primary consideration to the mother because her viability is not in doubt.
Using this approach, Lipschutz concludes – like Meir before him – that,
notwithstanding the fact that the baby becomes a *nefesh* at birth, there
is a cogent argument that the baby nevertheless may be sacrificed in a
case where the alternative would be a double loss. While Lipschutz does
not clarify his position on abortions earlier in pregnancy or in circumstances other than a threat to the mother's life, the "doubtful viability"
doctrine may well open the possibility for approval of abortions under
less extreme conditions. Lipschutz's approach, then, is plainly outside
the Maimonidean camp.[13]

The renowned Hungarian rabbi and *posek* (*halakhic* authority) Rabbi
Moses Schick (known as Maharam Schick, 1807–79), who was wholly a
product of the nineteenth century, takes Meir's tentative approach to this
matter of making choices, and applies it to the earlier stages of pregnancy.
In his *teshuvah* to Chayim of Munkatch, dated 1874, Schick responds to
the question of whether a doctor may dismember a fetus in order to save
the mother if both otherwise might die.[14] This is, of course, the classic
therapeutic abortion question, and Schick's reply traces many of the
prior positions on the matter. Schick agrees with those *Acharonim* who held
that without Maimonides' *rodef* argument Jews would be prohibited from
taking the life of the fetus. Interestingly, however, Schick does not seek
to explain Maimonides' use of the *rodef* to denote that the fetus simply
possesses certain characteristics in common with the *rodef*. Rather, he
maintains that in a case in which the presence of the fetus is threatening
the mother, what the fetus is doing is "an appurtenance of the spilling
of blood." As indicated above,[15] the "spilling of blood" is regarded as
one of the three "cardinal" sins that requires martyrdom. By extension,
any appurtenance of these three sins similarly dictates death in order to
avoid its commission. An "appurtenance of the spilling of blood" implies
that the act, while not murder *per se*, could be considered an extension
of the category of murder. This "appurtenance" is based in the rabbinic

---

[13] Though Lipschutz never explicitly refers to Meir's earlier *teshuvah*, a contemporary, Rabbi Akiva
Eger (1761–1837) of Posen, does. Despite the fact that Eger lived more than half his life in
the eighteenth century and, therefore, like Lipschutz, can be seen as a transitional figure, the
emerging landscape of modernity formed the backdrop to his writings. Nevertheless, Eger, citing
the *Panim Meïrot*, simply adopts Meir's cautious attitude that while there may be some reason to
save the woman's life if both will otherwise die, the matter requires further consideration. See
Tosafot R. Akiva Eger, *Ohalot*, 7:16.
[14] M. Schick, *Maharam Schick*, Muncacz, 1881, *Yoreh Deäh*, number 155.
[15] See above, chapter 3, p. 88, n. 109.

interpretation of the legal culpability of a Noahide for feticide (*Sanhedrin* 57b), which was extended to Jews by virtue of the principle that there is nothing that is prohibited for a non-Jew and permitted to a Jew.[16] Schick further contends that, as the fetus is the potential cause of the death of its mother, it is "like the appurtenance of a *rodef*," and ought to be treated as a *rodef*. It is unlikely, of course, that Lipschutz would have been much impressed with this argument.

Towards the end of his *teshuvah*, Schick turns to focus upon the issue of what is to be done if the baby has emerged and both mother and baby are in peril. He, too, advises that there is a good basis for saving the mother in such a situation, given the questionable viability of the child vis-à-vis the certainty of the mother's life. The last paragraph of his *teshuvah*, however, provides a limiting caveat to this notion that had not been mentioned before:

All of the above applies if we know with certainty that both will die. But we have only the doctors' word on that, and the Chatam Sofer ruled that a statement of doctors is subject to doubt.[17] However ... if the doctor says, "I am sure beyond a shadow of a doubt," and he is willing to act on his diagnosis, it would be permitted in the view of the sages, and it is conceivable that there would be no obligation on our part to prevent him ...

In Schick's view, as the doctor's opinion that both will die is uncertain, it would be improper to dismember this nascent being while in doubt. Only if the physician is prepared to convert this doubt to virtual certainty, and will take responsibility for such a position, might a procedure to save the mother become warranted. By stating "all of the above," Schick seems to imply that this proviso would hold true at an earlier stage of pregnancy, as well as for the baby whose "majority" had emerged. It is highly likely, of course, that were Schick's advice to be followed, it would have a restrictive impact on abortion. Schick closes his *teshuvah* by stating that this matter requires further deliberation.[18]

---

[16] See above, chapter 3, p. 62.

[17] Moses Sofer (1762–1839) in M. Schreiber, *Chatam Sofer*, Vienna, 1855, *Yoreh De'ah*, number 158. Bleich, "Abortion in Halakhic Literature," p. 360, n. 69, most succinctly synthesizes the Chatam Sofer's position: "The credence given to even a single witness in matters of halakhic proscription extends only to testimony of observed events. Diagnosis and treatment of medical conditions necessarily contain an element of subjective judgement; hence the judgement of a medical practitioner constitutes a *safek* rather than a certainty. As such, it cannot provide sufficient basis for sanctioning that which is forbidden in cases of 'doubt' ..."

[18] David Hoffman (1843–1921) in a brief *teshuvah*, *Melamed LeHo'il*, Frankfurt, 1932, *Yoreh De'ah*, number 69, cites Schick and the other relevant sources on this matter. He likewise concludes that when the "majority" of the baby has emerged grounds exist to save the mother.

Schick's contemporary and compatriot, Rabbi Yekutiel Teitelbaum (1808–83) of Sziget, provides almost the opposite outlook on abortion in a circumstance of doubt. Teitelbaum, one of the outstanding Chassidic scholars in Hungary, was asked about a woman in the sixth month of pregnancy, stricken with a dangerous illness, whose doctors had almost despaired of saving her.[19] Three non-Jewish experts subsequently concluded that if her pregnancy were terminated there would be hope that her life might be extended. Conversely, the potential existed that the abortion could be carried out and she might nevertheless die speedily. Is it permissible to perform such a procedure?

While the *halakhic* position that an abortion ought to be initiated in order to save the mother's life is unambiguous, in this instance, while the woman might be saved, it could only be the hoped for, rather than the expected outcome. The question asked of Teitelbaum is actually quite similar to the one previously submitted to Isaac Schorr,[20] the salient difference being that in the case before Teitelbaum there is little assurance that the abortion procedure will, in fact, save the woman. Teitelbaum begins his response by agreeing with Landau that but for the fact that the fetus is viewed as being like a *rodef*, no justification would exist for killing it. The reality that the fetus is not a *nefesh* hardly suffices as a reason to terminate its existence. In other words, both the "not a *nefesh*" and the "like a *rodef*" explanations are required to permit abortion. In what sense, though, does Teitelbaum regard the fetus as being "like a *rodef*?" Here Teitelbaum concurs with Jacob Schorr – in contradistinction to the view of Landau – that the fetus is *"ke-rodef"* in the sense that just as in the case of a *rodef*, we should not trouble ourselves to assure a *mitah yafah* (goodly death), and we should use whatever means are necessary in order to eliminate the threat posed by the fetus.

But Teitelbaum goes further. He proceeds to broaden the applicability of the *"rodef"* analogy beyond the scope envisaged by Schorr. Teitelbaum points out that basing the duty to save the mother in the laws of *rodef* places a similar requirement on a non-Jew to save her from the *rodef*, as a non-Jew is equally obligated to impede such a pursuer. This is, of course, no small matter. After all, given that abortion had been deemed by the rabbis to be a capital offense for non-Jews,[21] understanding the *rodef* principle as permitting a non-Jew to abort in cases that presented a threat to the mother's life represents a noteworthy development. Furthermore,

---

[19] Unless otherwise specified, all Teitelbaum references and quotations are from Y. Teitelbaum, *Avnei Tzedek*, Sziget, 1886, *Choshen Mishpat*, number 19.
[20] See above, chapter 3, p. 84.   [21] See above, chapter 2, p. 52.

the *rodef* laws also countenance the killing of the *rodef* in a situation where it is doubtful whether the pursued can be saved. Stating the principle that "any [law] that is set aside for the sake of saving a life, is also set aside in a case of doubt,"[22] Teitelbaum determines that a pertinent feature of the *rodef* analogy is that it would allow for an abortion even if the chances of the mother's survival were clouded.

At the end of the *teshuvah*, having already concluded that, even in such a case of doubt, the interests of the fetus can be set aside for the mother, Teitelbaum considers whether the interests of the mother can be set aside. Is it acceptable further to endanger, and perhaps to shorten, the life of such a woman in a case where success is so doubtful? Teitelbaum's affirmative reply is more germane to "end-of-life" inquiries than to the abortion issue, but it does point to a fundamental question relevant to abortion. Is the danger that is associated with any abortion an acceptable risk for the woman to take, particularly when the benefit to her may not be life-saving?

An answer to this inquiry was soon provided by a *teshuvah* written in 1850. Rabbi Solomon Drimer of Skole in Galicia ventured into the debate over the reason for the *Tosafists'* stance prohibiting abortion for Jews,[23] offering a new interpretation to add to the growing list.[24] According to Drimer, the issue underlying the prohibition on abortion when the mother's life is not at risk is actually the fundamental *halakhic* concern over placing oneself in danger. Deuteronomy 4:15 – "For your own sake, therefore, be most careful" – forbids a Jew from intentionally incurring unnecessary hazards. Drimer states unequivocally that "according to the *halakhah*, abortion is considered dangerous," even if the fetus has not yet attained forty days. It might be replied, of course, that – within the context of nineteenth-century medicine – an abortion was hazardous, but so too was the process of giving birth itself.[25] This is true, concurs Drimer, but the risks that come with labor and delivery are in the category of

---

[22] See above, chapter 2, p. 46.
[23] Drimer does not explicitly describe his approach as an underlying reason for the prohibition, but this is how it is apprehended by F. Rosner, "Abortion," in *Modern Medicine and Jewish Ethics*, New York, Yeshiva University Press, and Hoboken, Ktav Publishing House Incorporated, 1986, p. 148. Rosner's perception seems to accord well with the tenor of Drimer's remarks.
[24] All Drimer references and quotations are from S. Drimer, *Beit Shlomoh*, Lemberg, 1878, *Choshen Mishpat*, number 132.
[25] While evidence from mid-nineteenth-century Galicia is not available, in America, at the start of the twentieth century, "[c]hildbearing was dangerous, and pregnant women feared dying during childbirth." See L. J. Reagan, *When Abortion Was a Crime: Women, Medicine, and Law in the United States, 1867–1973*, Los Angeles, University of California Press, 1997, p. 77. Though abortion might be assumed to have been more dangerous than childbirth, Reagan can conclude no more than "[m]ost likely abortion was more dangerous than childbirth . . ." (*ibid.*). Her research suggests that the risk gap might not be as wide as commonly thought.

tivo shel olam (the way of the world),[26] whereas the dangers associated with abortion are not. Hence, according to Drimer, the essential concern behind the *Tosafists'* prohibition of non-therapeutic abortion was the worry that women would thereby subject themselves to dangers that were *halakhically* unacceptable.

Accepting Drimer's notion that all abortion is dangerous to some extent, what should be done if the doctors and the woman concerned are all of the view that the abortion presents no substantial danger to her? Drimer responds by pointing to the difference between this question and the situation in *Yoma* 82a in which permission is given for a pregnant woman to be fed on *Yom Kippur* and a sick person to be given sustenance on the advice of doctors.[27] That text conveys that if the sick individual indicates that he needs food but the doctors are of the contrary view, one follows the desire of the patient, because "the heart knows its own bitterness." If, however, the patient says that he does not need food and the doctors disagree, then one ought to feed him according to the experts' instructions. In those cases, Drimer points out, the patient or the doctors who request what might seem, at first glance, to be an undesirable intervention,[28] are listened to because potential *pikuach nefesh* is at stake. However, when abortion is not unequivocally required to save the life of the mother it does not represent *pikuach nefesh*, such that the danger involved in the procedure is not outweighed by a sufficient mitigating benefit. Hence, in such cases, we ought not to listen to the woman's or her doctors' protestations that the danger can be discounted. Only if there is reason to believe that there is a legitimate danger to the woman, so that proceeding with the pregnancy and the birth would be more risky than terminating the fetus, would an abortion be indicated. If, however, the abortion will not be life-saving for the woman concerned, then the rationale for the *Tosafists'* prohibition remains: the motivation behind such an abortion is always insufficient to overcome the *halakhic* objection to the danger that is involved. In Drimer's view, therefore, no matter what the details of the case, the greater danger is always to be avoided. If the mother's life certainly were threatened, an abortion would be indicated in order to save her; if, though, her life is possibly at risk, but the nature of the jeopardy is uncertain, a policy of *shev ve-ʾal taʿaseh* (take no intervening action) is preferable, given that the greater danger of the procedure outweighs the uncertainty of her current situation.

[26] I.e., part of the natural process.   [27] See above, chapter 2, p. 45.
[28] As it would be preferable, of course, for an adult who does not really require food to fast on *Yom Kippur*.

This subject of the acceptability of abortion when the mother's life is not at stake continued to arise in different ways. It is hardly surprising that this is so, given that this issue so epitomized the divide between Rashi and Maimonides. It surfaced afresh when Rabbi Joseph Babad (1800–74) of Poland, the author of the well-known *Minchat Chinukh*, confronted the theoretical problem of whether one could perform an abortion in order to save one's own life.[29] Babad's consideration of this matter was prompted by his contemplation of the *mitzvah* of *kiddush HaShem* (the commandment to sanctify God's name). As noted, one of the particulars of this *mitzvah* requires that one should rather give up one's own life than commit murder.[30] Given this requirement, if one is ordered to kill a fetus or be killed, and the fetus is not behaving as a *rodef*, may one kill the fetus or should one choose death? In pondering this matter, Babad notes the *Gemara*'s principled inquiry, "[W]ho is to say that your blood is redder than his?"[31] This is, of course, the abiding, unsolvable conundrum that conveys the impossibility of trying to rate one life more highly than another. However, in the case of a fetus, Babad contends, the very fact that the fetus is not a *nefesh* argues that its blood is, so to speak, "less red." Furthermore, Babad observes, the *Mishnah* envisages the destruction of the fetus for the sake of saving the life of its full-*nefesh* mother. It follows then, that as the mother's blood is "no more red" than that of any other *nefesh*, the fetus may be destroyed in order to save the life of any other born individual. This position of the *Minchat Chinukh*, which is in line with Rashi's subordination of the fetus, would eventually be opposed when the rabbis of the twentieth century came to confront this question in an actual, rather than a theoretical, guise.[32]

Yet another scholar in the latter part of the nineteenth century would offer an attempt to explain Maimonides' use of the *rodef* classification. Rabbi Shneur Zalman of Lublin (died 1902) provides an ingenious explanation using an alternative depiction of the *rodef* that is discussed in the Talmud.[33] Maimonides himself had previously encapsulated the sense of this Talmudic insight in this way:

---

[29] *Minchat Chinukh*, Vilna, 1912, number 296.   [30] See above, chapter 3, p. 88, n. 109.
[31] *Sanhedrin* 45b.   [32] See below, pp. 119–120, and chapter 5, pp. 138–139.
[33] *Baba Kamma* 117b. The Talmudic text uses the example of a donkey and declares its owner to be a *rodef*: "A certain man managed to get his donkey onto a boat before the people on the boat had got out. The boat was in danger of sinking, so a certain person came along and pushed the man's donkey into the river, where it drowned. When the case was brought before Rabbah, he declared him exempt [from having to make restitution for the animal]. Said Abaye to him [Rabbah]: 'Was that person not rescuing himself by means of another man's money?' He [Rabbah], however, said to him: 'That man [the owner of the donkey] was, from the beginning a *rodef* . . .'"

A boat is about to sink from the weight of its load. A passenger who steps forward and lightens the load by throwing [the baggage of another] into the sea is not liable [to make restitution], since the baggage is like a pursuer (*kemo rodef*) coming after them to kill them. He performed a great *mitzvah* by throwing the baggage overboard and saving them.[34]

According to Zalman,[35] it is this view of the nature of the *rodef* that explains why Maimonides insisted on utilizing *lo tachos einekhah* (one should have no pity) as the Toraitic foundation for the requirement to block the *rodef* in addition to the alternative *lo ta'amod al dam re'i'ekhah* (you shall not stand idle while your neighbor bleeds).[36] For, as Zalman frames it, the central issue in the law of *rodef* is that – even in the case of a seemingly innocent *rodef* – one first must set aside any pity for the *rodef* in order to save the pursued.

From this perspective, the essential matter to which the law sought to respond by requiring that the *rodef* be killed forthwith is not to punish the *rodef* – the transgression of being a *rodef* would no more call for a summary death than other heinous acts – but rather a desire to intervene in order to preserve the potential victim. Thus, even should the conduct of a supposed *rodef* be entirely involuntary, like that of the donkey or the luggage, the *rodef* nevertheless must be sacrificed immediately. Indeed, the only sense in which the donkey or the luggage could be considered candidates to be "like a *rodef*" at all is that each represents a "threat" to life on the boat, and each can be jettisoned before the human passengers come to any harm. The problem with this argument is that the people on the boat can equally be seen as "threats," and yet there is no suggestion that any of them ought to be thrown overboard. Zalman acknowledges this point, and holds that this is precisely why Rashi's argument that "it is not a *nefesh*," is also needed. Unlike the human beings, the donkey or the luggage can be jettisoned because, as non-*nefesh* entities, they constitute "the *rodef* to the *nefashot*." No innocent *nefesh*, though, may be cast overboard. Even if all the people will drown, an innocent *nefesh* may not be singled out for destruction, because – as guiltless *nefashot* – they are all equal in standing to each other, and have done nothing to warrant being chosen for death.

Effectively, then, Zalman identifies two different modes of *rodef*-type behavior: there is the *nefesh* who may become a *rodef* through "intention

[34] *Hilkhot Chovel UMazzik* 8:15.
[35] All Zalman references and quotations are from S. Zalman, *Torat Chesed*, Jerusalem, 1909, *Even HaEzer*, volume II, number 42.
[36] See above, chapter 3, p. 59, n. 3.

and malice," and there is the non-*nefesh* which is to be treated like a *rodef* insofar as it poses a mortal threat to a *nefesh*, even if no intent or malice is present. Consequently, according to Zalman's classification, the fetus – held to be a non-*nefesh* like the donkey and the baggage – ought to be sacrificed when its presence threatens a *nefesh* with death, even though harmful intent and malice on the part of the fetus may be entirely absent. The fetus is a non-*nefesh* functioning like a *rodef* – meaning that, in the opinion of Zalman, it should be designated as a *rodef* – and hence a failure to remove it would be a transgression of the Torah's *mitzvah* "*lo tachos.*" By dismissing any intent requirement for a non-*nefesh* to be considered a *rodef*, Zalman hereby neatly preserves the significance of both Rashi's and Maimonides' outlooks, while plainly parting company with viewpoints akin to the position of Lipschutz.[37]

Parenthetically, it is worth observing that an early-twentieth-century scholar, Rabbi Issar Meltzer (died 1953), would build a similar analogy to Zalman's within his own commentary to the *Yad*.[38] Meltzer, however, differed slightly from Zalman in viewing both the mother and the fetus as each being a *rodef* to the other. According to Meltzer, in the case of the overloaded boat it is not accurate to describe the luggage as being a *rodef* and the human passengers not. The human passengers are *rodfim* as well. So, too, in the case of the mother and fetus, the mother should also be seen as a *rodef*. The mother, like the fetus, behaves in an involuntary fashion, but, because she prevents the fetus from emerging, she is to be considered a *rodef* to the fetus. In Meltzer's view, then, the fetus is to be sacrificed not because it is any more a *rodef* than its mother, but because, until it is born, the life of the mother takes precedence over that of the fetus, given that both are *rodfim*. Plainly, Meltzer too effectively interweaves the need for both Rashi's and Maimonides' positions.

Zalman's *teshuvah*, however, is noteworthy not just for his perceptive approach to the *rodef* problem, but also for his analysis of the varying outlooks on the prohibition on fetal destruction. Zalman pursues this analysis through a comparison of a number of different texts, principally those of Maimonides and Rabbeinu Nissim. Maimonides, Zalman states, concurred with the attitude of the *Tosafot* to *Sanhedrin* 59a and *Chullin* 33a that a Jew is not permitted to kill a fetus, based on the principle that "there is nothing which is permitted to a Jew but prohibited to a non-Jew."[39]

---

[37] See above, pp. 95–98.
[38] All Meltzer references and quotations are from I. Z. Meltzer, *Even HaAzel*, Jerusalem, 1935, to *Hilkhot Chovel UMazzik* 8:15.
[39] See above, chapter 3, p. 62.

Maimonides, of course, had codified the view of R. Yishmael that a non-Jew is liable for capital punishment for such an act.[40] Hence, Zalman avers, Maimonides held that Jews are biblically enjoined not to take fetal life. Conversely, maintains Zalman, Nissim follows the *Tosafot* to *Niddah* 44b in viewing it as permissible to kill a fetus, even though the laws of *Shabbat* can be set aside to save the fetus in the name of *pikuach nefesh*. In Nissim's view, then, insofar as there is a ban, it must be of rabbinic origin.[41]

Zalman proceeds to tie this divergence over the biblical or rabbinic nature of the prohibition to the question of whether the fetus is *yerekh imo* or *lav yerekh imo*.[42] From his reading of the *Arakhin* source, Nissim had inferred that the *lav yerekh imo* notion is more cogent.[43] Zalman, recapitulating Nissim's argument, explains that if the fetus were *yerekh imo*, then, in a case where the mother is condemned to death, the fetus would be concomitantly condemned and, therefore, ought to be executed along with its mother. In fact, given the prohibition against fetal destruction, the only justification for killing the fetus in such a case would be because it is the *yerekh* of a condemned woman. There is, however, another possible way to look at the *Mishnah's* instruction to kill a woman subject to capital punishment forthwith. The position that the fetus is actually *lav yerekh imo* combined with the stance that it is permitted to kill the fetus,[44] comports well with the view of the *Arakhin* text. As Nissim indicates, the combination of these two positions permits the fetus to be sacrificed not because of some sentence that has been applied to it by extension from its mother, but because of the overriding concern of the woman's *innui ha-din* (suffering associated with delay of sentence).[45] Thus, according to Zalman, one way of making sense of the sources is to couple the idea of *lav yerekh imo* with a sufficiently flexible understanding of the *Tosafists'* prohibition such that permission to kill the fetus can be obtained in certain pressing instances. For the prohibition to be malleable in this way means that it must have been a rabbinic ban.

---

[40] See above, chapter 2, p. 52, and chapter 3, p. 62. From a historical perspective, Maimonides could not have been familiar with the actual completed writings of the *Tosafot*, so his "agreement" with them is conjectural. Nevertheless, given the other evident similarities in approach, this is a reasonable suggestion.

[41] See above, chapter 3, p. 66.   [42] See above, chapter 2, pp. 32–33.

[43] See above, chapter 3, p. 65–66.

[44] Rabbi Zalman describes the *Tosafot* to *Niddah* 44b as conveying that "there is no prohibition on the killing of the fetus." Plainly, according to this view, if a prohibition were in place, it could only have been rabbinic, given the apparent ease with which it is brushed aside.

[45] See above, chapter 2, pp. 37–38.

The contrary position, Zalman points out, as expressed by Maimonides, conveys both that the prohibition was biblical and that the fetus was *yerekh imo*.[46] Seen this way, the biblical ban on killing an innocent fetus is only set aside in *Arakhin* because the fetus is condemned as a consequence of being *yerekh imo*. Were the fetus not included in its mother's guilt by means of the *yerekh imo* provision, there would be no possibility to override the ban – unless, of course, the fetus was behaving like a *rodef*. If, then, the ban is actually biblical in nature, either the *yerekh imo* or the *rodef* approach becomes necessary in order to make sense of the circumstances in which the Talmud permits fetal destruction. Zalman posits that any Toraitic prohibition on fetal destruction would be operational only after the fetus has been in existence for forty days, because a non-Jew was not killed for causing fetal destruction prior to forty days – the basis from which the Toraitic prohibition for Jews was derived.

Zalman is of the view that there exists an intrinsic connection between attitudes on the matter of *yerekh imo* or *lav yerekh imo* and the debate over whether the ban is, at root, Toraitic or rabbinic. While acknowledging the plausibility of both views, Zalman indicates that he tends towards regarding the prohibition as rabbinic, a conclusion which would plainly make the consequences of transgression far less serious. The prohibition, posits Zalman, is in place "because one ought not to kill a fetus that, in the future, is destined to be a *nefesh* from [the household of] Israel."[47] Thus, like Nachmanides before him, Zalman offers a defense of the need for the prohibition based on the potential that is inherent in the fetus.

All of this leads Zalman to conclude that destruction of the fetus is "permitted" if it is done *le-to'elet ve-refu'at imo* (for the benefit and [medical] healing of its mother).[48] This is certainly true, he maintains, for those who view the prohibition on fetal destruction as rabbinic. But even those who see the ban as Toraitic have a basis to allow for fetal destruction. Given that they hold to *ubar yerekh imo*, killing the fetus without cause would be unwarranted, while it would be acceptable to do so "for the benefit and healing of its mother," because the fetus is "like a limb of its mother that it is permitted to sever in the name of her [medical]

---

[46] Maimonides does not state explicitly that the fetus is *yerekh imo*. Nevertheless, his ruling on how to deal with an individual who tries to treat the fetus of a pregnant slave differently from its mother in terms of grants of freedom (*Avadim* 7:5) has been understood as implying that this is his view. See *Ravad ad loc.* See also *Shulchan Arukh, Choshen Mishpat, Hilkhot Geneivah* 2:12.

[47] Zalman was by no means alone among nineteenth-century rabbis in regarding the killing of the fetus as a rabbinic rather than a Toraitic transgression. To cite but one further example, Chayim Pallagi (*Chayim VeShalom*, Smyrna, 1872, volume 1, number 40) is emphatically of this view.

[48] This is not a term that Zalman defines with any precision.

well-being." That is why, Zalman explains, Maimonides needs the *rodef* argument for a woman who is having difficulties while in labor. For once she is "on the birthstool" the fetus is no longer *yerekh imo*, and hence some other justification must be adduced in order to kill it. Before the onset of labor, however, while the fetus is yet *yerekh imo*, "the benefit and healing of its mother" would suffice to call for its destruction.

Zalman, then, contributes a composite set of ideas which suggests that there would be few obstacles to an abortion prior to forty days, that destruction of the fetus after forty days might be countenanced provided that a genuine case of "the benefit and healing of its mother" could be made, and that upon the onset of labor the fetus would have to be a *rodef* in order to warrant termination. Zalman, it must be said, provides a very effective and legally sound rendering of the manner in which the views of Rashi and Maimonides might be harmonized.

There are, of course, few cases in which "the benefit and healing of its mother" becomes a more poignant consideration than in the instance of rape. A contemporary of Zalman, Rabbi Yehudah Perilman of Minsk, authored an 1891 *teshuvah* which, while it does not deal with abortion directly, provides a significant precedent for a possible *halakhic* approach to abortion following rape.[49] While discussing the circumstances in which the use of a *mokh*[50] is acceptable, Perilman raises the Talmudic discussion between Rabbi Yehudah and Rabbi Yossi about the length of time that a woman who has been raped or seduced must wait until she may marry.[51] R. Yehudah is of the view that she must wait the statutory Talmudic period of three months so that there is no doubt about paternity. R. Yossi, however, permits immediate marriage on the basis that a woman in such circumstances would use the post-coital *mokh*. This led Perilman to infer that while women are normally not permitted to destroy seed, R. Yossi's position indicates that, in the case of rape, such destruction would be acceptable. Feldman succinctly explains Perilman's logic in this regard: "The reason she may is that while woman is said to be a vehicle for reproduction (*karka olam*), as a human being she differs from 'mother earth' in that she need not nurture seed implanted within her *against her will*; indeed, she may 'uproot' seed illegally sown."[52] Perilman clearly intends that the "uprooting" be done as swiftly as possible, in the manner of post-coital contraception. Nevertheless, if the swift "uprooting" of seed is permitted in the case of rape, then, presumably such "uprooting" might

---

[49] All Perilman references and quotations are from Y. Perilman, *Or Gadol*, Vilna, 1924, number 31.
[50] See above, chapter 3, p. 81.   [51] *Yevamot* 35a and *Ketubot* 37a.
[52] Feldman, *Birth Control*, p. 287.

be permissible at a later point as well. This is certainly the conclusion that Feldman draws from Perilman: "More specific references to abortion of a conceptus resulting from rape seem to be lacking in the available Responsa. What the Rabbis would have ruled, however, can safely be surmised from the sentiment reflected here . . ."[53]

It is clear that by the twilight of the nineteenth century, abortion deliberations still remained much more of a theoretical *halakhic* matter than a regular, practical concern. Abortion also remained an area in which frank disagreement could still be aired. Thus Rabbi Yechiel Epstein (1829–1908) of Belorussia, in his well-known *halakhic* summation of the 1890s, *Arukh HaShulchan*, took issue with the Maimonidean *rodef* classification.[54] Epstein, in a succinct comment, begins by quoting Maimonides, which he follows with *Mishnah Ohalot*. He then elucidates the *Mishnah*'s permission to kill the fetus as being based in the notion "that the fetus is not yet a *nefesh*, and not because it is a *rodef* – and this is 'the way of the world.'" "Furthermore," Epstein inquires, "if it were for the reason of being a *rodef* [that the fetus could be killed], what difference is there between the head having emerged and it not having emerged?"[55] While by no means the first time that Maimonides' reasoning had been called into question, Epstein is perhaps unusually explicit in rebuffing the *rodef* explanation.

However, precisely the opposite view is expressed by Epstein's contemporary, Rabbi Chayim Soloveitchik (1853–1918). Soloveitchik, who was a highly respected Talmudist, head of the Volozhin yeshiva, and rabbi of Brisk, had a renowned sense of compassion for others and a lenient tendency in applying the law.[56] However, when addressing the subject of the fetus – as he did in his *chiddushim* (novel insights) to Maimonides' *Mishneh Torah*[57] – it was not so much the lenient application of the law as its construction that was the focus of his thinking.

[53] *Ibid.*

[54] Epstein's reputation for leniency is not in dispute. He is quoted as having instructed his student, Rabbi Maimon, "When any problem in connection with the prohibitions of the Torah comes before you, you must first presume it is permitted, and only after you have carefully studied the *rishonim* and can find no possibility of leniency are you obliged to rule that it is forbidden." It should be noted that although *Arukh HaShulchan* was not completed until the first decade of the twentieth century, the *Choshen Mishpat* section was finished in 1893. See Y. Horowitz, "Epstein, Jehiel Michael Ben Aaron Isaac HaLevi," in *Encyclopaedia Judaica*, Jerusalem, Keter Publishing House, volume VI, pp. 831–832.

[55] *Arukh HaShulchan, Choshen Mishpat* 425:7.

[56] M. Hacohen, "Soloveitchik, Hayyim," in *Encyclopaedia Judaica*, Jerusalem, Keter Publishing House, volume XV, pp. 129–130.

[57] *Chiddushei Chayim HaLevi* (1936) to *Hilkhot Rotzeiach* 1:9.

Just as in Epstein's case, his starting point is not a *shëeilah* (question), but rather a conceptual difficulty within the *halakhah* itself.[58] It should be noted that Soloveitchik was considered a "giant" in the type of Talmudic analysis that has come to dominate much of the world of traditional learning.[59] Consequently, his perspective would prove highly influential for significant *poskim* of the twentieth century.[60]

Soloveitchik makes particularly effective use of his *shnei dinim* method[61] when analyzing the laws applicable to the destruction of the fetus. By applying this technique to the *rodef* precept, Soloveitchik discerns that two essential ideas are critical to the *rodef* principle: first, saving the one being pursued, and second, stopping the *rodef* – even if it means killing the *rodef*. In the case of the fetus, however, the Talmud never designates the fetus as a *rodef*, stating only that the mother "is being pursued from heaven."[62] As Soloveitchik explains it, this statement conveys that, *prima facie*, while one is obligated to save the mother, the requirement to stop the *rodef* may not be carried out by killing the fetus, as heaven is the real *rodef*. However, if this is so, how can the fetus be killed in the name of saving the mother? Washofsky succinctly encapsulates Soloveitchik's solution:

The answer flows from a similar "*shnei dinim*" analysis of the concept of *pikuah nefesh*. The duty to preserve life also consists of two rules: the equal status of all persons, so that "one life does not override another," and the permission to set aside virtually all the commandments of the Torah in order to save human life ... [B]y ruling that the fetus "is like a pursuer," Rambam declares it is indeed a *nefesh* under the first rule and enjoys a claim to equal protection. Its life may not be set aside on behalf of another except in a case of dangerous childbirth, when it can be considered a *rodef*. It is the fetus, and not the mother, who is the

---

[58] Washofsky, "Abortion and the Halakhic Conversation," p. 48 writes of the approach that was championed by Soloveitchik: "Problems in *halakhah* are studied not so much in terms of their real-world settings and circumstances as by means of the basic concepts said to underlie them. Drawing fine logical distinctions between aspects of a basic concept, the analyst seeks to dispose of a problem which had occupied the minds of Talmudists for generations."

[59] For a succinct overview of Soloveitchik's approach, see Washofsky, "Abortion and the Halakhic Conversation," p. 48.

[60] Unterman and Feinstein (see chapter 5, below), in particular, would rely upon Soloveitchik.

[61] L. Jacobs, *A Tree of Life: Diversity, Flexibility, and Creativity in Jewish Law*, Oxford, Oxford University Press, 1984, pp. 60–61. According to the *shnei dinim* (two laws) theory, *halakhic* precepts generally are composed of two fundamental ideas. Apparent conflicts between *halakhic* authorities, therefore, are not the outcome of disputes in which one is "right" and the other "wrong." Rather, they emerge because each is operating on the basis of a different one of the two ideas contained within the precepts. The disputes, therefore, do not reflect contradictions, they are simply the result of differing orientations.

[62] See above, chapter 2, p. 49.

aggressor in this case because she, a "full legal person" (*nefesh gamur*) to whom *pikuah nefesh* pertains in both its aspects, takes precedence over the incomplete *nefesh* of the fetus.[63]

It follows from this that the laws of *pikuach nefesh* apply to a fetus just as to a full *nefesh*. The only exception to this rule occurs when the fetus poses a threat to the mother, in which case the fetus is to be treated as if it were a *rodef*. According to Soloveitchik, the fetus is susceptible to such treatment in a way that the mother is not, because the fetus is not a "full" *nefesh*, whereas the mother is.

Effectively, then, Soloveitchik's understanding delimits Rashi's position. Although Rashi had said that the fetus could be killed because it is "not a *nefesh*," Soloveitchik holds that this is only meant to apply when the behavior of the fetus causes it to be stripped of the protection that it would otherwise enjoy, that is, when it is conducting itself as a *rodef*. This means that it is only insofar as the fetus is the direct cause of a threat to its mother's existence that its life can be taken. If it is not "like a *rodef*" – if some other causal agent is pursuing the mother – the fetus must remain inviolate. Soloveitchik, then, clearly demonstrates why the positions of both Maimonides and Rashi are necessary, and offers a relatively restrictive reconciliation of their approaches.

While Soloveitchik's outlook would be seen as foundational by some leading *halakhic* authorities, he also has been criticized for straying from the sense of the Talmud. Washofsky writes:

Soloveitchik's *shnei dinim* method draws conceptual distinctions, which, if intellectually stimulating, have the most tenuous roots in legal reality. In our case, for example, he quite literally invents two *halakhic* institutions: the "semi-*rodef*" and the "semi-*nefesh*." These are unprecedented concepts of Jewish law, for while the Talmud and the *posqim* speak at length of the "pursuer" and the "person," never before has it been suggested that one can be "a pursuer who is not a full pursuer" or "a person who is not a full person." Soloveitchik's *hiddush* may resolve this particular ruling of Rambam, but it is patently artificial, forcing the Talmudic texts into interpretations that do not correspond to their plain or obvious meaning. It is a weak reed upon which to support a *halakhic* decision of the gravest import.[64]

Washofsky acknowledges, however, that notwithstanding the apparent innovation, Soloveitchik's construction "works" in the sense that it creates a clear answer to the problem, an answer that is adjudged to be acceptable within the *halakhic* system. That solution, of course, effectively defines any

---

[63] Washofsky, "Abortion and the Halakhic Conversation," p. 49.   [64] *Ibid.*, pp. 50–51.

more lenient positions as being untenable on the basis that they permit the unthinkable destruction of a "semi-*nefesh*."

Washofsky's objection that Soloveitchik has produced "unprecedented concepts" represents an important insight. Given, though, that the *shnei dinim* method is hermeneutically sound, that these "concepts" harmonize Maimonides with the Talmud, and that they produce what Soloveitchik obviously regards as the "correct" outcome, their *halakhic* cogency and usefulness have clearly come to outweigh concerns over their "artificiality." After all, Soloveitchik's alleged "artificiality" or "innovation" is only different in degree – not manner – from some of Soloveitchik's predecessors who essentially built "partial *rodef*" arguments based on the fetus being "*like* a *rodef*." As Washofsky would agree, then, while Soloveitchik's solution might well require considerable *halakhic* creativity, it is by no means beyond the *halakhic* pale.

Soloveitchik's *shnei dinim* technique represented an unusual methodological approach. But the response to the abortion issue of Soloveitchik's *Sefaradi* contemporary, Rabbi Yosef Chayim ben Elijah Al-Chakam (1835–1909), is remarkable because of its lack of a methodological approach altogether. Al-Chakam lived in Baghdad and, although he never served as official rabbi of the city, he was a popular preacher, wrote about both *halakhah* and *Kabbalah*, and edited the text of the *Sefaradi* prayer book. His responsa include answers to queries from Baghdad, Iraq, and all over the Far East.[65] Al-Chakam confronted the abortion issue through a question almost identical to those previously dealt with by Bacharach and Ya'avetz. In the case of a married woman who has become pregnant as the result of an adulterous affair, and is now faced with the prospect of giving birth to a *mamzer*, "is it permissible [for her] to drink something that will abort the fetus, given that [the fetus] is already formed and has been inside her for five months? Is it permissible for others to assist her in this matter by bringing her to the doctor so that he may give her the drugs, or by bringing her the drugs from him?"[66]

Al-Chakam's answer is brief. He immediately states that he will not be providing any definitive response to the inquiry: "In this matter I do not want to provide an actual ruling, neither to prohibit nor to permit, but only to copy for you that which I have found in the responsa of the *Acharonim*..." Al-Chakam proceeds to describe the positions of

---

[65] A. David, "Joseph Hayyim Ben Elijah Al-Hakam," in *Encyclopaedia Judaica*, Jerusalem, Keter Publishing House, volume x, pp. 242–243.

[66] All Al-Chakam references and quotations are from Y. Al-Chakam, *Rav Pa'alim*, Jerusalem, 1905, *Even HaEzer*, volume 1, number 4.

Bacharach and Ya'avetz, reiterating Bacharach's opposition to such an abortion and Ya'avetz's approval. He concludes by offering what he considers to be the salient element of the views of Maharit, which is instructive, given the general uncertainty over the manner in which Maharit's two *teshuvot* ought to be understood.[67] Al-Chakam makes explicit reference to both Maharit's *teshuvah* number 97 and *teshuvah* number 99, leaving no doubt that he had taken both into account. The essential message that Al-Chakam distills from these two *teshuvot* is that, in the case of a Jewish woman, "it is permitted to intervene medically in order to cause her to abort, if there is [some] *tzorekh* [need] on the part of the mother." This stance, Al-Chakam posits, could provide that, in the case before him, "there is a family defect and disgrace and *chillul HaShem* if the fetus remains and is not aborted, [that would make one] consider this a [case of] great need." Al-Chakam desists from any further exploration of this idea, and closes his *teshuvah* with these words: "And I have already said that I shall not add my own [insight] in this matter, and I will not reveal my view, and my only advice for the questioner is that he should bring these issues to a scholar (*chakham*) and he [the *chakham*] will instruct him what to do."

There are two noteworthy aspects of Al-Chakam's succinct *teshuvah*. First, Al-Chakam's interpretation of Maharit's position is significant. Despite the fact that Al-Chakam refers to both of Maharit's *teshuvot*, he makes no mention of Maharit's acceptance of the abortion prohibition, or of Maharit's *chabbalah* explanation. Rather, he stresses the lenient element of responsum number 99 that advocates permitting abortion for Jews based on maternal need. Al-Chakam certainly was aware that Maharit's views could be read in a far more restrictive fashion, but he elected to focus exclusively on the less limiting reading. It is appropriate to infer from this that Al-Chakam regarded this understanding of Maharit's tendency as the more convincing one.[68] After all, had he held this reading of Maharit to be possible but weak, Al-Chakam most certainly could have relied simply on Bacharach and Ya'avetz – whose insights were directly relevant to the question at hand – without utilizing Maharit,

---

[67] See above, chapter 3, pp. 69–71.

[68] Sinclair, "Legal Doctrine and Moral Principle," p. 27, n. 113. Sinclair writes of Al-Chakam, "his emphasis of the lenient *responsum* is clearly an indication of his objective preference for a source closer to, rather than distant from the classical Rabbinic doctrine on feticide." Sinclair may be correct about this, but there is no evidence that his assertion is right, anymore than there is evidence that Bacharach "preferred" sources that were further removed from "classic Rabbinic doctrine." All that can be known with certainty is that Al-Chakam thought it more appropriate to place emphasis on the more lenient source; the reason he did so is a matter of speculation.

whose arguments were not specifically germane to the matter of adultery. Al-Chakam, of course, does not only opt to concentrate on Maharit's leniency, but goes even further in opining that an abortion in the case of adultery might constitute the type of "need" to which Maharit refers. Given that Al-Chakam states from the start that he does not intend to rule on the question before him, he certainly provides a strong hint that there is textual support for a permissive response to this inquiry. He also indicates that it is possible to perceive maternal "need" in cases that are less than life-threatening in nature.

The second aspect of Al-Chakam's *teshuvah* that deserves comment is his most unusual decision to provide a review of the legal history of the subject under consideration without giving a ruling. His proposal that the questioner should take this matter to some local authority for a ruling is, after all, a reversal of the normal responsa process. Normally, a local rabbi would submit a difficult question of this type to a sage like Al-Chakam for authoritative adjudication, not the other way around.[69] If Al-Chakam did not regard this matter as one that was appropriate for him to decide, then why did he think it important to write a *teshuvah* that was essentially a non-*teshuvah*? Why did he not simply refer the matter to the local rabbi for decision without troubling to record his own unwillingness to rule? Sinclair offers this explanation for Al-Chakam's enigmatic strategy:

Yosef Hayyim's approach in this case is highly uncharacteristic both of his own halakhic writings and of the *responsa* genre in general. Indeed, it is the specificity of the definitive reply to a factual situation which endows the Rabbinic *responsum* with its unique normative status.[70] Presumably, the reason for Yosef Hayyim's deviation from the generally accepted method of responsa writing lies in the need to express the tension between halakhic doctrine and the moral issue of preserving fetal life, especially where the mother is not in any direct physical danger. Yosef Hayyim does, indeed, cite Bachrach's remark regarding the conflict between *Torah* law and conventional morality in his brief reference to the latter's *responsum*. In Yosef Hayyim's eyes it is evident that the best solution

---

[69] Elon, *Jewish Law*, volume III, p. 1460. Elon writes: "Complex problems that local courts could not resolve, and fundamental questions transcending the immediate parties and involving the wider public, ultimately reached one of the recognized respondents active in the various centers of the diaspora . . . In this role, the respondents also contributed to the preservation of a certain measure of uniformity of decision and to the maintenance of close ties among the diaspora communities within each Jewish center and between one center and another." Even if the local rabbi might have been able to handle the problem passed to him by Al-Chakam – and this is questionable – Al-Chakam's action hardly would have aided any "uniformity of decision" on this type of issue.

[70] Here, Sinclair refers his reader to Elon, *Jewish Law*, volume III, pp. 1457–1459.

for this type of tension is to desist from writing a definitive legal *responsum* and to leave the actual decision in the hands of a local rabbi who will, presumably, be in a position to assess the moral aspects of the case on a first-hand basis and rule accordingly. Yosef Hayyim does not specifically refer to conventional morality except insofar as he does cite Bachrach on this point. The tension between halakhic doctrine and his very evident desire to avoid making a definitive ruling is, however, a very palpable one and may, presumably, be explained on the basis of the moral ramifications of sanctioning the abortion of a five month fetus for no reason other than it being a *mamzer*.[71]

Sinclair's position is that Al-Chakam was persuaded of the textual validity of allowing this abortion, but had moral reservations about actually proceeding, particularly given that the pregnancy was so well advanced. According to Sinclair, it was Al-Chakam's hope that the local rabbi would be better equipped to deal "first-hand" with this difficult conundrum.

But Sinclair's position is itself problematic. After all, if Al-Chakam is so troubled by the "moral ramifications" of allowing such an abortion, then why does he cite the *halakhic* record selectively in a way that appears to encourage this type of procedure? Had Al-Chakam wanted to give the local rabbi the maximum latitude to rule against this abortion as being morally deficient, he could simply have cited Bacharach alone, or he could have cited Bacharach and Ya'avetz, while questioning the true "need" involved in this instance. Al-Chakam, however, does neither. Instead, he ventures beyond citations that deal directly with the adultery issue and chooses to supplement Bacharach and Ya'avetz with the most lenient reading of Maharit, when he equally well could have opted to include restrictive views, such as those of Maimonides or Landau. Then Al-Chakam adds even more credence to the lenient perspective by volunteering that the instance before him might indeed be held to be an example of "need." At the very least, Al-Chakam skews his presentation towards a presumption that such an abortion could find *halakhic* support. Had he really wanted to communicate his concerns over the "moral ramifications of sanctioning the abortion" to the local rabbi, this *teshuvah* would not have served him well. Even if, then, we accept Sinclair's thesis that much of the responsa literature on abortion expresses "the tension between halakhic doctrine and the moral issue of preserving fetal life,"[72] in the case of Al-Chakam, this is not the most logical explanation of his reticence. Given that the plain tendency of the *teshuvah* is to support what Sinclair terms "halakhic doctrine," the local

---

[71] Sinclair, "Legal Doctrine and Moral Principle," p. 23.
[72] For further explanation and analysis of Sinclair's position see below, chapter 7, pp. 243–251.

rabbi would have been better off without Al-Chakam's answer if the rabbi's intention were to provide a more "moral" answer than "halakhic doctrine" might otherwise suggest.

In truth, we will never know with any sense of assurance why Al-Chakam declined to issue a judgment. Perhaps the simplest explanation is that Al-Chakam thought that it was more appropriate that a local rabbi, who could become more familiar with the particulars of the case, should rule. Alternatively, perhaps he regarded this issue, as a genuine case of "*teyku*," that is, an instance in which he could, with a true sense of equanimity, have ruled either way. Perhaps the fact that Al-Chakam left his *teshuvah* in an unresolved state should be seen as symbolic. For, in actuality, his unsettled position accurately reflected the unbridged differences on this matter that continued unabated.

The nineteenth century ended, therefore, without conspicuous con-currence having emerged on almost any aspect of the abortion issue. While all affirmed that a woman whose life is threatened by her fetus has permission to destroy the fetus, there was no clear-cut view as to whether this was because the fetus was a *rodef* or simply because it lacked *nefesh* status. No coherent understanding had crystallized concerning what be-ing "like a *rodef*" connoted, or over the reason behind the *Tosafists'* prohi-bition. No agreement was evident over the standards of medical certainty that were required before an abortion could proceed. No consensus had coalesced around which – if any – circumstances, short of imminent danger to the mother's life, might be acceptable grounds for abortion. Moreover, seven hundred years after the divergent views of Rashi and Maimonides had become apparent, their inheritors still had arrived at no clear method for resolving the differences between them.

THE TWENTIETH CENTURY DAWNS

The arrival of the twentieth century was not, of course, a turning point that called for any particular *halakhic* rethinking. Nevertheless, while the effects of modernity would need to ripen still more before their impact would become truly evident, profound changes would arise in the na-ture of the response to abortion as the century progressed. One trend, however, was already evident from early on: the *teshuvot* of the twentieth century began to revolve far more around matters of practical concern than had previously been the case.

The *teshuvot* of Rabbi Mordecai Winkler presented an early example of this phenomenon. Winkler was asked about the case of a pregnant woman who was bringing up blood and was suffering from generalized weakness.[73] The doctors offered an alternative: either they would immediately begin using drugs in order to induce a miscarriage, or they would perform a surgical abortion at some future point. The woman sought guidance from Winkler regarding the most appropriate choice. It is clear from the facts that the woman's life, while at some risk, was not in imminent danger. Indeed there seems little doubt that, had this question been asked of Drimer in the nineteenth century,[74] he would have advocated a *shev ve-àl tàaseh* approach, arguing that the danger involved in either proposed procedure was unacceptable, given that the woman was not in direct peril. Winkler's reasoning, however, differs markedly from that of Drimer, and the divergence seems to stem mainly from a practical, rather than a textual origin. Winkler maintains that, while the dangers to any woman in the circumstances of a spontaneous miscarriage – such as the one in Exodus 21:22–23, or the one that might have resulted from hunger had the woman not been fed in *Yoma* 82a – are doubtless significant, this is arguably not the case when modern medicine is available. When such procedures "are performed by doctors and by use of drugs, it is possible that it is known to them [the physicians] that by these means there is no suspicion of danger..." Even acknowledging, writes Winkler, that some amount of danger exists in any serious medical intervention, this danger may well be acceptable if its purpose is to prevent a more serious danger.[75] The danger of the procedures themselves, then, would only be a factor if – through improper or insufficient care – a likelihood existed that going ahead with one of them would be more risky than doing nothing. Thus, in principle, Winkler would agree with Drimer that the "greater danger" indeed is to be avoided. In practice, however, Winkler comes up with the opposite response to that of Drimer: in circumstances in which appropriate medical assistance is in attendance, avoiding a therapeutic abortion or induced miscarriage on account of danger is not the correct path. Consequently, Winkler does not rule out either procedure, but rather advises the woman concerned to evaluate the relative dangers of the two suggested courses with the help of her doctors.

---

[73] References and quotations concerning this Winkler *teshuvah* are from M. Winkler, *Levushei Mordekhai, Mahadurah Tinyana*, Budapest, 1924, *Yoreh Deàh*, number 87.

[74] See above, pp. 101–102.

[75] Winkler illustrates this notion of relative danger by citing a responsum in which a young boy was required to undergo surgery for a serious condition. While the surgery was dangerous in and of itself, it was permitted in order to alleviate the "great danger" in which the lad found himself.

But Winkler's interaction with the abortion issue extended to yet another, even more complex, issue. In a *teshuvah* dated 1913, Winkler was
asked about the case of a woman, who had been advised by her doctor
that, should she become pregnant, she would face a real and present
threat to her mental well-being. Could she, under such circumstances,
undergo an abortion?[76] In his answer, Winkler cites a late-seventeenth-
century *teshuvah* in which Rabbi Israel Meir Mizrachi was asked whether
non-kosher chicken soup could be given to a mentally troubled individual who, as a result of his belief that the soup had medicinal qualities,
appeared to be calmed by the consumption of this *tareif* broth.[77] In reply,
Mizrachi – noting that individuals with mental illness are at risk of suicide,
or injuring themselves, or putting others at risk[78] – expressed the unambiguous view that serious mental illness is a danger that may be equated
to a threat to one's physical well-being. Based on this ruling by Mizrachi,
Winkler infers that, because mental-health risk has been considered to
be akin to physical-health risk, this woman could be permitted to abort
in the event that she became pregnant. Winkler's response is significant.
While it is likely that his permissive reply is predicated on the assumption
that the mental-health risk under discussion is a life-threatening one, his
reply suggests that mental-health concerns should be seen to be just as
serious potential triggers for abortion as their physical counterparts.

A *teshuvah* by Rabbi Yitzchak Oelbaum, penned in the very same year,
also displays a practical and permissive approach while replying to a
question that had arisen before.[79] Like Rabbi Ayash in the eighteenth
century,[80] Oelbaum was asked about a case in which a pregnant mother
had an existent "weak" child who, according to the doctors, would not
live unless it was breast-fed by its mother. The woman had noticed a
change in her milk around the fourth week of pregnancy that seemed
like it might be threatening to the nursing child. The mother wanted
to know if she could abort the fetus in order to save the existent child.
Oelbaum, while questioning whether the doctors were accurate in their
assessment, concludes that an abortion would be permitted if the experts
were of the view that the existing child indeed would be in danger. It
is worth noting that Oelbaum, like Ayash, allows for the consideration

---

[76] References and quotations concerning this Winkler *teshuvah* are from *Levushei Mordekhai, Choshen Mishpat*, number 39.
[77] M. Mizrachi, *Peri Ha-Aretz*, Jerusalem, 1899, *Yoreh De'ah*, volume III, number 2.
[78] This view was founded in the earlier position of Nachmanides.
[79] All Oelbaum references and quotations are from *Shéeilat Yitzchak*, Prague, 1931, number 64.
[80] See above, chapter 3, pp. 83–84.

of the needs of an individual other than the mother in weighing the abortion decision. Unlike Ayash, however, Oelbaum does not make his permission contingent on the proposed abortion technique. It should be made clear that Oelbaum provides a warrant for abortion in this circumstance only as a last resort to save the child's life: his approval is dependent upon every other option for saving the child having been exhausted. Oelbaum's judgment in this matter was, however, the subject of great caution among other *poskim*, who continued to view the sole *halakhic* justification for abortion as the mother being *in extremis*.[81]

If, however, Oelbaum's *teshuvah* seemed exceptional, it appears almost conventional when compared to a wrenching question that arose from the First World War. The conundrum, reported in the literature by Rabbi Issar Yehudah Unterman,[82] dealt with a real instance of the question that Babad had earlier examined in theory.[83] Unterman recounts the circumstances in this way:

This question once arose in practice during the period of the German occupation of Poland and Lithuania in the First World War. It happened that in the ranks of the German soldiers and officers stationed in Jewish towns, one of the officers had intimate relations with a Jewish girl. When she revealed to him that she was pregnant and asked that he take responsibility for the results of his actions, he requested that she go to a doctor for an abortion in order to get out of this situation. They turned to a Jewish doctor in the town in order to carry out the abortion, and even though the girl did not desire it [the abortion], [the officer] pressed her to agree. However, the doctor refused [to carry out the abortion] because it was forbidden according to the law of the Torah (and also, according to the law of the state, such an act was regarded as a criminal transgression). Thereupon the officer threatened [the doctor's life] with a drawn revolver (for they [the Germans] regarded themselves as having absolute dominance over the lives of the inhabitants). The doctor requested the postponement of his decision [as to whether he would choose to perform the abortion or be killed] in the matter for one day, and, in the mean time, he brought the question to a rabbi. The rabbi gave serious contemplation to this problem of the "appurtenance of spilling blood," and could not come to a decision.

Unterman does not report how this harrowing saga was eventually resolved. But what is clear from this account is just how much was yet unclear as the twentieth century began. According to Unterman's

---

[81] See M. Stern, *HaRefu'ah L'Or HaHalakhah*, Jerusalem, 1980, p. 104.
[82] I. Y. Unterman, "*B'Inyan Pikuach Nefesh Shel Ubar*," *Noam*, volume 6, 1963: 5. Unterman's reaction to this extraordinary dilemma will be explored below. See chapter 5, pp. 138–139.
[83] See above, p. 103.

description of the case, the rabbi whom the doctor consulted was unable to decide whether feticide was an "appurtenance of murder" – in the face of which the doctor might be asked to give up his life rather than commit such an act – or a less serious infraction, which would dictate that the doctor should carry out the abortion in order to preserve his own life.[84] Plainly, as Unterman relates it, this rabbi could find no firm foundation on which to base a view on such a fundamental issue as whether an abortion ought to proceed under such circumstances or not. It is possible, of course, that this rabbi was not sufficiently expert in this area of the *halakhah* to make a pronouncement on the matter. If, however, greater expertise was required, it only underscores that the response to questions of abortion in which the mother's life was not threatened was anything but straightforward and simple.

Into this rather undetermined picture stepped the great Lithuanian Talmud scholar, Rabbi Chayim Ozer Grodzinsky (1863–1940). Grodzinsky, the leading *dayan* (judge) of Vilna, and a "vehement opponent of Zionism and of secular education for Jews," saw the growing Reform movement in the West as destructive, and held that the *yeshivot* of the East were the "strongholds of Judaism."[85] In essence, then, he was decidedly unenthusiastic about some of the Jewish products of modernity. Grodzinsky's three volumes of *teshuvot* entitled "*Achiezer*" appeared during the turbulent years between the Wars, in 1922, 1925, and 1939. Grodzinsky twice deals directly with issues relevant to abortion. In one *teshuvah*, he ventures into the discussion of whether or not the prohibition on fetal destruction is biblical or rabbinic.[86] Grodzinsky

---

[84] The "appurtenance of murder" argument is clarified above, p. 98. If the abortion were an "appurtenance of murder," then it might be subsumed within one of the three sins for which the doctor ought to surrender his own life. If not, then he has a duty to preserve his own life at the expense of that of the fetus. For one response to this matter, see Unterman's view in chapter 5, pp. 138–139, below.

It is important to note that this is the first time that the "appurtenance of murder" argument is applied to abortion. Unterman would later be the first major proponent of this approach (see chapter 5, below). Unterman, though, provides no primary reference for this incident. Hence, it is possible that the rabbi to whom this problem was brought contemplated the issue in quite different terms from those of Unterman, and Unterman retroactively applied his own construction to the rabbi's thinking.

It is also worth observing that the woman's expressed wish not to have an abortion is not in any way seen to be germane to this *halakhic* discussion. As the doctor's life hangs in the balance, if abortion is not an "appurtenance of murder" then the procedure might be deemed necessary in order to save him, regardless of the woman's preferences. This ought not to be understood as implying that the woman's desires were insignificant, but that, in these circumstances, they were not the paramount concern.

[85] H. H. Ben-Sasson, "Grodzinski, Hayyim Ozer," in *Encyclopaedia Judaica*, Jerusalem, Keter Publishing House, volume VII, pp. 928–929.

[86] Grodzinsky, *Achiezer*, volume III, number 65, section 14.

states that – notwithstanding the wording of the *Tosafot* to *Niddah* 44b –
the *Tosafot* were of the view that the ban was Toraitic, by extension of the
prohibition on the Noahide. Conversely, Grodzinsky points out, the reasoning of Nissim indicates exactly the opposite, namely that there is no
Toraitic prohibition. Grodzinsky concludes that there is a real possibility that there is no Torah-based prohibition, but advises that the matter
"requires study." Grodzinsky deals with the tradition that drew a distinction between the first forty days of gestation[87] and the rest of pregnancy
but exhibits scarcely greater certainty: "It appears that a Noahide is not
put to death for this and, even with regard to an Israelite it is possible
that there is no Toraitic prohibition." Yet again, a fundamental issue
remained the subject of unresolved *halakhic* indeterminacy.

In his other pertinent *teshuvah*, Grodzinsky was asked about a woman
suffering from a serious lung disease who had become pregnant, and according to the doctors, her well-being necessitated performing surgery
and destroying her fetus.[88] The doctors further advised that there was a
real danger that if the surgery were not carried out, the woman would die
in childbirth. Should she heed the doctors and proceed with the abortion? Grodzinsky begins his answer by referring to Maimonides' *rodef*
classification. Plainly, states Grodzinsky, while this fetus might become a
rodef, it is not a *rodef* at present. Does this imply that Maimonides would
not permit the killing of the fetus in the circumstances described? In the
view of Grodzinsky, it does not imply anything of the sort. Grodzinsky
echoes the notion, succinctly stated in Landau's *Nodah bi-Yehudah*, that it
is unthinkable to sacrifice a *tereifah* in the name of an individual who is
not afflicted.[89] Hence, if the fetus were not designated as a *rodef*, there
certainly would exist no justification for killing it. Grodzinsky, however,
then takes this logic a step further than had Landau: Maimonides, avers
Grodzinsky, would apply this argument only when the woman is in trouble during the birth process itself. For it is only once she is "on the
birthstool" that the fetus becomes a separate body, ceases to be *yerekh
imo*, and is subject to being considered a *rodef*. Indeed, at the point that
the fetus becomes a "separate body," regarding it as a *rodef* is a *sine qua
non* of being able to kill it. Conversely, however, so long as the woman
has not gone into labor, even Maimonides would agree that the fetus is
yerekh imo and, hence, is "like one of her limbs." "Of course," emphasizes
Grodzinsky, "one is obligated to sever a limb in order to save the life of
the whole body..."

---

[87] During the first forty days, of course, some held that the fetus was to be regarded as "mere fluid."
See above, chapter 2, pp. 33–34.
[88] Grodzinsky, *Achiezer*, volume III, number 72, section 3.   [89] See above, chapter 3, p. 90.

As Grodzinsky sees it, then, the paramount rabbinic ideas applicable to this instance are those of the Talmud – that "she is being pursued from heaven" – and of Rashi, that the fetus is not a *nefesh*. Hence, conveys Grodzinsky, before the onset of the birth process, both Rashi and Maimonides would regard it as appropriate to sacrifice the fetus in order to save the mother from her own "limb." Once the birth process is underway, they still would concur that the fetus ought to be killed to save the mother, albeit invoking their respective reasons to support their positions. Grodzinsky concludes that there is essentially no real dispute between the positions of these two great *Rishonim*, but that the most important aspect – certainly in the case before him – is that the fetus was not yet held to be a *nefesh*.

Grodzinsky, then, is of the view that this woman does not need to wait until the fetus becomes a *rodef*. The termination of her pregnancy on the advice of her doctors is consistent with the idea of being saved from a limb that otherwise would threaten her entire being. Grodzinsky's approval, however, carries with it the condition that the woman should rely only upon physicians who are experts in such procedures and should not go ahead with any surgery that is accompanied by unwarranted danger. Despite this minor constraint, it seems plain that Grodzinsky takes a relatively lenient approach to therapeutic abortion. Unlike some of his predecessors, he is prepared to countenance therapeutic abortion even when the mother is not the subject of an "immediate pursuit," and even when the fetus is not the direct cause of the threat to her.

If, however, Grodzinsky seems relatively lenient, this is perhaps even more true of his contemporary, Rabbi Ben-Zion Ouziel (1880–1953). Far from the *Ashkenazi* milieu of Grodzinsky, Ouziel was born in the land of Israel, became chief rabbi of Tel Aviv in 1923, and served as *Sefaradi* chief rabbi of Israel from 1939 until his death.[90] In his three-volume collection of *teshuvot*, *Mishpetei Ouziel*, Ouziel deals with two separate questions on abortion.

In the first, dated 1938, Ouziel was asked whether a woman who is at risk of permanent deafness if her pregnancy continues could have an abortion.[91] Ouziel begins his answer by rejecting any suggestion that the fetus could have *nefesh* status. The fetus is not like a *goses be-yedei shamayim*,[92]

---

[90] I. Goldshlag, "Ouziel, Ben-Zion Meir Chai," in *Encyclopaedia Judaica*, Jerusalem, Keter Publishing House, volume XII, pp. 1527–1528.

[91] All references and quotations to this first *teshuvah* by Ouziel are from B. Ouziel, *Mishpetei Ouziel*, Tel Aviv, 1935, *Choshen Mishpat*, volume III, number 46.

[92] See above, chapter 3, p. 63, n. 20. One who kills a *goses be-yedei shamayim* is liable for the death penalty.

he writes, because, in the case of a *goses*, "there was a *nefesh*, and something of that *nefesh* remains," but for a fetus, there is not even the slightest trace of a *nefesh*. Plainly, Ouziel and Soloveitchik disagree profoundly on this fundamental issue. Ouziel proceeds to echo the language of the *Tosafot* in *Niddah* when he states, "since it is not called a *nefesh* at all, it is permitted to kill it." Ouziel, however, is mindful that there were those, like Ya'avetz, who had maintained that this *Tosafot* text, because of its apparent inconsistencies with the two other *Tosafot* selections, was "not precise, for who would permit the killing of a fetus without reason?"[93] Ya'avetz had also stated that one could not bring proof that it is permitted to kill a fetus from the *Arakhin Gemara*'s concern over the woman's dishonor.[94] Ouziel counters this by contending that it is, in fact, Ya'avetz's words that are not precise. While it is true that concerns over the dishonor of the woman do not allow for the killing of a fetus once labor has commenced and the fetus has become a "separate body," this was not the case with a woman who was to be executed at an earlier point in her pregnancy. The *Gemara*'s call to kill the fetus on account of the possible – but by no means certain – "dishonor" that may result is further proof to Ouziel that the fetus is not a *nefesh* and that it is permitted to kill it.

If, however, it is permitted to do away with the fetus, then why would it be appropriate to contravene the *mitzvah* of *Shabbat* by carrying a knife through a public thoroughfare, in order to extract a being that is not considered a *nefesh* and that may appropriately be killed? After all, if the fetus is not a *nefesh*, then preservation of the *Shabbat* certainly ought to take precedence, given that fetal destruction is acceptable. Ouziel deals with this problem by alluding to the potential of such a "trapped" fetus to become a *nefesh*. While it is true that there is no requirement to override the *Shabbat* on behalf of the fetus, one does so based on the hope that, if one acts with sufficient speed, one might be able to reach the fetus before it dies, and thereby allow it to live and become a *nefesh*. This is the reason, writes Ouziel, why the *Tosafot* in *Niddah* employs the *goses* analogy. Even though, as the Talmud puts it, "the majority of *gosesin* die,"[95] we still transgress the *Shabbat* to save a *goses*. So, too, with a fetus: we transgress the *Shabbat* in order to give life to the minority of fetuses that can be saved.

Hence, in Ouziel's view, the fact that it is permitted to kill the fetus hardly dictates a cavalier attitude to fetal existence. In fact, Ouziel is not

[93] See above, chapter 3, p. 63.
[94] *Hagahot Ya'avetz* to *Niddah* 44b. The "dishonor" refers to the potential for the fetus to be discharged in a disgracing fashion. See above, chapter 2, p. 39.
[95] *Gittin* 28a.

only concerned to save a fetus if at all possible, but is also emphatic that it is not permitted to kill a fetus in just any circumstance:

> In any case, it is very clear that the killing of fetuses is not permitted unless there is a need, even if it is for a *tzorech kalush* (thin need), such as to prevent the *nivul* (dishonor) of the mother. But without a need it is certainly prohibited because of the destruction [involved] and the prevention of the possibility of life for a *nefesh* in Israel.

Thus, Ouziel recognizes that there is a prohibition on abortion unless there is at least some acceptable need for it. Indeed, in the lines that follow, Ouziel holds that there is actually no contradiction between the *Tosafot* statement in *Niddah* and those in *Sanhedrin* and *Chullin*. There is, he conveys, an extant prohibition on fetal destruction, but where there is a reason for killing the fetus, the prohibition does not apply. Were this not the case, Ouziel suggests, it would be impossible to kill any fetus.

This is precisely why, Ouziel continues, Maimonides required the *rodef* designation. For, in the case of a woman having difficulty in labor, the fetus, while not yet a *nefesh*, has become a "separate body." While it would not be in the category of murder to kill it, it nevertheless would be a transgression of a Torah-based prohibition. How, then, can it be said that, in such a circumstance, the mother's life takes precedence over that of the fetus? Given that the fetus has become an independent being, which the *halakhah* prohibits from being killed without reason, the fact that the fetus is not yet a *nefesh* is insufficient to explain why it should be sacrificed on its mother's behalf. There are, after all, separate Torah-based prohibitions on killing both the mother and the fetus, and the status of inequality between them hardly mitigates these prohibitions. Hence, this would appear to be a case of "who is to say that your blood is redder than his?" were it not for the *rodef* classification. As the fetus is acting "like a *rodef*," we are commanded to save the pursued from the pursuer, even at the cost of the pursuer's life. The woman's life takes precedence, then, because she is being pursued; without this reason, the fetus could not be killed.

Ouziel is even more specific when it comes to explaining why Maimonides held that a fetus – that had become a "separate body" – could be a *rodef* until birth, but not thereafter. In the instance of a woman having difficulties prior to birth, the fetus is a *rodef* because it is struggling against her: "The Rambam thought that the difficulty experienced by any woman in the birth process, before the fetus had emerged, was caused by the fetus, as it was turning over in its mother's womb in order not to come out of her, and was fighting against the strength of the woman's push during the birth process." However, after the fetus crowns, this changes:

With the emergence of its head, the fetus ceases to be a *rodef* as it [now] wants to come out completely in order to aspire to a new life and to escape strangulation, since the Creator of the universe implanted in all created beings an instinctive sense to seek the spirit of life, and to flee from anything which might cause death. And this natural tendency is also found in the fetus; so that when the mother is in difficulty after the fetus crowns, it becomes clear that the fetus is not the cause of her difficulty in birth, but, rather, natural reasons – that are not connected to the fetus – are the causes. And, as there is no *rodef* and no pursued, we do not set aside one *nefesh* for another.

Put differently, Ouziel maintains that if the mother is still in trouble once the fetus emerges, then there must have been other forces that were pursuing her all along, so it is no longer tenable to continue with the prior assumption that the fetus is the *rodef*. This neat explanation accounts well for Maimonides' use of the *rodef* classification, as well as for its cessation. Its problem, of course, is that it requires the acceptance of two premises: first, that a fetus that is within a woman having difficulty in labor must have been the cause of her difficulty, and second, that the fetus then ceases to be the potential cause of her trouble if her difficulties persist following its birth. These premises, although *halakhically* elegant, cannot always be said to accord with medical reality. It is important to recall, however, that Ouziel, like Grodzinsky, understands Maimonides only to be applying the *rodef* designation to circumstances in which the fetus has become a separate body during the birth process. Before this point, Ouziel reiterates, there is no *mitzvah* to save the fetus, and it is permitted to kill it, so long as there is some "compelling reason."

Ouziel proceeds to show that not every reason that might be proposed for an abortion is actually compelling. Ouziel offers the example of levirate marriage: a childless widow who was pregnant at the time of her husband's death does not enter into a levirate marriage, because, if she subsequently produces a viable child, her deceased husband will not be childless.[96] What would happen, however, if the widow were to consummate a levirate marriage and only later discover that she had, in fact, been pregnant from her deceased husband? Ouziel replies that, in

---

[96] Levirate marriage – *yivum* – was a requirement of the Torah that the rabbis later ameliorated. It demanded that the brother of a man who died without children marry the deceased's widow in order to "build up the name" of his dead brother. Clearly, however, if the dead brother had offspring, this would be unnecessary. See Deuteronomy 25:5–6.

such a case, *halakhah* would direct that her levirate marriage should be annulled, and a sin offering should be brought for the unwitting infraction. Ouziel, however, then goes on to pose a further question. Given that the prohibition on fetal destruction is rabbinic in nature, why not simply abort the fetus that was conceived with her deceased husband to avoid having his child, and to eliminate, retroactively, the possibility for transgressing the Toraitic laws of levirate marriage? Ouziel answers his own inquiry by asserting that the widow may not abort the fetus because the fetus is her husband's property, and nobody is permitted to cause him loss. Exodus 21:22–23, after all, already had instructed that the husband is due financial compensation for fetal loss. Hence, the widow certainly may not destroy her husband's property – that property being the fetus who will "continue his name in Israel" – in order to obviate infraction. Hence, even though she has a substantial reason for an abortion, it is not one that could be considered to be sufficient.

As the *teshuvah* draws to a close, Ouziel critiques two of the explanations previously put forward for the prohibition on abortion. Echoing Ya'avetz, Ouziel opines that the prohibition on the wanton destruction of male seed only applies to improper acts of spilling seed and, therefore, cannot form the basis for the abortion ban. Nor, in Ouziel's view, is the prohibition on self-endangerment a sensible foundation for the ban. Were self-endangerment really an issue, writes Ouziel, many medical procedures would become problematic. Jews are, however, commanded to heal, even though danger may be involved. In place of these two rejected explanations, Ouziel suggests an alternative: *periah ureviah* (the commandment to be fruitful and multiply). Quoting rabbinic sources that convey the notion that one who refrains from producing children keeps God's indwelling presence (*Shechinah*) away from Israel,[97] Ouziel posits:

> If such things are said in regard of one who does not engage in *periah ureviah*, who does nothing in practice, how much the more so [would they be said] of one who takes action that would diminish the possibility of life and growth of one *nefesh* in Israel. And there is no doubt that this is what the *Tosafot* intended when they said that Israel was prohibited from killing fetuses . . .

Ouziel, then, advances the theory that the prohibition on intentional abortion – without sufficient reason – stems not so much from technical concerns, but rather from the tradition's desire to maximize reproductive results.

---

[97] *Yevamot* 63b–64a.

Ouziel concludes his *teshuvah* by ruling that a woman threatened by permanent deafness certainly may have an abortion. Ouziel repeats that even for a *tzorekh kalush* an abortion would be permissible, and reiterates his understanding of the *Arakhin Gemara* that in a case in which "dishonor" for the woman is possible, fetal destruction would be acceptable. In this context, there is, states Ouziel, no greater "dishonor" than permanent deafness, for it would affect the woman's whole life, bring her misery, and make her debilitated in the eyes of her husband. An abortion at the hands of expert and skilled doctors would definitely be indicated.

In his subsequent abortion *teshuvah* Ouziel was asked two distinct questions. First, could a woman who, according to the doctors, was experiencing a dangerous pregnancy but was not yet close to the onset of labor have an abortion? Second – the same question, previously answered by Bacharach and Ya'avetz – could a fetus that was conceived in adultery to a repentant single or married woman be aborted?[98] Ouziel takes lenient stance in his replies to both matters. In response to the first question, Ouziel begins by positing that *Mishnah Ohalot*, together with Maimonides' use of the *rodef* idea, might lead one to conclude that an abortion would be permitted only in a case of immediate, pressing danger in the birth process, and not if the danger is more remote. However, after discussing the literature, Ouziel rules in exactly the opposite way. As the Torah does not punish one who kills a fetus, and as the magnitude of the danger is a matter of doubt, "in an instance of danger, it is permitted to bring about the death [of the fetus]." Moreover, because Ouziel holds that *ubar yerekh imo*, it is clearly acceptable, in his view, to sacrifice one's own limb in order to save oneself, even if the nature of the danger is dubious. After all, Ouziel recalls, Ya'avetz permitted the killing of a fetus before labor in order to save a woman from an "evil that could cause her great pain." In the case of danger in pregnancy, therefore, it is "plain" that an abortion can be allowed.

Ouziel also follows in Ya'avetz's footsteps in the matter of the fetus conceived through adultery, albeit preferring a completely different line of reasoning to that of his predecessor. In drawing a connection between adultery and offspring, Ouziel turns his attention to the Talmudic teaching of Shimon ben Lakish:

The whole section [of the blessings and curses] refers to none other than the adulterer and the adulteress. [It states,] "Cursed be the man that makes a graven

---

[98] All references and quotations to this second *teshuvah* by Ouziel are from *Mishpetei Ouziel, Choshen Mishpat*, volume III, number 47.

or molten image . . ." (Deuteronomy 27:15). Does it suffice merely to pronounce, "cursed" with such a person? It refers to one who has immoral intercourse, and begets a son who goes to live among heathens, and worships idols; cursed be the father and mother of this man, as they were the cause of his sinning.[99]

Expanding upon Rashi's explanation of this text, Ouziel elucidates that the terrible parental curses alluded to here are actually the outcome of two separate acts: the improper intercourse itself – even if no birth results – and the arrival of a child who, because of his shame at being a *mamzer* and not finding a wife,[100] will go to dwell among the heathen and worship their gods. Logically, therefore, while the adulterous parties cannot "undo" their intercourse, they can avoid the deep transgression of being considered to be individuals who, effectively, have made "a graven or molten image." They can evade this fate by not allowing the child to be born. There is, of course, no death penalty for a Jew who might kill a fetus. Hence, Ouziel avers, in the case of a *mamzer*, "the killing of whom would circumvent the prohibition of 'cursed is the man who makes a graven or molten image,' it is permitted to kill [the *mamzer*] before its head emerges . . ."

The corollary, however, of this explanation is that – taking into account the *halakhic* principle *ain shaliach lidevar aveirah* (one may not appoint an emissary to carry out a transgression) – Ouziel contends that an abortion may be carried out only by one of the parents. A *shaliach*, after all, cannot perform an action for which he, himself, cannot be obligated. The possibility of avoiding "cursed is the man . . ." therefore, can apply only to those who conceived the *mamzer*: the parents. Nor, states Ouziel, may the parents circumvent this provision by going to a non-Jew to perform the abortion. A non-Jew is subject to the death penalty for killing a fetus, so that a request for assistance from the non-Jew would be a transgression of the biblical injunction that one may not "place a stumbling block before the blind." The desire to avoid "cursed is the man . . ." on the part of the parents would not make such a biblical transgression acceptable. Hence, Ouziel rules that, in the case of a married woman, the couple may take steps to abort a bastard fetus in order to escape the serious infraction of "cursed is the man . . ." In the case of a single woman, however, whose relationship is not technically adulterous, and whose child, consequently, would not be a *mamzer*,[101] Ouziel holds that an abortion could not be countenanced.

---

[99] *Sotah* 37b.   [100] This is Rashi's explanation for the young person's departure.
[101] For the legal response to single women and adultery, see above, chapter 3, p. 79, n. 82.

It is difficult to guess what motivated Ouziel to rule in this fashion. He could have taken the Bacharach approach and simply forbidden the abortion of a fetus destined to be a *mamzer*. Conversely, he could have embraced Ya'avetz's reasoning for permitting such an act. The fact that he did not adopt Ya'avetz's logic suggests that he may well have been uncomfortable with Ya'avetz's controversial determination that the mother's life was effectively forfeit, such that her suicide would not be a cause for serious opposition.[102] If, however, Ya'avetz's position was disturbing, Ouziel's approach requires a considerable stretch of imagination. After all, one would be hard-pressed to find contemporary evidence that the mere reality of *mamzerut* is inevitably the cause of departure from the Jewish community, much less that it leads to idol worship. Hence, to ground permission to kill the fetus in the avoidance of a transgression that is almost certain not to materialize is a rather problematic intellectual proposition. It is possible, of course, that Ouziel himself was aware that his approach, while textually elegant, had weaknesses. If this is so, then the fact that he nevertheless maintained this approach may be an indication of how far he was prepared to reach in order to sustain as lenient a position as possible on this subject. This understanding at least would be consistent with his apparent general response to abortion, which permits an abortion to proceed in almost all the cases before him for which *halakhah* provided an opening.

One more instance of leniency merits particular attention. It is impossible to think of the period during which Ouziel served as Chief Rabbi of Israel without considering the Holocaust of European Jewry that consumed one-third of the Jewish people between 1939 and 1945. It is a truism that the landscape of the Holocaust bore no parallel to any other experience, such that rabbinic rulings from within that world cannot be seen, in any way, as creating precedents for *halakhic* rulings in "normal" times. Nevertheless, it is important to record that, as modernity reached its nadir, we have at least one example of a reasoned *teshuvah* on the subject of abortion even from the depths. Rabbi Ephraim Oshry, one of the few *poskim* who remained alive in the Kovno ghetto in Lithuania,[103] recorded the following question put to him in August 1942, in the wake of

---

[102] See above, chapter 3, p. 80.
[103] I. J. Rosenbaum, *The Holocaust and Halakhah*, New York, Ktav Publishing House Incorporated, 1976, p. 14. Rabbi Oshry was one of the few rabbinic authorities who was able to pen relatively complete *teshuvot* under conditions of such overwhelming adversity. Rosenbaum describes how this came to be: "He committed his responsa to writing on whatever scraps of paper he could find, and buried them in the ground, confident that someday redemption would come. He was in a unique position to determine the requirements of the Halakhah, not only because of his

the SS decree of May 1942, that any Jewish woman found to be pregnant would immediately be put to death: "I was asked [concerning] a woman who became pregnant in the ghetto, whether it is permissible for her to abort, in order to stop the pregnancy, given that the *tmeïim* [Nazis] have decreed that they will kill any Jewish woman who becomes pregnant, [together] with her fetus, and, if so, there is an amount of danger to her life."[104]

In reply, Oshry cites *Mishnah Ohalot*, as well as the *Shulchan Arukh*'s codification of Maimonides' position on the *rodef*. Though Oshry does not state it, the *rodef* argument was inapposite, because the Nazis were the true *rodfim* in this instance, and while the fetus could be considered part of the causative chain, it was most certainly not the instigator of the woman's precarious plight. Instead, Oshry cites the views of Lipschutz, Eger, and Schick on the desirability of saving the mother in an instance where the alternative is that both will die.[105] Given that the fetus can be held to be of "doubtful viability," Oshry concludes that in the case before him it is "of course" appropriate to permit an abortion in order to save this woman's life. While Oshry's answer is most certainly *halakhically* significant, it is a response that plainly is limited to the unique circumstances of the Holocaust, in which the extraordinary extremes of Nazi behavior frequently called for rabbis to give the best possible answer from within the worst possible conditions.

As the twentieth century approached its midpoint, then, the *halakhic* process pertaining to abortion hardly appeared to be a conversation that was leading to any focused outcome. In fact, it hardly appeared to be a conversation at all. Rabbis employing accepted standards of *halakhic* reasoning could be found taking opposite points of view with firm assuredness concerning their correctness and without any noticeable attempts at convergence. Thus, Zalman, Epstein, Al-Chakam, Ouziel, and Grodzinski all could formulate relatively lenient rulings on abortion and the application of the *rodef* principle, while Schick and Soloveitchik could take much more stringent stances. Indeed, an analysis of Jewish attitudes to abortion issues within the first century and a half of modernity leads to two conclusions: first, different *poskim* dealt with these matters

---

scholarship, but also because he was appointed for a time by the Nazis as one of the custodians of the warehouse of Jewish books which they had set up in Kovno. Rabbi Oshry thus had access to at least some of the major works of Rabbinic literature necessary in formulating his *teshuvot*."

[104] All Oshry references and quotations are from E. Oshry, *ShuT MiMaâmakim*, New York, 1959, number 20, pp. 126–127.

[105] See above, pp. 95–99.

in varied and sharply contrasting ways, and, second, those who tended towards more lenient interpretations of the law outnumbered those who took a stricter approach.

The fact that there were more rabbis who trod the path of relative leniency ought not, however, to lead to the inference that the Jewish attitude to abortion was, relatively speaking, more relaxed during this period. For, in actuality, there was no such thing as a "Jewish attitude" that can be said to have coalesced in any coherent manner. The existence of a plurality of rabbis who provided somewhat lenient answers to the infrequent questions asked on the subject only indicates that a more lenient approach continued to have a capacity to garner significant adherents; for these rabbis, the lenient reply seemed to offer a more logical response to the cases under their consideration. Largely, then, the *sheʾelot* on abortion that surfaced in this period could be judged on their merits, without concerns about broader ramifications that might need to be considered. Few in number and essentially disconnected from each other, these inquiries said nothing statistically or philosophically significant about any overall Jewish response to abortion. Indeed, a response of this type had neither been sought nor had it been contemplated.

There was, after all, little call for such an encompassing view. Abortion in the late nineteenth and early twentieth centuries in most emerging nation states was a practice that was restricted legally, that was normally handled behind a veil of secrecy, and that allowed for little discussion.[106] Countries like the United States and Britain, which had – in their pre-modern incarnations – no formal proscriptions on abortions early in pregnancy, enacted restrictive anti-abortion laws in the nineteenth century.[107] In many countries, abortion was prohibited on pain of imprisonment. Still, there were some places where abortion was allowed under certain circumstances.[108] Clearly, therefore, while women regularly might have wanted and obtained unsanctioned abortions, abortion was publicly either forbidden, or was possible in a few locations under very specific conditions.

---

[106] See L. Breitenecker and R. Breitenecker, "Abortion in the German-Speaking Countries of Europe," and R. E. Hall, "Commentary," in D. T. Smith (ed.), *Abortion and the Law*, Cleveland, The Press of Western Reserve University, 1967, pp. 206–234.

[107] C. Tietze, *Induced Abortion: A World Review*, 1981 (4th edition), New York, A Population Council Fact Book, 1981, pp. 8–10.

[108] The Swiss Code, for example, forbade abortion, but granted "impunity" so as "to obviate danger to the life and health of a pregnant woman." See Breitenecker and Breitenecker, "Abortion," pp. 216–217.

For the most part, then, the statements of the rabbis of the nineteenth and early twentieth centuries did not move far beyond the relatively restricted range of issues that were under consideration in the societies in which they lived. Given the increasing criminalization of abortion in the nineteenth century, it is probably not surprising that the number of *teshuvot* written on the subject during this span is relatively small. Jews were hardly likely to seek rabbinic permission for procedures that, from a legal viewpoint, could not be carried out openly. What is perhaps more noteworthy, however, is the fact that the restrictive tendency of the surrounding legal structures was not reflected in any discernible way in the responses of the rabbis. To the contrary, the rabbis appeared to be tilting more towards leniency at the very time that civil mores were heading in the opposite direction. As, however, the rabbinic evidence from this period is sparse, this paradoxical analysis can only be described as speculative, not conclusive. What is certain, though, is that the conditions that might call forth the crystallization of a more defined, broad, or generalized position on abortion simply were not yet present.

Had this picture continued to be the societal backdrop to the *halakhic* process, the established rabbinic pattern of providing varied, individual answers to discrete, diffuse questions might well have continued indefinitely. But this was not to be the case. Societal developments were about to emerge that would refuse to be ignored. And just as the *halakhic* positions of centuries past had been influenced by external forces, so, in the middle of the twentieth century, outside events would permeate the *halakhic* world-view and would stimulate internal reactions. It would not be long before these influences would result in depictions of abortion within Judaism in far starker tones than had been evident previously. In the process, a true *halakhic* conversation, lacking until now, would soon be underway.

CHAPTER 5

The struggle returns: Jewish views begin to take form

The advent of the second half of the twentieth century brought with it a sweeping revolution in societal attitudes to abortion. In nation after nation the call for abortion-law reform became irresistible. Profound and widespread legal liberalization began to shape the landscape in a way that would make this period entirely discontinuous from that of the nascent nation states of the nineteenth century. Liberalization, it must be stressed, did not always imply that abortion was available without restrictions, but, in every place in which the liberalization process arose, it wrought dramatic changes, allowing for abortion under a broad range of circumstances that previously had been the subject of prohibition. Thus, in the quarter century from the mid 1950s to the early 1980s, an unprecedented avalanche of abortion-law reform – never contemplated in the first half of the century – touched the lives of approximately 60 percent of the world's population.[1]

A number of contributing forces propelled these tectonic shifts. The horror of the loss of women's lives through improper care that too often accompanied illegal abortion was undoubtedly an important

[1] The first country to legalize abortion was Soviet Russia in 1920, but, due to low birth rates, this legalization was reversed until it was legalized again in 1955. The first lasting and "definitive steps towards the liberalization of abortion laws" came in Scandinavia: Iceland in 1935, Sweden in 1937, and Denmark in 1938. Japan liberalized its laws in 1948, the socialist countries of Eastern Europe (with the exceptions of Albania and East Germany) followed the USSR in liberalization in 1956–57, and the People's Republic of China liberalized in 1957. Between 1966 and 1981, Australia, Austria, Canada, Cuba, Finland, France, East Germany, West Germany, India, Italy, the Republic of Korea, Norway, Singapore, Sweden, Tunisia, the United Kingdom, the United States, Vietnam, and Zambia all legislated liberalized statutes. During this same period, Iran, Israel, and New Zealand liberalized their laws, before imposing new restrictions. Meanwhile, "[o]fficial alarm at declining birth rates and soaring abortion rates" prompted Bulgaria, Czechoslovakia, Hungary, and Romania, which had liberalized in the 1950s, once again to adopt more restrictive laws. By the 1980s, abortion remained either illegal or substantially restricted in Belgium, Ireland, Malta, Portugal, Spain, and in most of the Arab, African, Central Asian, and South American countries. See Tietze, *Induced Abortion*, pp. 7–17 and J. Van der Tak, *Abortion, Fertility, and Changing Legislation: An International Review*, Lexington, Lexington Books, 1974, chapters 2–5.

133

factor.[2] The burgeoning of more relaxed attitudes towards sexuality and reproductive functioning was another cause, the impact of which cannot be underestimated. These new attitudes themselves were intertwined inextricably with the arrival of safe and reliable birth-control methods, which, for the first time in human history, allowed for a great deal of control over procreation. Given that unwanted pregnancies could now largely be avoided, there can be little doubt that many women who, in earlier generations, might have been forced into a position where they desired an abortion, were able to avoid this outcome by utilizing contraception. Conversely, the atmosphere of reproductive freedom engendered by effective birth control, may well have encouraged the idea that even when contraception was not used, or was ineffective, a woman's decision to abort ought to be respected.[3] Hence, the availability of contraception and its concomitant facility to manage family planning was, most likely, an important factor in creating an environment in which a relaxing of abortion-law restrictions came to be demanded.

In some places though, an entirely different issue provided the critical spark that lit the reform flame. It was not contraception – which ultimately would affect billions of people directly – but rather, the prospect of fetal deformity – which actually would affect but a tiny proportion of the population – that provided a substantial push towards legal amelioration of abortion limitations as a whole. In the United States, which represented but one example of this phenomenon, the major thrust for abortion reform followed two episodes that occurred in the early 1960s:

1962: Abortion makes national headlines in the case of Sherry Finkbine, an Arizona mother of four who had decided to have an abortion after learning of the possible effects of thalidomide, which she had taken in early pregnancy. The day before her scheduled abortion, Mrs. Finkbine seeks publicity to warn

---

[2] Reagan, *When Abortion Was a Crime*, pp. 209–215. Reagan, citing a study by C. Tietze, "Mortality with Contraception and Induced Abortion," in *Studies in Family Planning*, September, 1969, writes: "At the end of the 1920s, abortion-related deaths accounted for 14 percent of maternal mortality. By the early 1960s, abortion-related deaths accounted for nearly half, or 42.1 percent, of the total maternal mortality in New York City. Furthermore, when skilled practitioners performed this procedure, the mortality rate was lower than that for childbirth. Abortion deaths were almost completely preventable."

[3] Van der Tak, *Abortion, Fertility, and Changing Legislation*, pp. 2–4. Van der Tak writes: "*[W]hen societies and individuals are motivated to begin the effort to control their fertility abortion and contraception can rise simultaneously*. If contraception fails or the demand exceeds supply, women thus motivated will resort to abortion to terminate unwanted or untimely pregnancies that they now find unacceptable . . . Thus, abortion and contraception are complementary rather than competitive means to control fertility."

other pregnant women of the dangers of thalidomide; as a result the abortion is cancelled by the hospital, which refuses to perform it (despite a judge's recommendation) out of fears of legal prosecution. Mrs. Finkbine eventually obtains an abortion in Sweden; the embryo is severely deformed.

1962–1965: An outbreak of German measles (rubella) leads to births of 15,000 congenitally abnormal babies; in some states, physicians who perform abortions on pregnant women who have the disease risk losing their licenses. The rubella outbreak adds impetus to the medical profession's growing shift toward favoring liberalized abortion laws.[4]

These incidents provided the primary stimulus for Colorado to become the first state in the nation to reform its abortion law in 1967.[5] By the time of the 1973 US Supreme Court ruling in *Roe* v. *Wade*,[6] fourteen US states had already amended their statutes to allow for abortions in cases where the pregnancy resulted from rape or incest, the fetus may be born malformed physically or deficient mentally, or the mother's life or health are threatened.[7] Elsewhere in the world, concerns for the fetus also led to deep public consternation.[8] Societal anguish over fetal abnormality then, was an important catalyst towards the legalization of abortion.

This anguish over fetal abnormality was, furthermore, an important catalyst in the shaping of Jewish attitudes within this unprecedented phase of abortion history. In the *halakhic* heritage, fetal abnormality had never before received any detailed attention. With very few exceptions, permissive *teshuvot* usually had based their conclusions exclusively on considerations of maternal pain, and not on the future potential life of the fetus or any other person.[9] It was the mother's mental or physical anguish that had to be weighed, and which was acknowledged to be the salient factor in determining whether an abortion might be permissible. The impact of a potential handicap or defect in the fetus was not ordinarily a consideration, in the absence of considerable maternal suffering. True,

[4] M. Costa, *Abortion: A Reference Handbook*, Santa Barbara, ABC-CLIO Incorporated, 1991, p. 11. I. Jakobovits, "Review of Recent Halakhic Periodical Literature," *Tradition*, volume 5, number 2, 1963: 267–270, p. 267, n. 1, notes that the German measles problem was a relatively newly discovered challenge: "The incidence of abnormalities following German measles, particularly in epidemic form, was first pointed out in an Australian medical journal in 1941, and the right to resort to abortion in such cases has been discussed in medical literature, with mostly negative conclusions, ever since."
[5] Costa, *Abortion*, p. 13.   [6] See *Roe* v. *Wade*, 410 US 113 (1973).   [7] Costa, *Abortion*, pp. 13–20.
[8] See, for example, the Liège trial, referred to on p. 143, below. Though the trial did not lead directly to legal reform in Belgium, its reverberations were most significant indeed.
[9] The two clear exceptions already cited are the *teshuvah* of Yehuda Ayash (see above, chapter 3, pp. 83–84) and that of Yitzhak Oelbaum (see above, chapter 4, pp. 118ff.).

some scholars, at previous junctures, had dealt with the matter of whether it was acceptable to kill an abnormal "monster" baby upon birth.[10] However, the subject of aborting a fetus to avoid potential disabilities had only been an issue when it threatened to result in severe disability to the mother as well.

The usual approach of the tradition to this type of challenge was expressed elegantly in a 1940 Romanian *teshuvah* in the case of an epileptic mother who was concerned that she might give birth to an epileptic child:

> For fear of possible, remote danger to a future child that maybe, God forbid, he will know sickness – how can it occur to anyone actively to kill the fetus because of such a possible doubt? This seems to me very much like the laws of Lycurgus, King of Sparta, according to which every blemished child was to be put to death...Whatever the author of *Teshuvot Levushei Mordekhai* wrote in order to permit an abortion was only because of fear of mental anguish for the mother. But for fear of what might be the child's lot? – The secrets of God are not knowable.[11]

The rare reference to non-Jewish annals in this *teshuvah* provides an eloquent articulation of the Jewish abhorrence of killing an innocent being, no matter what its impairment. Indeed, the author skillfully creates a connection between abortion and the deeds of the cruel Spartan regime. In fact, of course, the law of Lycurgus dealt with infanticide, not abortion. The *teshuvah* clearly blurs the *halakhic* distinctions between infanticide and abortion, suggesting that the author is keen to promote an abhorrence of this type of abortion. The attempt to make such abortion appear to be of the utmost gravity would soon become even more pronounced. However, the fundamental point made by this *teshuvah* is a traditional one: abortion could only be considered if the mother were *in extremis*, and as, in the instance under discussion, the mother could have no more than vague fears concerning the child's possible disabilities, such a reaction over an uncertain future was unwarranted.

By the mid twentieth century, however, the "secrets of God" were becoming more knowable, and developing medical experience was providing greater certainty about the nature of what lay ahead within a variety of different conditions. With more cases of fetal abnormality becoming the subject of public discussion, the unfolding debate inevitably

---

[10] Jakobovits, "Recent Halakhic Periodical Literature," provides a synopsis of two important sources: the twelfth-century *teshuvah* in *Sefer Chasidim* (ed. Zitomir, 1879, number 186), and the 1807 *teshuvah* of Rabbi Eleazar Fleckles of Prague.

[11] Sperber D., *Afrekasta D'Anya*, Satmar, 1940, number 169.

found its way into rabbinic *teshuvot*. Thus, within a few short years of each other, a number of rabbis in different parts of the world began to respond to this heretofore unexplored issue of the permissibility of abortion when faced with potential birth defects.[12]

Rabbi Issar Yehuda Unterman (1886–1965) was among the first to answer such a question. Born in Brest-Litovsk, Belorussia, Unterman served in Lithuania and England, before holding the *Ashkenazi* offices that Ouziel had occupied for the *Sefaradim*: Unterman served as chief rabbi of Tel Aviv from 1946 and as chief rabbi of Israel from 1964.[13] Unterman's approach to legal matters was once characterized in these terms: "While he insisted on unflinching loyalty to the minutiae of the *halakhah*, he approached public issues with moderation and understanding."[14]

In the late 1950s, Unterman was asked about the permissibility of an abortion for a woman who, after a "number of weeks" of pregnancy, had become ill with German measles, leading to the fear that her baby would be born with substantial physical or mental deficiencies. At the stage that the question was asked, the woman concerned had not yet passed the fortieth day of pregnancy, leading to the request for an urgent response if the fortieth day were deemed to be a significant turning point in such an instance.[15] In the formal *teshuvah* – written after the event – Unterman wastes no time in giving a negative answer to the question. He begins by reviewing the discussion of the *Halakhot Gedolot* and *Nachmanides* as to whether one overrides the *Shabbat* in order to save a fetus whose mother

[12] The responsa that are discussed in this chapter come from Orthodox, Conservative, and Reform rabbis. In the nineteenth century, as Jews came to perceive their place in the modern world in different ways, various ideological responses emerged that eventually gave rise to the contemporary Reform, Conservative, and Orthodox movements (see Seltzer, *Jewish People, Jewish Thought*, chapter 13). The responsa penned by Conservative, Orthodox, and Reform rabbis differ little in style from the responsa of previous centuries. The one salient difference between Reform responsa and those of Orthodox and Conservative Judaism is a functional rather than a stylistic matter: while the rulings provided by Orthodox and Conservative rabbis are – at least in theory – binding upon the questioner, Reform responsa are not.

There is considerable debate among the partisans of the different movements as to the *halakhic* authenticity of responsa from the various streams of Judaism. This work does not take a position on that dispute. The decision to include responsa, and other writings on Jewish legal matters, from all Jewish sources is not intended as a validation of their authenticity or of their authoritative standing within *halakhah*. Rather, it is an attempt to include the full spectrum of Jewish writings insofar as they seek to fashion Jewish responses to abortion that are based in *halakhah*.

From the beginning of modernity, the responsa cited herein can be considered to be the work of Orthodox rabbis unless otherwise indicated.

[13] J. Goldman, "Unterman, Isser Yehuda," in *Encyclopaedia Judaica*, Jerusalem, Keter Publishing House, volume XV, pp. 1688–1689.

[14] *Ibid.*

[15] Unless otherwise indicated, all Unterman references and quotations are from I. Y. Unterman, "B'Inyan Pikuach Nefesh Shel Ubar," *Noam*, volume 6, 1963: 1–11.

has died.[16] The fact that one does, opines Unterman, demonstrates that the laws of *pikuach nefesh* are operative for the fetus, a view with which Maimonides would have agreed.[17] Consequently, already in his second paragraph, Unterman declares killing a fetus like the one in question to be forbidden by the Torah. However, in explaining his stance, Unterman goes further than had any of his predecessors in the direction of negatively depicting abortion: "In any case, we see from this that without the *rodef* reason, it would be forbidden to kill the fetus, even if this would lead to the saving of a dangerously ill woman, for [the reality of her condition] does not make [an abortion] any less an appurtenance of murder, and this [concern] is not rejected in the name of saving a life." Whereas Schick had held that a fetus that threatens its mother's life is guilty of "an appurtenance of the spilling of blood,"[18] Unterman now declares abortion itself to be an "appurtenance of murder," where the mother's life is not directly threatened. Notwithstanding the fact that, in the case of a fetus, killing it would not make one liable for capital punishment, in Unterman's view a "grave prohibition" could be said to exist because of the "appurtenance of murder" that would be involved in such an act.[19]

Indeed, Unterman finds support for his view in the language of the *Tosafot*. Concurring with Ya'avetz that the words of the *Tosafot* in *Niddah* which say that "it is permitted to kill [the fetus]" can be dismissed as being linguistically imprecise, Unterman holds that the *Tosafists'* comparison to the *goses* is, however, most apposite.[20] Quoting the *mishnah* that states "[O]ne who closes the eyes when the soul is departing, is as one who sheds blood,"[21] Unterman maintains that this is why killing a fetus is likened to killing a *goses*. In the case of a fetus, too, one who kills it engages in an element of spilling blood. Does this, then, imply that if asked to kill a fetus one should prefer to die rather than engage in such an "appurtenance of murder," as was mooted in the case of the doctor instructed to perform an abortion at gunpoint?[22] No, avers Unterman: unless there is a specific Toraitic negation of an action deemed to be an "appurtenance," one is

---

[16] In this situation, of course, the intervention is undertaken purely for the sake of the fetus. See above, chapter 2, pp. 47–48.

[17] This position is made most explicit in I. Y. Unterman, *Shevet MiYehudah*, Jerusalem, 1983, p. 25. Unterman does not claim that the implication of the laws of *pikuach nefesh* applying to the fetus is that the fetus is to be regarded as a *nefesh*.

[18] See above, chapter 4, p. 98.

[19] The actual laws of murder – with possible capital penalty – do not apply, of course, to the fetus since it is not a *nefesh*. This, however, would not prevent its killing from being an "appurtenance of murder."

[20] See above, chapter 3, pp. 62–63.   [21] *M. Shabbat* 23:5.

[22] See above, chapter 4, p. 119.

not required to give up one's life to avoid it, despite the seriousness of the act that one is being required to commit. As Unterman could not locate a direct Toraitic negation of feticide, one ought not, from his perspective, to give up one's life if one is required to carry out an abortion on pain of death. Thus, Unterman's description of feticide as an "appurtenance of murder" ought not to mask the reality that there still remained a distinct difference between homicide and feticide: one is required to die rather than commit homicide, but not when it came to feticide.[23]

To perceive abortion as an "appurtenance of murder," Unterman needed to maintain a fairly restrictive understanding of Maimonides' *rodef* principle. For the only instances in which Unterman might countenance abortion would be those in which no "appurtenance of murder" could be involved. Clarifying this position in a separate *halakhic* article, Unterman explains that the law concerning the *rodef* has two unusual features. First, as an outgrowth of the *"lo tachos einekhah"* (have no pity)[24] text, there is no duty to save the life of a *rodef*. Second, the killing of a *rodef* is permitted and does not involve the slightest sense that it is murder.[25] According to Unterman, however, the two laws are independent of one another. Thus, in the case of a *rodef* whose pursuit is unintentional – the result of *tivo shel olam* (the way of the world)[26] – the second law does not apply but the first one does. Hence, when a fetus is behaving like a *rodef*, the law states that it is not "permitted" to kill it – because there is no intentional pursuit – but neither is there a duty to save it. There is, though, a duty to save the mother, and, given that there is no corresponding duty to save the pursuing fetus, if the only way of saving the mother is by sacrificing the fetus, then this duty must be fulfilled for one should "have no pity."

---

[23] This distinction between homicide and feticide was evident in an altogether different context within a 1934 *teshuvah* written by Yosef Rozin (1858–1936) of Rogatchev – Y. Rozin, *Tzofnat Pa'aneach*, Warsaw, 1935, number 59. Rozin was asked whether an abortion on the part of a wife could constitute grounds for a husband to divorce her. In Jewish law, of course, had the wife committed murder, it might establish grounds for divorce (on the basis of "transgressions of the Laws of Moses," see *Ketubot* 72a). Rozin rules that while the wife should be informed that this is a serious transgression "within the bounds of the spilling of blood," the husband nevertheless does not have grounds for divorce. Plainly, here too, the distinction between homicide and feticide holds in the area of divorce: while Rozin is of the view that feticide is a matter of great gravity, it is not homicide, and it represents insufficient foundation for a divorce.

In many ways, Rozin paved the way for the rhetoric that Unterman later would enshrine as *halakhic* principle. Rozin's position that this woman's individual abortion is "within the bounds of the spilling of blood," can be seen as a precursor of Unterman's later stance that non-therapeutic abortion in general should be regarded as an appurtenance of murder.

[24] See above, chapter 3, p. 59, n. 3.   [25] Unterman, *Shevet MiYehudah*, p. 25.
[26] See above, chapter 4, p. 102.

Unterman further explains this approach by referring to the *Yerushalmi*'s stance that when it comes to the struggle between mother and fetus, we do not know who is killing whom.[27] Unterman is undeterred by the fact that the *Yerushalmi* never declares the fetus to be a *rodef* and is normally perceived to be discussing an issue of *pikuach nefesh* with respect to the birth process itself. "Just as the fetus is regarded as a *rodef* because it is pressing to get out, and [thereby] endangers the mother," writes Unterman, "so we also ought to say the opposite: the mother, whose closure is preventing the one about to be born from emerging, is a type of *rodef* to it [the fetus]."[28] Both the mother and the fetus, therefore, are *rodfim* to each other. Such a situation, Unterman contends, is analogous to the instance of the sinking boat, where there are multiple humans and non-humans that are *ke-rodfim*.[29] Just as in the case of the sinking boat where we get rid of the luggage first because it is "not a *nefesh*," so here, too, we get rid of the fetus first because its existence is not as "complete" as its mother's until it emerges.

As Unterman stated from the outset, it follows from all this that Maimonides ought to be understood as conveying that the *rodef* argument is a *sine qua non* for abortion to proceed: if the fetus is not behaving as a *rodef*, there exists no mandate whatsoever to kill it. Unterman, consequently, is prepared to declare that Rashi and Maimonides disagree on this matter, and cannot be reconciled neatly: Rashi, and others among the *Rishonim*, are indeed open to the possibility that the fetus might be killed in order to heal the mother. However, in the *Mishneh Torah*, Maimonides draws a clear distinction between killing for purposes of healing another, and killing when no other alternative exists.[30] The latter, Maimonides rules, is not punished, but the former is. In their rulings on feticide, Unterman posits, Rashi and those who share his outlook fail to make this distinction, whereas Maimonides does so. Hence, implies Unterman, Maimonides appropriately discerns that it is only when one is "forced" into performing an abortion that it is acceptable to proceed, that is, when the fetus is behaving as a *rodef*.[31] It comes as no surprise, then, that Unterman rejects Yaʿavetz's permission to abort a fetus conceived in adultery,[32]

[27] See above, chapter 2, pp. 50–51.   [28] Unterman, *Shevet MiYehudah*, p. 28.
[29] See above, chapter 4, p. 104.
[30] The phrase "no other alternative exists," implies that it is the only way to save somebody who will otherwise die. See *Hilkhot Yesodei HaTorah* 5.
[31] Unterman, *Shevet MiYehudah*, p. 27. Unterman, "*B'Inyan Pikuach Nefesh Shel Ubar*," 6.
[32] Unterman, "*B'Inyan Pikuach Nefesh Shel Ubar*," 3. Beyond Unterman's objection that such a fetus is not a *rodef*, he has other concerns with Yaʿavetz's reasoning. These reservations are based in Unterman's understanding of *Mishnah Arakhin* that when an accused woman is known to be

and Grodzinsky's tentative acceptance of abortion for fetuses less than forty days old.[33]

It should be observed, however, that in the matter of fetuses less than forty days old, Unterman's concerns go well beyond the *rodef* issue, and provide for an unusual differentiation between Jews and non-Jews.[34] Unterman refers to the rather strange report that had been brought by Maharit, in one of his *teshuvot*, about Rashba's account that Nachmanides had once rendered medical assistance to a gentile woman, first in order to help her conceive, and then to have an abortion.[35] While Unterman states that he searched in Rashba's *teshuvot* for this reference but could not find it,[36] he nevertheless proceeds on the basis that the *teshuvah* is authentic. Three aspects of this report surprise Unterman. First, if true, it suggests that Nachmanides transgressed the biblical law of "do not place a stumbling block before the blind."[37] Second, Maharit's comments, appear to ignore the gentile woman's culpability for the killing of her fetus. Third, Rashba seems to be trying to convey something by recording this event, but it is unclear what it is.

Unterman resolves these difficulties as follows: a fetus under forty days old is described in the *Gemara* as being "mere fluid."[38] The *Gemara*'s description notwithstanding, however, according to Nachmanides' own interpretation of the *Halakhot Gedolot*, the laws of *pikuach nefesh* dictate that one should override the *Shabbat* even for a fetus that has existed for less than forty days.[39] The reason for overriding the *Shabbat* at such an early stage is that even a fetus less than forty days old is, in the future, destined to become a *nefesh*, and, therefore, action should be taken on its behalf with an eye towards that future. Hence, despite the fact that, at this early juncture, the fetus is described as "mere fluid," it is "even now thought of as a living being that it is forbidden to injure."[40] However, avers Unterman, this outlook – based as it is in Torah law – applies to Jews but does not apply to non-Jews. Consequently, there is no requirement upon non-Jews to save such nascent life for the sake of future

---

pregnant, her trial is postponed until after she has given birth (see above, chapter 2, p. 38, n. 42). Consequently, as Bleich, "Abortion in Halakhic Literature," p. 365, explains, Unterman maintains a position that is contrary to that of Ya'avetz: "The status of an adulterous woman in our times is always that of a woman prior to trial. Accordingly, there is no justification for the destruction of a fetus illicitly conceived."

[33] Unterman, *Shevet MiYehudah*, p. 27.   [34] Unterman, *"B'Inyan Pikuach Nefesh Shel Ubar,"* 7ff.
[35] See above, chapter 3, p. 70.   [36] Unterman, *"B'Inyan Pikuach Nefesh Shel Ubar,"* 8.
[37] For other references to "do not place a stumbling-block before the blind," see above, chapter 3, p. 72.
[38] See above, chapter 2, pp. 33–34.   [39] See above, chapter 2, p. 48.
[40] Unterman, *"B'Inyan Pikuach Nefesh Shel Ubar,"* 8.

potential, as there is for Jews. Non-Jews are only required to act upon
the conditions they encounter in the present. It is true, of course, that
according to the rabbinic understanding of "whoever sheds the blood
of man in man," a non-Jew is liable to receive capital punishment for
killing a fetus. However, asserts Unterman, the law against shedding the
blood of "man in man" only applies when a fetus actually has form and
limbs and blood, and can be considered a "man in man" that has blood
to shed. If, before forty days, the fetus is "mere fluid," then it cannot
have these requisite characteristics, and as a non-Jew is not required
to take future potential into account, a non-Jew could kill such a fetus
even though a Jew could not. In Unterman's view, then, Rashba is most
certainly referring to a fetus that is less than forty days old, and it is this
differentiated approach of the Jew vis-à-vis the non-Jew that Rashba was
trying to convey. Moreover, if the fetus is less than forty days old, and if
Unterman's analysis is correct, then clearly both Nachmanides and the
gentile woman were conducting themselves properly. Nachmanides was
not guilty of "placing a stumbling block," because under forty days there
is no transgression over which a non-Jew could stumble, and the gentile
woman bore no culpability whatsoever.

Unterman, furthermore, brings an even more compelling argument
why concerns over future potential should make stages of fetal development irrelevant for Jews. In his commentary to *Sanhedrin* 85b, Rashi
explains that one who steals a fetus with the intention of selling it is guilty
of having stolen a *nefesh*.[41] Clearly, maintains, Unterman, the fetus is not
considered a *nefesh* at the time that it is stolen, but the law nevertheless
takes account of its future status. As the fetus in the vast majority of cases
is destined to become a *nefesh*, the thief is obligated for the theft of a *nefesh*
even before birth.[42] It is obvious that if future considerations are considered primary, it makes no difference whether the fetus has attained forty
days. It is small wonder, then, that Unterman declares that "already from
the beginning, a fetus in its mother's womb is regarded as '*kadam*' – like
a person – and it is forbidden to interfere with its life since it is destined
to be [an *adam*] and we regard him [the fetus] as if he had independent
existence."[43]

---

[41] Unterman explains that kidnappers captured pregnant women in order to obtain children at
birth that would not know they were stolen. The woman would be released after she gave birth.
At the time of the woman's capture, then, the thieves had every intention of "possessing" the
fetus, but not the woman. For a fuller exposition, see Unterman, *Shevet MiYehudah*, p. 10.

[42] Unterman, "*B'Inyan Pikuach Nefesh Shel Ubar*," 4ff., and Unterman, *Shevet MiYehudah*, pp. 9ff.

[43] Unterman, "*B'Inyan Pikuach Nefesh Shel Ubar*," 4.

This perspective on fetal standing is, moreover, wholly consistent with declaring the killing of a fetus that is not a *rodef* to be "an appurtenance of murder." Unterman concludes, therefore, as he began, by declaring that there is a "grave prohibition" of abortion under the circumstances described in the question before him. This would be true even if there were some certainty about the projected deformities, but because, in this instance, fears exist without firmness, it is impossible to override the prohibition on this "type of murder" in order to ease the burden of care on the prospective parents.[44]

It would be inaccurate, of course, to describe Unterman's position as, in any way, discontinuous with those scholars of the past who understood Maimonides in a fairly literal fashion. But use of language – especially in such a delicate and finely balanced area – can be highly significant. It is, therefore, important to observe that Unterman was the first prominent *posek* explicitly to reject abortion in terms that placed it within the category of murderous acts. This is a particularly important linguistic shift. It is one thing, after all, to speak of a serious prohibition on abortion, the contravening of which involves transgression. It is, however, quite another degree of magnitude – one that might arguably be deserving of a far more vigorous response – to connect abortion, however loosely, to murder. It is likely, of course, that, more than just increasing the stakes linguistically, Unterman's rhetoric was aimed at defining a very narrow range of acceptable abortion procedures. It is beyond speculation, however, that this shift in terminology, which Unterman's writings exemplify so clearly, would change the nature of the *halakhic* response to abortion in the second half of the twentieth century.[45]

A contemporary of Unterman, Rabbi Moshe Yonah Zweig of Antwerp (died 1965), took an approach that, while similar, was less stringent than that of the chief rabbi. Zweig, like Unterman, was asked to respond to issues surrounding the continued gestation of a fetus that was presumed to be abnormal. A widely followed trial in the Belgian city of Liège had acquitted a mother who had killed her baby because of substantial deformities brought on by thalidomide. The specific question put to Zweig was whether, according to *halakhah*, a woman who has taken thalidomide can abort a fetus that, in the doctors' estimation, will be born without some of its limbs.

---

[44] *Ibid.*, 9.

[45] This, it might well be contended, is the very substance of the responsa process: rhetorical moves, produced through persuasive argumentation, eventually evoke new categories of legal thought.

Zweig provides an extensive review of the issues salient to the case. Early in his response he reveals the approach he intends to take through an "untraditional" reading of Rashi's position in *Sanhedrin* 72b. From Zweig's perspective, the fact that Rashi declares the fetus not to be a *nefesh* is not an indication of lesser fetal standing of a type that could raise the issue of the potential circumstances – short of a threat to the mother's life – that could justify sacrificing the fetus. Rather, Zweig reads Rashi's statement that "it is not a *nefesh* and it is permitted to kill it and to save its mother" as signifying that "even though it is not called a *nefesh*, it is, in any case, forbidden to dismember it – unless to save its mother."[46] Put differently, Zweig reads Rashi as saying that despite the fact that the fetus lacks *nefesh* standing, the law effectively protects it from being killed in all situations except the one that would require its death in order to save its mother's life. In fact, avers Zweig, it was probably for this reason that Rashi chose the case of a woman in difficulty during labor to discuss the parameters of fetal destruction; Rashi intended that his words should apply only to a woman who is in such a threatened circumstance. In actuality, of course, since Rashi was simply dealing with the Talmudic material before him, this understanding might be more a reflection of Zweig's ingenuity.

Given Zweig's reading of Rashi, it is easy to see how the positions of Rashi and Maimonides could be harmonized from his vantage point. Zweig understands both to be saying that the fetus can be killed only if there is a real and present danger to the mother's life. This apparent correspondence between the two outlooks raises the question of why Maimonides needed to utilize the *rodef* argument at all, if the law effectively could be defined in the same way without it. Zweig has a ready response for this challenge: We know, writes Zweig, that "in the killing of a fetus in its mother's womb, there is no sense of murder attached, as it is not called a *nefesh*, and there is permission to kill it…"[47] We do not need the *rodef* argument in order to gain authorization to kill the fetus when the mother's life is in danger. However, a significant feature of the *rodef* classification that emerges from the Torah is that one who has the opportunity to save an individual who is being pursued, and fails to save that individual, actually transgresses one positive and two negative *mitzvot*.[48] Hence, when the *rodef* argument is invoked, it is not

---

[46] M. Y. Zweig, "*Al Hapalah Melakhutit*," *Noam*, volume 7, 1964: 38.

[47] *Ibid.*, 52. It should be noted that Zweig, unlike Unterman, continues the historic trend of explicitly rejecting any connection between the killing of the fetus and "murder."

[48] The two negative *mitzvot* associated with the *rodef* (as seen above chapter 3, p. 59, n. 3) are "*lo tachos einekhah*," "you shall show no pity" (Deuteronomy 25:12), and "*lo ta'amod al dam rei'ekhah*,"

just that one is allowed to take all appropriate means to save the person being pursued, but, in fact, one is *required* to save him or her. Therefore, contends Zweig, Maimonides needed to provide the *rodef* argument not in order to permit one to save the mother by killing the fetus – for such permission was already a given. Rather the *rodef* argument is necessary to compel one to do so,

> For example, [in the case of] a woman who refuses to kill her fetus at the time when she is having difficulty in the birth process and is hovering in danger – out of the love of a mother for her offspring – or in a case where her husband will not agree under any circumstances to the dismemberment of the fetus even though she [the mother] is in danger.[49]

In such instances, the *rodef* argument is necessary in order to inform us that killing the fetus to save the mother is not an optional possibility, but rather a Torah-based demand.

In Zweig's view, then, the prohibition of the *Tosafot* is firmly in place, unless the mother's life is under threat. Zweig, moreover, advances two rationales for explaining the *Tosafot* prohibition. Which rationale is the more appropriate depends upon whether the fetus is regarded as *yerekh imo* or *lav yerekh imo*. While Zweig seems to hold that the fetus ought to be seen as *yerekh imo*, his outlook on the question makes little difference, as he sees the prohibition as being unbending no matter which position might be favored. Thus, if the fetus is held to be *yerekh imo*, Zweig concurs with Maharit that the most cogent reason behind the prohibition is the concern over *chabbalah*.[50] If, conversely, the fetus is held to be *lav yerekh imo*, then the *chabbalah* explanation becomes inapposite because the fetus is no longer part of its mother. Consequently, from the *lav yerekh imo* vantage point, Zweig appeals to the explanation previously offered by Nachmanides, that one is forbidden to kill a fetus "without any need" because of the future potential for life and observance that the fetus portends.[51]

Zweig is adamant, then, that without a quantifiable threat to the mother, abortion would constitute a serious transgression. He underscores this point by making a philosophical retort to a *halakhic* position on maternal suffering that is raised within the *Mishneh Torah*.

"you shall not stand idle while your neighbor bleeds" (Leviticus 19:25). The positive *mitzvah* is based on the first part of the Deuteronomy 25:12 verse, "*ve-katzotah et kappah*," "you shall cut off her hand," and, in the current context, signifies that one is required to take even the most radical measures to save the pursued. See Zweig, "*Al Hapalah Malachutit*," 51–52.

[49] Zweig, *ibid.*, 52.

[50] *Ibid.*, 41 ff. It is worth observing that on p. 45 Zweig acknowledges that the *chabbalah* explanation may not prevent a woman from self-aborting. See above, chapter 3, p. 71.

[51] *Ibid.*, 45.

When considering the responsibilities of a husband to provide for a wife who is experiencing food cravings during pregnancy, Maimonides ruled:

> If a certain amount were set aside for her support, but she has a desire to eat more, or to eat "other foods" because of the sickness that comes from the craving that she has in her stomach, she may eat from that which is apportioned to her whatever she wants. Her husband may not stop her, saying if she eats too much or eats wrong food she might miscarry; for *tzaʾar gufah kadim* – her physical pain is to be considered first.[52]

According to Zweig, the principle of *tzaʾar gufah kadim* implies that her bodily pain takes precedence over the life of the fetus. This notion, avers Zweig, is consistent with the instruction in *Arakhin* that conveys that the fetus ought to be killed before the execution of a condemned woman in order to prevent her disgrace.[53] However, Zweig is quick to add, the ruling that a pregnant woman's bodily pain should be considered ahead of the life of the fetus is only true when her life is in imminent danger or when it is possible that she may well be in such danger.[54] From Zweig's perspective, when a threat of this type is not present, *tzaʾar gufah kadim* most certainly would not apply.

Why, though, would it not apply in such circumstances? After all, the *Mishneh Torah* certainly utilizes *tzaʾar gufah kadim* in a context in which the threat to life is minimal. Zweig illustrates the problem that is caused by allowing a principle like *tzaʾar gufah kadim* to be invoked in cases in which the mother's life is not at stake: the views of Yaʾavetz notwithstanding,[55] were the appropriateness of an abortion primarily to be measured according to the quantification of "great pain" experienced by the mother, then the abortion decision would become an entirely subjective evaluation on the part of the woman concerned. For who, besides her, can say "if the fetus is causing her great pain or little pain"?[56] Moreover, Zweig recalls, the *Tosafot* maintain that there is no pain or affliction greater than shame,[57] a fact that – if the woman's pain were to be considered the pivotal criterion – would allow for abortion on the word of the woman that the presence of the fetus is bringing her humiliation. In Zweig's view, such an approach would raise so many "obstacles," that it is plain that the woman's physical suffering should only be taken into account, when determining whether or not to kill the fetus, if her life is also at stake.

[52] *Hilkhot Ishut* 21:11.   [53] See above, chapter 2, p. 39.
[54] Zweig, "*Al Hapalah Malachutit*," 47–48.
[55] Zweig points to the fact that Yaʾavetz conceded that his views "require further investigation"; *ibid.*, 53.
[56] *Ibid.*, 54.   [57] *Tosafot* to *Shabbat* 50b, s.v., "*bishvil*."

In his analysis, Zweig makes explicit reference to the first forty days of pregnancy as a distinct period. He maintains that an abortion during this initial time would be prohibited were it "for no reason," but would be acceptable, if, in the opinion of expert Jewish physicians, there were an "urgent need" for such a procedure.[58] Zweig does not specify exactly what would constitute an "urgent need." He indicates, though, that allowing abortion before forty days in cases of "need" is the best reading of the *Acharonim*.[59] After forty days, however, abortion would be prohibited with the exception of the "need of healing the mother." Presumably, therefore, if there is to be a logical differentiation between the ruling that applies prior to forty days and that which is in force thereafter, the "urgent medical need" that would permit abortion before day forty cannot be, in Zweig's thinking, necessarily congruent with the "need of healing the mother." Hence, before forty days, a more lenient standard must be in effect.

Not surprisingly, then, Zweig's response to the question before him is to reject any suggestion that an abortion would be acceptable in the case of a potentially malformed fetus. Even if there were absolute certainty of the deformities, Zweig writes, this has nothing to do with any urgent "need of the mother," or her "healing," and so an abortion could not be acceptable. Zweig forcefully repels the idea that such an abortion could even be considered a merciful act: "Any attempt on the part of the mother to abort the fetus would be exclusively on account of self-love and egotism, wrapped, as it were, in the cloak of compassion for this unfortunate being, and this is not designated the 'need of the mother' at all."[60] Without a life-threatening maternal crisis, therefore, fetal abnormality in and of itself would never render an abortion permissible. Zweig concludes that abortion can be countenanced only on the advice of two expert Jewish physicians, who both contend that the abortion is an urgent matter out of fear for the "health of the body" of the mother.[61]

---

[58] Zweig, "*Al Hapalah Malachutit*," 48.

[59] Zweig cites Bacharach (see above, chapter 3, pp. 73ff.), Drimer (see above, chapter 4, p. 101), and Rozin (see above, p. 139, n. 23), as being of the view that there is no prohibition operative at less than forty days. Bleich ("Abortion in Halakhic Literature," p. 340, n. 31) is surely correct in his critique of Zweig for misunderstanding Bacharach in this regard. Zweig's assertion ("*Al Hapalah Malachutit*," 53) that Bacharach sees no prohibition on abortion during the first forty days is patently at odds with the reality of Bacharach's position.

[60] Zweig, "*Al Hapalah Malachutit*," 55.

[61] Zweig's use of the term "health of the body" is probably a carefully deliberated choice. While it is possible that he has the idea of *tza'ar gufah kadim* in mind, his usage here is more likely an attempt to emphasize that an abortion because of a threat to the mother's physical well-being would be acceptable, unlike one justified by an emotional condition.

Perhaps a little more surprising, though, is Zweig's final argument, which he advances after having already given his answer. Clearly mindful of the circumstances of the Liège case, Zweig points out that it is not just eminent doctors and jurists who hold objections to abortion in this type of situation, but that leaders of the Church also have voiced their opposition. There is, then, in Zweig's view, a further reason to prohibit abortion for reasons of fetal abnormality: it would be a *chillul HaShem* (desecration of God's name) were Jews to permit abortion in such an instance.[62] The Jewish stance on abortions like these, contends Zweig, is not a private matter, but one that involves taking a public position. Consequently, it would be a blatant and public *chillul HaShem* if, as the result of a permissive ruling, Jews effectively made others appear to be more elevated – more an *am kadosh* (holy people) – than Jews themselves.

While Zweig offers *halakhic* support for this position, his reasoning seems more apt to weaken his case than to strengthen it. Tacked on, almost as an afterthought, this strategy suggests that if his previous arguments were not sufficiently persuasive, Jews should at least be concerned that permitting such abortions would make Jews and God "look bad." Zweig ignores the reality that many, both within the Church and without, would abhor those abortions to which he would accede for the sake of acute maternal need. For those inclined to view matters in this light, a greater "holiness" most certainly would attach to groups prepared to avoid those abortions that Zweig would regard as legitimate. Hence, even if Jewish legal considerations ought to be influenced by "how things look" to non-Jews – and this is a problematic proposition – Zweig's own stance would probably be regarded by numerous non-Jews as lacking in holiness. Consequently, the *chillul HaShem* that Zweig denotes seems more reflective of a subjective evaluation of the type of abortion under discussion than any compelling piece of *halakhic* reasoning.[63] Compelling *halakhic* reasoning or not, there can be no doubt that this argument occupies a place of some importance in Zweig's rejection of abortion for reasons of fetal impairment.[64]

Writing in the early 1960s, the minister of the Fifth Avenue Synagogue in New York City, who was soon to become the chief rabbi of the

---

[62] Zweig, "*Al Hapalah Malachutit*," 56.
[63] *Chillul HaShem*, it should be noted, does have *halakhic* implications. Nevertheless, since there is no specific circumstance that can be said to demand its application, invoking it is a subjective decision.
[64] For further consideration of the reasons that Zweig might have found this strategy persuasive, see below, chapter 7, pp. 243–245.

British Commonwealth, Rabbi Immanuel Jakobovits (1921–99), successfully encapsulated the thrust of the position of Rabbis Unterman and Zweig on the matter of deformed fetuses. After reviewing the strict *halakhic* prohibitions on killing babies born with abnormalities, Jakobovits continues:

While these cases deal only with malformed persons already born, they clearly establish the principle that physical or mental defects in no way compromise the claim to life, and once there is no distinction between normal and abnormal persons in the laws of murder applicable after birth, it follows that no such legal distinction can be made in respect to *foeticide* before birth either. Moreover, in regard to the destruction of an unborn child suspected *possibly* to be deformed, there is always the chance that a potentially healthy child may in fact be destroyed. And in matters of life and death the usual majority rule does not apply; any chance, however slim, that a life may be saved must always be given the benefit of the doubt. Hence, even if the abortion of a *definitely* deformed foetus could hypothetically be sanctioned, the possibility that a normal child might be destroyed would militate against such a sanction.[65]

Cautioning that a competent rabbinic authority is the only one who can make definitive rulings in actual cases, Jakobovits offers the following general statements on the appropriate *halakhic* attitude to abnormal fetuses:

1. A physically or mentally abnormal child, whether before or after birth, has the same claim to life as a normal child.
2. Whilst only the killing of a born (and viable) child constitutes murder in Jewish law, the destruction of the foetus too is a crime and cannot be justified except out of consideration for the mother's life.
3. Consequently, the fear that a child may (or will) be born deformed is not in itself a legitimate indication for its abortion, particularly since there is usually a chance that the child might turn out to be quite normal.
4. Such an abortion may only be contemplated if, on reliable medical evidence, it is genuinely feared that allowing the pregnancy to continue would have such debilitating effects (whether psychologically or otherwise) on the mother as to present a hazard to her life, however remote such danger may be.[66]

It is important to note that in his last point Jakobovits is clearly of the view that the only psychological conditions sufficient to warrant an abortion are those that would pose a threat to the mother's survival. Here he appears to take a view on this subject consistent with that of Winkler before him.[67]

---

[65] Jakobovits, "Recent Halakhic Periodical Literature," 269.   [66] *Ibid.*, 270.
[67] See above, chapter 4, p. 118.

Jakobovits does not go as far as Unterman in describing abortion without appropriate justification as an appurtenance of the shedding of blood. In fact, elsewhere Jakobovits explicitly states that when abortion lacks acceptable grounds, "the destruction of an unborn child is a grave offense, although not murder."[68] In the above passage, however, Jakobovits does take the original approach of designating such abortion as a "crime." Of course, if Jakobovits is correct, then, as has been demonstrated, a number of his rabbinic predecessors had approved of deeds that he would deem "criminal." Jakobovits, like Unterman before him, effectively recast "unjustified" abortion as being not merely a "wrong," but a transgression of the acceptable boundaries of civilized society.

However, not all the *teshuvot* concerning abortion for the sake of potential deformities are wholly dismissive of the idea. A clear example of a different mode of thinking on the subject was penned in 1950, although not published until 1966. Authored by Rabbi Yehiel Ya'akov Weinberg (1885–1966), it is addressed to the rabbis of England. Weinberg, educated in the *yeshivot* of Mir and Slobodka, received his doctorate from the University of Giessen and served as a rabbi in Berlin. After emerging from the concentration camps, he lived in Montreaux, Switzerland, where his scholarship and teaching acted as a significant bridge between modern scholarship and the Talmudic tradition, as well as between Eastern and Western Jewry: his *Seridei Eish* collection contains *Wissenschaft*-style studies, typical of the Western approach, alongside the *chiddusim* and *teshuvot* that were characteristic of the East.[69] Weinberg, like Unterman, was asked about rubella, but this time from the perspective of the physician. Given that the law in England permitted abortions for German measles to be carried out after three months of pregnancy, may a Jewish doctor perform an abortion for either a Jewish or non-Jewish patient under such circumstances? The individual who submitted the question also informed Weinberg that since the government employed the doctor concerned, the doctor had reason to be apprehensive about flouting government directives in this regard.[70]

Weinberg lays to rest any thought that all the ways of explaining the differences between the viewpoints of Rashi and Maimonides had been

---

[68] I. Jakobovits, "Jewish Views on Abortion," in F. Rosner, and J. D. Bleich (eds.), *Jewish Bioethics*, New York, Sanhedrin Press, 1979, p. 121.

[69] M. Hacohen, "Weinberg, Jehiel Jacob," in *Encyclopaedia Judaica*, Jerusalem, Keter Publishing House, volume XVI, pp. 399–400.

[70] Y. Weinberg, "*Hapalat HaUbar B'Ishah Cholanit*," *Noam*, volume 9, 1966: 193. See also Y. Weinberg, *Seridei Eish*, Jerusalem, 1966, volume III, number 127.

exhausted, by offering a new insight. In the *Mishneh Torah*, Weinberg observes, Maimonides rules that one may only appropriate the property of another in order to save one's own life, if the value of the property is subsequently repaid to its owner.[71] The exception to this rule, however, which appears in the very same chapter of the *Yad*, is when the property itself is the source of the threat. The classic example of this exception is that of the overloaded boat, in which an individual steps forward to lighten the boat by throwing luggage overboard. That person will not later be liable to repay the owners for the value of the luggage that has been lost, as the luggage was functioning as a *rodef*. The general principle that follows from this is that, insofar as the property is acting as a *rodef*, its owner is not recompensed when it is destroyed. This, maintains Weinberg, is the reason why Maimonides invokes the *rodef* principle in the case of the fetus. It is not to permit the killing of the fetus; Rashi's explanation that the fetus is not a *nefesh* suffices to allow this. Rather, Maimonides uses the *rodef* explanation to demonstrate that Exodus 21:22's requirement that financial compensation be paid to the husband for fetal destruction is not operative in this type of procedure. According to this interpretation, then, the views of Rashi and Maimonides are not at odds with each other; both would have agreed that fetal destruction is permissible on the basis that the fetus is not a *nefesh*.[72]

While Weinberg has a definite and distinctive conception of the way in which Rashi and Maimonides are to be understood, the same decisiveness is not evident in many of the other issues that he discusses. Though Weinberg critiques Bacharach's reason for the prohibition,[73] approvingly mentions Maharit's *chabbalah* explanation,[74] and discusses

---

[71] *Hilkhot Chovel UMazzik* 8:4.

[72] Weinberg, "*Hapalat HaUbar B'Ishah Cholanit*," 204–205.

[73] *Ibid.*, 206. Bacharach (see chapter 3, p. 77) had maintained that although women are not obligated by the "be fruitful and multiply" commandment, they are required to fulfill God's aim: "He formed it to be inhabited." Weinberg, however, holds that this injunction is like the "be fruitful and multiply" commandment, at least in the respect that it is seen to apply only to one's own children. Hence, writes Weinberg, this would lead to the view that a woman could perform an abortion for any woman other than herself, a conclusion not imagined by any *posek*, including Bacharach.

[74] Weinberg understands the *chabbalah* involved to refer to the wounding of the fetus rather than the mother. Since he regards a fetus less than forty days old as akin to "mere fluid," *chabbalah* would not apply to such a fetus. Bleich ("Abortion in Halakhic Literature," p. 341) critiques Weinberg's position for ignoring the mother: "Despite the cogency of Rabbi Weinberg's reasoning regarding 'wounding' of the fetus, his reasoning is inapplicable in cases of abortion by means of dilation and curettage which certainly involves 'wounding' of the mother as well, irrespective of the stage of pregnancy at which this procedure is initiated. Following this line of thought, it should be forbidden other than for therapeutic considerations which constitute licit grounds for 'wounding.'"

the "appurtenance of murder" consideration as a motivating factor for the ban, he acknowledges that "we still do not know the reason for the prohibition on a Jew killing a fetus..."[75] – it requires "further study."

Weinberg also places in the "requiring further study" category Grodzinsky's notion that when a fetus is considered *yerekh imo* it is obvious that one is obligated to sever a "limb" in order to save the body as a whole. Basing his position on a *Tosafot* to *Sanhedrin* 80b, Weinberg holds that *yerekh imo* does not apply if the mother has become a *tereifah*. The fact that the mother's life hangs in the balance does not imply that the fetus, which possesses independent "animation," necessarily is similarly threatened. Put another way, her becoming a *tereifah* does not *ipso facto* make the fetus a *tereifah*. Hence, writes Weinberg, "[I]t is doubtful if we are permitted to destroy the fetus in order to save the mother, even though we are, of course, mandated to destroy a limb in order to save the body, since the fetus possesses independent animation."[76] Notwithstanding the fact that the fetus is not to be considered a *nefesh*, Weinberg is doubtful, then, that the fetus may be destroyed to save the mother if the fetus is not the cause of its mother's difficulties.

Even when Weinberg appears to have found an area in which he seems determined to be unequivocal, equivocation emerges. Weinberg takes the forceful position that, in the case before him, it certainly would be acceptable to abort a fetus threatened with deformities if the fetus were less than forty days old.[77] Thus, Weinberg embraces the stance of those of his predecessors who held that before forty days the standing of the fetus should be regarded as relatively less substantial, and hence, an abortion for this cause most certainly would be warranted. In a later note to his published *teshuvah*, however, Weinberg cautions that, having become aware of Unterman's contrary view on this matter, he cannot arrive at a conclusion on this subject without further *halakhic* conferring.[78]

Even Weinberg's final answer ends up being more a statistical "best bet" than a determined argument for a position. Discussing the availability of abortion after forty days, Weinberg quotes Ya'avetz's contention that abortion should be allowed for the mother's pain or "great need" even in the case of a healthy fetus. It is this stance of Ya'avetz that returns in the last lines of Weinberg's answer, albeit without strong conviction. Weinberg writes:

[75] Weinberg, "*Hapalat HaUbar B'Ishah Cholanit*," 215.   [76] *Ibid.*   [77] *Ibid.*, 213–214.
[78] Weinberg, *Seridei Eish*, p. 350, n. 7.

It is my duty to comment that all that we have written concerning the permission to abort a fetus in order to save the woman from sickness is only according to the method of those *Rishonim* who think that the permission of the *Mishnah* in the case of one who is in difficulty in childbirth is because of the fact that the fetus is not called a *nefesh* . . .[79]

Weinberg then points out that there are, nevertheless, other *Rishonim* who employ Maimonides' interpretation of the *Mishnah* to forbid abortion unless the fetus is acting as a *rodef*. He proceeds to resolve this conflict as follows: "But since the majority of the *Rishonim* differ with Maimonides, as was shown above, it is possible that [one ought] to permit and to rely on Ya'avetz."[80]

Weinberg, then, unlike his contemporaries who grappled with this problem, seems to give tentative permission for an abortion – even be-yond forty days – in the case of a fetus threatened with severe deformities, based on the pain that it would cause the mother. As has been seen, how-ever, Weinberg is by no means resolute in his leniency. Perhaps, though, his repeated uncertainty should not be the cause of reproof: Weinberg is, after all, one of the inheritors of an indeterminate tradition. He is certainly faithful to this ethos. Another possible reason for Weinberg's tentativeness may lie in the fact that a lenient position is always harder to sustain than a stringent one: the Talmud eloquently expresses this notion when it observes that it is harder to permit, since permitting requires true courage of conviction, while a more rigid opinion can be the result of doubt.[81]

A far more determined lenient stance on the question of fetal abnor-mality, however, appeared in the American writings of Rabbi Solomon Freehof (1892–1990). Unlike the other twentieth-century rabbis whose responsa have been reviewed up to this point, Freehof replied to a fetal abnormality inquiry that arose from within the Reform, rather than the Orthodox, community. Indeed, through much of the 1900s, Freehof was known as the preeminent author of responsa for *halakhic* inquiries from Reform Jews.[82] Freehof was asked about the permissibility of an abortion for a young woman who contracted German measles in the third month of her pregnancy, where there were various medical opinions as to the probability of the child being deformed.[83]

---

[79] Weinberg, "*Hapalat HaUbar B'Ishah Cholanit*," 215.   [80] *Ibid.*

[81] *Beitzah* 2b and Rashi, "*de-hetirah adif*."

[82] W. Jacob, "Solomon B. Freehof," in E. Stevens (ed.), *Central Conference of American Rabbis Yearbook*, New York, Central Conference of American Rabbis, 1991, volume C, pp. 190–191.

[83] W. Jacob (ed.), *American Reform Responsa: Collected Responsa of the Central Conference of American Rabbis 1889–1983*, New York, 1983, # 171, p. 541.

In reply, Freehof undertakes a concise review of several of the Jewish texts relevant to abortion, noting in particular the *teshuvot* of Bacharach, Ya'avetz, and Ouziel. Freehof then concludes:

In the case which you are discussing, I would, therefore, say that since there is strong preponderance of medical opinion that the child will be born imperfect physically and even mentally, then for the mother's sake (i.e., her mental anguish now and in the future) she may sacrifice this part of herself. This decision thus follows the opinion of Jacob Emden and Ben Zion Uziel against the earlier opinion of Yair Chaim Bachrach.[84]

Freehof's appeal to the "preponderance of medical opinion" seems to represent a perception of the prevailing medical view rather than a direct response to the questioner's uncertainty whether to heed "her doctor" or the contrary view of the other doctors. The wording of the question seems to indicate that a number of doctors suspect that the child may be born undamaged. Freehof's willingness to look beyond this disagreement and to rule in the most lenient way possible, probably demonstrates his determination to avoid even the smallest prospect of maternal "mental anguish now and in the future." Indeed, by invoking Ya'avetz and Ouziel as his primary textual supports – without explaining how their views relate to the question before him – Freehof seems to be indicating that leniency ought to be the preferred path when making abortion decisions. It is noteworthy that, in this *teshuvah*, Freehof employs the historic criterion of permitting abortion solely for the "mother's sake." It is only when she is threatened with "mental anguish" that an abortion can be contemplated.

But Freehof was not alone in ruling decisively in a lenient direction when confronted with potential fetal abnormalities. Rabbi Shaul Yisraeli, an Israeli, also found reasons to be permissive. In a responsum published in 1966, Yisraeli, like Zweig, was asked about the permissibility of abortions for women who had taken a particular medicine – in this instance a relaxant – which was known to stunt fetal development.[85] Yisraeli was informed that the consequence of the medication was that the majority of affected infants were born with physical deformities or mental incapacity that "make their deaths better than their lives."

Yisraeli begins by positing that there are at least two possible reasons for the *Tosafists'* prohibition on fetal destruction for Jews: one, following

---

[84] *Ibid.*, p. 543.
[85] All Yisraeli references and quotations are from S. Yisraeli, *Amud HaYemini*, Tel Aviv, 1966, number 32.

Maharit, is the potential *chabbalah* that the mother might undergo. The other is the issue of *"baʾal tashchit,"* the injunction against wanton destruction of property.[86] In this case, the property referred to is the fetus, which technically "belongs" to the husband. Yisraeli, however, advances arguments explaining why both reasons are inapposite to the circumstances before him. In the case of *chabbalah*, Yisraeli, citing *Sanhedrin* 84b, points out that the text provides permission for wounding that is performed for the purposes of healing, and that the rabbis connected this permission to the Torah's verse, "you shall love your neighbor as yourself (Leviticus 19:18)."[87] Just as you would want such wounding performed upon yourself, the rabbis convey, so, if necessary, it can be performed upon another. Yisraeli argues that such wounding is indeed necessary. As regards *baʾal tashchit*, Yisraeli maintains that as the purpose of the proposed abortion is not destructive, *baʾal tashchit* is not a concern. Just as a mourner who rends garments (*keriah*) at a funeral does not transgress *baʾal tashchit*, because the destruction has a constructive aim, so too in this type of abortion there is a constructive aim.

Yisraeli, then, is of the view that, as neither reason for the prohibition applies, abortion of deformed fetuses would be permitted, so long as the intent of the *Tosafists* was not to prohibit abortion on account of it being an appurtenance of murder. If this were their intent, such abortion would be prohibited. Through the course of his *teshuvah*, however, Yisraeli proceeds to show that the fetus is not considered a *nefesh*, and that spilling of blood is not involved in this type of abortion. Indeed, Yisraeli goes even further: he invokes the deaths of King Saul and Rabbi Haninah ben Teradion to hint that in instances where extreme suffering is the alternative, the tradition might approve of an action which, at first glance, appears to be an improper taking of life. Rabbi Haninah was martyred by the Romans for teaching Torah.[88] While being burnt at the stake, he refused his students' advice to commit suicide by opening his mouth so that the flames could enter and kill him more quickly. However, he did permit the executioner to hasten the cessation of his suffering by increasing the flames and by removing the woolen mats around his body that had been placed there as impediments, to prolong his suffering. King Saul, whose arms-bearer refused King Saul's request to kill him when they were surrounded by the Philistines, fell on his own sword rather than

---

[86] This principle is founded in Deuteronomy 20:19.
[87] *Sanhedrin* 84b allows a son to perform bloodletting, a form of wounding, in the name of healing, for his father.
[88] See *Avodah Zarah* 18a–b.

allow the enemy to "make sport" with him.[89] These two accounts have been used in the past as justifications for taking life *in extremis*.[90]

Yisraeli understands Haninah's executioner to have intervened properly to advance Haninah's death and to release the rabbi from suffering. His was an act committed within the bounds of the *Sanhedrin* 84b understanding of "you shall love your neighbor as yourself." The same argument could be utilized to explain why King Saul's act of self-*chabbalah* was acceptable.

As Yisraeli's position is not dissimilar to that of Maharit, it is not surprising that Yisraeli quotes Maharit approvingly, and finds "no contradiction" between Maharit's two *teshuvot*. *Chabbalah*, not murder, was Maharit's concern as well, and Maharit allowed feticide for the "need" of the mother, a "need" that certainly could include a sickness that was not immediately life-threatening. All of this leads Yisraeli to conclude that it is permitted to kill the fetus when the continued existence of the fetus is inextricably bound up with the suffering of another, such as the *innui ha-din* (suffering associated with delay of sentence) caused to the mother in tractate *Arakhin*. This is true even if the fetus is not the cause of the suffering, but its presence interferes with the possibility of alleviating the torment.

Yisraeli, however, ventures even further. He proceeds to raise the question of whether consideration should not also be given to the likely future suffering of the fetus as well. As has been seen, this is a controversial step because introducing the concerns of anybody except the mother goes beyond the parameters of the normative *halakhic* focus.[91] Nevertheless, Yisraeli asks why one would not be allowed to kill the fetus in order to alleviate its suffering, given that one might kill it in order to relieve the suffering of others. Anticipating the reply that such an act would be unthinkable on the basis of the notion that every moment of life is precious and because of the future potential for observance that is inherent in the fetus, Yisraeli again points to the cases of King Saul and Haninah. The fact, Yisraeli contends, that King Saul's life was about to be enveloped by suffering led to a preference for hastening his death. Haninah's executioner was rewarded with the world to come for helping to hasten his death at the stake. Moreover, Yisraeli points out, issues of future potential are not raised in circumstances involving substantive distress.

---

[89] See 1 Samuel, chapter 31.
[90] On Haninah, see Tosafot, *Avodah Zarah* 18a, "*ve-'al yachbol atzmo*." On King Saul, see Radak on 1 Samuel 31:4.
[91] See above, pp. 135–136.

Yisraeli not only introduces concerns about the future prospects for the fetus, but raises considerations about the parents as well. These go well beyond anything that legitimately might be subsumed under maternal "need." Yisraeli states that the suffering of the parents, who will see their offspring afflicted with such limitations that its life will be "no life," should be taken into account. Furthermore, Yisraeli contends, if the fetus is indeed born with impaired mental capacity, then one of the reasons for preserving its life – namely that its life will offer the possibility for the preservation of *mitzvot* – is no longer operative. Combining this reality with the "great pain of the parents and family members," leads Yisraeli to conclude that "for all these reasons it appears that abortion would be permitted in such instances."

There can be no doubting the courage of Yisraeli's position. He surely was well aware of the starkly contrary views that had been expressed on the subject of abortion in cases of fetal abnormality. He was certainly acquainted with the tradition's emphasis on only taking into account the consequences for the mother of continuing the pregnancy, to the exclusion of concern for others. Yet he looks at the textual heritage in a quite different way, admitting the possibility of abortion in circumstances in which suffering is at stake, and acknowledging a wider circle of concern than had usually been taken into account. It is critical to recall, however, that while taking this path, Yisraeli still regarded himself as remaining firmly within the *halakhic* tradition.

Yisraeli was not the sole Orthodox voice of leniency. He was joined by Rabbi Eliezer Waldenberg (born 1917). Rabbi Waldenberg, who later became a member of Israel's Supreme Rabbinical Court, authored the voluminous responsa collection *Tzitz Eliezer*, and has written extensively on contemporary *halakhic* problems, particularly medical issues. Within *Tzitz Eliezer*, Waldenberg deals in detail with the subject of abortion on no fewer than six occasions. In the first instance, in volume VII, Waldenberg responds to the problem of a dispute between a husband and wife. The woman's doctor had advised her to have an abortion on the basis that her continued pregnancy, which was then at an early stage, would be a danger to her health, though not life-threatening. This hazardous circumstance had arisen in some measure because of her becoming pregnant shortly after giving birth. The husband, however, objected to the prospective abortion. Should the abortion proceed or not?[92]

---

[92] References and quotations concerning this Waldenberg *teshuvah* are from E. Waldenberg, *Tzitz Eliezer*, Jerusalem, 1963, volume VII, number 48, p. 190.

Waldenberg first advises that the couple should get a second medical opinion. The first doctor, Waldenberg points out, was not "religious," and, therefore could not be expected to make Torah considerations a part of his medical judgment. In suggesting that the couple should consult a religious doctor, Waldenberg implicitly conveys that only a religiously ob- servant doctor has the competence to make the medical decision whether an abortion might be indicated, based on the doctor's commitments to the tenets of Jewish law. Waldenberg then contends that if a religious doctor says that an abortion under these circumstances would be war- ranted, solid *halakhic* support exists to allow an abortion to go forward. Specifically, Waldenberg invokes Maharit – citing only Maharit's lenient *teshuvah* number 99 – and Ya'avetz, to the effect that it is permitted to abort for the "healing," or the "need" of the mother, even if it is not to save the mother's life. If no such "need" exists, writes Waldenberg, abortion would be a serious transgression indeed. This having been said, how- ever, the abortion prohibition is, in Waldenberg's view, clearly rabbinic, and "everybody agrees" that it contains "no element of actual murder." Waldenberg also derives support for his approach from the *teshuvah* of Ayash, who had permitted an abortion in the case of a nursing mother where fears were held for the well-being of the suckling infant.[93] In such instances, opines Waldenberg, when the mother is experiencing great suffering because of the pregnancy, there is reason "to be lenient" in ruling on the appropriateness of an abortion. Waldenberg concludes by stating that it would be preferable if the abortion were carried out be- fore the fortieth day of pregnancy, since abortion is a much less serious matter during this early period, given that the fetus still comes under the definition of being "mere fluid."[94]

Plainly, Waldenberg takes a view that is starkly different from that of Unterman. Seeing not the slightest trace of "actual murder" involved in this type of abortion, Waldenberg is comfortable in authorizing an abortion for reasons of maternal health. He is quite prepared, moreover, to invoke the Talmud's forty-day period as a foundation for declaring fetal status to be of relatively less significance during this initial stage. Waldenberg certainly does not rule out an abortion of this nature even

[93] See above, chapter 3, pp. 83–84.
[94] See above, chapter 2, pp. 33–34. Among the sources that Waldenberg cites for the fetus being "mere fluid" is Bacharach's *teshuvah* in *Chavvot Ya'ir*. In this regard, however, Waldenberg presents a misleading picture in much the same way as had Zweig (see above, p. 147, n. 59). Bacharach had held that the turning points to which one might allude during pregnancy are all essentially meaningless from a practical point of view (see above, chapter 3, pp. 73ff.). Within this *teshuvah*, Waldenberg clearly states a quite different position.

beyond the fortieth day; he only states that it would be "preferable" if the abortion could take place sooner.

In the same year that Waldenberg wrote his first abortion *teshuvah*, Waldenberg's Israeli colleague Rabbi Ovadiah Yosef (born 1920), who was later to serve as *Sefaradi* chief rabbi of Israel, also ruled in favor of abortion for the sake of maternal health, but limited it to the first three months of pregnancy. Yosef was asked about a woman who had already undergone three deliveries by Caesarian section, was now at the conclusion of the second month of yet another pregnancy, and her doctors were advising her that if she did not abort there was a danger to her life.[95] Despite the fact that the woman's life was not at immediate risk, Yosef clearly had more compelling reasons to permit an abortion than did Waldenberg, given that the woman's life ultimately would be threatened. At the end of his *teshuvah*, Yosef advises that two Jewish doctors should be independently consulted and, if both are persuaded of a threat to her life, an abortion could proceed on the dual basis that the fetus is behaving as a *rodef* and the mother's life takes precedence. Quoting the Talmudic proposition that a fetus is "recognizable" at three months,[96] Yosef holds that it is likely that up to this point, there is no Toraitic prohibition on abortion. If the prohibition is rabbinic, it certainly may be set aside in cases of sickness, even when no immediate danger is involved. Yosef is, however, evidently of the view that beyond three months an abortion could only be countenanced if the mother's life were in the balance.

It is clear from his *teshuvah* that Yosef was very conscious of the tradition's equivocation on the question of whether abortion is forbidden "from the Torah" or "from the rabbis." Yosef sought clarification of this conundrum from Waldenberg. Replying in volume VIII of *Tzitz Eliezer*, Waldenberg reiterates his previous view that the prohibition is wholly rabbinic.[97] Waldenberg cites, among others, the views of the early twentieth-century scholar Rabbi Shmuel Engel (1853–1935) of Germany. Engel held that one who kills a fetus transgresses a rabbinic prohibition, not one of the Torah, and also maintained that killing a fetus could in no way be subsumed within the "appurtenances of the spilling of blood."[98] Waldenberg also makes reference to a *teshuvah* by the Russian *Acharon*

---

[95] All Yosef references and quotations are from O. Yosef, *Yabi'ah Omer*, Jerusalem, 1964, *Even HaEzer*, volume IV, number 1.

[96] *Yevamot* 37a.

[97] References and quotations concerning this Waldenberg *teshuvah* are from *Tzitz Eliezer*, Jerusalem, 1965, volume VIII, number 36, pp. 218–219.

[98] S. Engel, *Maharash Engel*, Bardiov, 1926 and on, *Choshen HaMishpat*, number 89.

Rabbi Aaron Shmuel ben Israel Kaidonover (1614–76). In his *Emunat Shmuel*, Kaidonover wrote that even the prohibition on fetal destruction is no more than *ketzat issur* (a bit of a prohibition) thereby implying that its prohibitive standing is by no means strong.[99] Finally, Waldenberg mentions the stance of the nineteenth-century *halakhist* Rabbi Solomon ben Judah Aaron Kluger (1785–1869). In the context of a *teshuvah* dealing with breast-feeding, Kluger points out that if the woman in *Arakhin* could be executed because of *innui ha-din* (the suffering associated with delay of sentence), then, given that the fetus does not have the standing of a living human being, this surely means that the mother's *tzaàrah de-gufah* (bodily suffering) is sufficient to permit the destruction of the fetus.[100] From this, Waldenberg concludes that "there are reasonable positions in the *halakhah* that instruct towards leniency, even in an instance when imminent danger to the woman is not anticipated, but when her health condition is undermined, such that it causes her suffering of the body and soul to the point where a faithful doctor decides that there is a need to perform an abortion." Waldenberg, then, not only confirms that the prohibition is rabbinic rather than Toraitic, but he also communicates that no transgression would be involved if serious *tzaàrah de-gufah* were at stake, even in a non-life-threatening circumstance. In this regard, Waldenberg opposes the position of Zweig, who did not consider *tzaàrah de-gufah* to be a worthy justification for abortion unless the mother's life hangs in the balance.[101]

Waldenberg's third *teshuvah* dealing with abortion directly addresses the subject of potential fetal abnormality. Found in volume IX of *Tzitz Eliezer*, this *teshuvah* is essentially an extensive overview of his thinking on the subject of abortion generally.[102] The question to which Waldenberg responded concerned the permissibility of rendering abortion assistance to a non-Jew, but the answer to this inquiry is not the central feature of the *teshuvah*. Rather, the more significant aspect of the *teshuvah* is Waldenberg's ruling regarding the acceptability of aborting fetuses with potential deformities.

Regarding this issue, Waldenberg rules in a similar way to his earlier response to the woman whose health was threatened: "Hence it appears that if there is a grounded fear that the child will be born with a defect or with restrictions, one ought to encourage [a ruling] to permit an abortion

---

[99] A. Kaidonover, *Emunat Shmuel*, Jerusalem, 1970, number 14.
[100] S. Kluger, *Sefer Tzlota D'Avraham*, Lemberg, 1868, number 60.   [101] See above, p. 146.
[102] References and quotations concerning this Waldenberg *teshuvah* are from *Tzitz Eliezer*, Jerusalem, 1967, volume IX, number 51, pp. 233–240.

prior to the completion of forty days of pregnancy, and even to extend this until three months, [provided that] fetal movement is not yet [detected]." What is different in this instance from his ruling in volume VII is that here Waldenberg not only states that an abortion would be acceptable up to forty days, but explicitly extends the window of permissibility until the end of the first trimester, given that fetal movement has not been sensed.

In reaching this conclusion, Waldenberg again relies heavily on the *teshuvot* of Maharit, Bacharach, and Ya'avetz. Citing, on this occasion, both *teshuvot* of Maharit, Waldenberg points out that Maharit based the abortion prohibition in the *chabbalah* explanation, but that *chabbalah* is acceptable for healing purposes.[103] Hence, following the line of Al-Chakam, Waldenberg understands Maharit to permit abortion in cases of real maternal need. From Bacharach and Ya'avetz, Waldenberg adopts the notion that the abortion prohibition is based in the purposeless destruction of seed. While expressing no small measure of surprise at Ya'avetz's reasoning process, Waldenberg nevertheless relies on Ya'avetz's position that the destruction of seed is not "purposeless" if it is carried out for a "great [maternal] need." It is from his understanding of Bacharach, however, that Waldenberg extends leniency for abortion until the end of three months. Citing an early-twentieth-century *teshuvah* of the Hungarian Talmudist Rabbi Eliezer Deutsch (1850–1916), Waldenberg comes to the view that the three-month stage has precedent in cases of maternal need.[104] Deutsch, in turn, had based his views on these differing stages of pregnancy on his perception of Bacharach's writings in *Chavvot Ya'ir*. As has already been shown, however, the difficulty with this position is that while Bacharach indeed discussed these stages of pregnancy, he rejected the notion that any of them should be seen as practical turning points of any type.[105] Hence, while Waldenberg has a basis for leniency in the area of abortion for fetal deformities, and has a solid precedent for favoring the first forty days of pregnancy, his recognition of a three-month turning point has less firm *halakhic* support.

In this *teshuvah*, Waldenberg reiterates the rabbinic nature of the abortion prohibition, and reemphasizes that the killing of a fetus cannot be regarded as an "appurtenance of spilling of blood." Beyond accentuating these important issues he also opens up a hitherto unexplored area.

[103] See above, chapter 3, p. 71.
[104] Deutsch had allowed for abortion only until three months in cases of direct danger to the mother and preferred that the mother self-abort by drinking some type of abortifacient drug.
[105] See above, chapter 3, pp. 73ff., and p. 147, n. 59.

Naturally, Waldenberg maintains that he has opted for the correct *ha-lakhic* path in determining that abortion is permissible in a variety of circumstances short of a direct threat to the life of the mother. Nevertheless, Waldenberg points to the fact that there are obviously a number of responsa that take the position that abortion can be condoned only in an instance of urgent peril for the mother. While this is not the approach that Waldenberg generally favors, he acknowledges that there are occasions when invoking this more strict approach can bring a measure of "salvation and saving" if confronted with certain difficult *halakhic* problems. By way of example, Waldenberg cites the case of a pregnant woman suffering from a cancer that will kill her "sooner or later." The doctors are of the view that continuation of her pregnancy will shorten her life. The woman's response to the doctors is that she wants to complete the pregnancy and bear the child, even if it has the effect of hastening her death. How ought the law to respond in such a circumstance? Waldenberg indicates that if one were to adopt the position on abortion of the more lenient *poskim* – like him – one would be forced to demand that the woman undergo an abortion in order to extend her life, whether or not this was in accordance with her wishes. After all, Waldenberg observes, it is an act of *pikuach nefesh* even if the woman's life is prolonged for just a short time, and, hence, the demands of *pikuach nefesh* for the woman most certainly would override any desire to protect the fetus. The interpretation of the abortion law preferred by the lenient *poskim* would lead to the conclusion that an abortion would be required of a woman in a circumstance such as this as soon as practicable.

Following the outlook of the stricter *poskim*, however, no such requirement would pertain. According to their perspective, there exists an unyielding Torah-based prohibition on abortion unless the woman's life is in imminent danger. Hence, from the vantage point of the stricter *poskim*, an abortion in this instance would be forbidden until the point was reached when the abortion became an indispensable intervention in the course of saving the mother's life. Plainly, therefore, the mother's reasonable desire to continue with her pregnancy under these tragic circumstances could only be *halakhically* accommodated by means of the stricter construction of the abortion provisions. Displaying considerable *halakhic* broad-mindedness, Waldenberg consequently holds that, while the lenient path is generally the one to be followed, there are instances in which the stricter legal understanding ought to be applied in the name of "heavenly compassion."

Waldenberg concludes this third *teshuvah* on abortion with a lucid, eighteen-point summary of the *halakhah* on the subject. In this review he further demonstrates his lenient reading of the sources by contending that there is a basis to permit abortion for a nursing woman, or a married woman who has committed adultery, or for one who has been raped. Also noteworthy in this extensive synopsis is Waldenberg's stance, based on Exodus 21:22–23, that it is important to make every attempt to obtain the agreement of the husband to an abortion because of his "property interest" in the fetus. Waldenberg, however, does not suggest that, if grounds for an abortion exist, the procedure ought in any way to be impeded by the husband's refusal to grant his consent. Furthermore, while Waldenberg does not go as far as did Ayash in prohibiting abortion by "physical means,"[106] he does exhibit a clear preference for an oral medication in carrying out the procedure. In these areas, Waldenberg seeks to perpetuate traditions with strong textual basis.

In the final point of his summary, Waldenberg exhorts Jews to refrain from abortion for any other than the most compelling of reasons. He describes the *halakhic* strictures in this area as "placing a boundary against licentious behavior." There can be little doubt that Waldenberg would be concerned about "licentious behavior" in any context. But he, like Zweig,[107] argues on the grounds that because such "licentious behavior" has been outlawed by the surrounding nations, Israel might look less worthy on the scale of holiness were it to permit such activity. It is plain that the *halakhah* has internal reasons for wanting to curb licentiousness and its own mechanisms for coping with it. It is significant, therefore, that both Zweig and Waldenberg decide that it is important to make an argument based on external considerations. Implicitly, they both seem to be suggesting that if internal arguments for cleaving to abortion strictures are not sufficiently compelling, then the *halakhah* must at least conform to some external yardstick of morality. Of course, the reality that surrounding nations may have "established a boundary" cannot determine the appropriateness of a *halakhic* boundary. This raises a difficult question: if indeed it is acceptable to look beyond the *halakhah* for criteria by which *halakhic* behaviors might be measured, who will determine which scale of morality is appropriate, and in which circumstance it will be required?[108]

---

[106] See above, chapter 3, pp. 83–84.   [107] See above, p. 148.
[108] This matter will be explored further in chapter 7.

THE TAY-SACHS CONFRONTATION

Eight years would pass between the publication of Waldenberg's *teshuvah* in volume IX and his next foray into the abortion arena in 1975. In that year, Professor David Meir, Director of the Sha'arei Tzedek Hospital in Jerusalem, posed a question to Waldenberg about the devastating genetic illness, Tay-Sachs disease. Professor Meir, who was familiar with Waldenberg's previous opinions in the abortion area, indicated to Waldenberg that, while it had become possible to test a fetus for Tay-Sachs disease, it was not possible to obtain the results of such tests before the conclusion of the third month of pregnancy. Hence, Professor Meir inquired, given that the consequences of Tay-Sachs disease are so serious and so certain,[109] would an abortion be warranted even beyond three months of pregnancy? Alternatively, is the three-month stage "absolute," such that, in the second and third trimesters, no reason short of a direct threat to the mother's life would be sufficient to permit an abortion?[110]

Before turning to Waldenberg's reply, it is important to place the problem of Tay-Sachs disease within its immediate *halakhic* context, given that in the early 1970s, a number of rabbis had begun to discuss the issue. Bleich, in a 1972 *halakhic* article, indicated his understanding that *halakhah* opposed abortion for any type of genetic fetal abnormality:

> The fear that a child may be born physically malformed or mentally deficient does not in itself justify recourse to abortion ... Since the sole available medical remedy following diagnosis of severe genetic defects is abortion of the fetus, which is not sanctioned by Halakhah (Jewish law) in such instances, amniocentesis, under these conditions, does not serve as an aid in treatment of the patient and is not *halakhically* permissible ...[111]

Bleich was in good company in holding this view. Rabbi Moshe Feinstein (1895–1986), head of *Yeshivat Tiferet Yerushalayim* in New York City and the rabbi considered to be the leading light of the American

---

[109] Dorland's Illustrated Medical Dictionary describes Tay-Sachs disease as follows: "[T]he most common ganglioside storage disease, occurring almost exclusively among northeast European Jews. Tay-Sachs disease is ... specifically characterized by infantile onset (3–6 months), doll-like faces, cherry-red macular spot (90+ percent of the infants), early blindness, hyperacusis, macrocephaly, seizures and hypotonia; the children die between 2 and 5 years of age"; *Dorland's Illustrated Medical Dictionary* (27th edition), W. B. Saunders Company, Harcourt Brace Jovanovich Incorporated, Philadelphia, 1988, p. 493.

[110] References and quotations concerning this Waldenberg *teshuvah* are from *Tzitz Eliezer*, Jerusalem, 1975, volume XIII, number 102.

[111] Bleich, as cited in F. Rosner, "Tay-Sachs Disease: To Screen or Not to Screen," *Tradition*, volume 15, number 4, 1976: 107.

traditional Jewish community, whose "rulings were accepted as authoritative by Orthodox Jews throughout the world," had a similar outlook.[112] In a 1973 *teshuvah* on the advisability of screening for Tay-Sachs carriers, Feinstein ruled that abortion for Tay-Sachs disease is forbidden.[113] Dr. Fred Rosner, a noted expert on *halakhah* pertaining to medical matters, added specific detail to the stance taken by Bleich and Feinstein in an article penned in 1975:

> The various objections to amniocentesis and abortion in Jewish law are predicated on considerations surrounding the fetus. Extreme emotional stress in the mother leading to suicidal intent might constitute one of the situations in which abortion might be sanctioned by even the most Orthodox Rabbi. If a woman who suffered a nervous breakdown following the birth (or death) of a child with Tay-Sachs disease becomes pregnant again, and is so distraught with the knowledge that she may be carrying another child with the fatal disease that she threatens suicide, Jewish law could allow amniocentesis. If this procedure reveals an unaffected fetus, the pregnancy continues to term. If the result of the amniocentesis indicates a homozygous fetus with Tay-Sachs disease, rabbinic consultation should be obtained regarding the decision of whether or not to abort. No general rule of permissiveness or prohibition can be enunciated in regard to abortion in Jewish law. Each case must be individualized and evaluated on the basis of its merits . . .[114]

Rosner's encapsulation of the *halakhic* position on this type of abortion cannot be characterized as tending towards leniency. Nobody would disagree with Rosner that Jewish law insists on judging each case of abortion individually. But Rosner – who presumably is concerned that a fetus be a *rodef* if abortion is to be permitted – suggests that a mother, who has already suffered with one experience of Tay-Sachs disease, would need to demonstrate that her own life is at risk by threatening suicide, before amniocentesis would be allowed. Even then, he does not counsel that there is basis in Jewish law to support such an abortion, but stipulates that a rabbi would have to decide "whether or not to abort." Rosner, then, portrays the *halakhic* stance on Tay-Sachs disease as effectively dismissing lesser examples of maternal "need," and only contemplating abortion if the consequence of the disease is an actual threat to the mother's life.

A viewpoint contrary to that of Bleich, Feinstein, and Rosner was articulated by Rabbi Aryeh Grossnass, *Dayan* of the London *Beit Din*, in

---

[112] "Feinstein, Moses," by editorial staff, in *Encyclopaedia Judaica*, Jerusalem, Keter Publishing House, volume VI, p. 1213.
[113] Feinstein, as cited in Rosner, "Tay-Sachs Disease," 106.
[114] Rosner, "Tay-Sachs Disease," 108.

a *teshuvah* published in 1973.[115] Within his *teshuvah*, Grossnass ponders the idea that one ought to override the *Shabbat* in order to save a fetus because of the fetus' future standing as a *nefesh*. Grossnass, who relies heavily on Landau,[116] is apparently of the view that an individual only attains *nefesh* standing if that individual is indeed viable. This being the case, Grossnass argues that if medical experts state that the fetus is certain to die within several years, as is definite in an instance of Tay-Sachs disease, it is possible that there is no prohibition on killing such a fetus, since the fetus cannot become a viable *nefesh*.[117] While Grossnass is tentative on the matter, his *teshuvah* provides some evidence that the opposition to the abortion of a fetus with Tay-Sachs disease, whose mother is not in a life-threatening situation, was not universal.

Given this background, Waldenberg's response to the question before him can only be seen as both bold and decisive:

> In this special case in which the consequences are so grave if the pregnancy and childbirth are allowed to continue, it is permissible to terminate the pregnancy until seven months have elapsed, in a way in which no danger will befall the mother. Beyond seven months, the issue is more serious . . . since at the end of seven months the fetus is often fully developed.

Waldenberg proceeds to cite Maharit and Ya'avetz concerning the permissibility of abortion for the "healing of the mother" or for "great need" in order to save the mother from "great pain." Waldenberg notes that in the adultery case discussed by Ya'avetz, permission for an abortion is grounded in emotional pain rather than any physical threat. He then returns to the case before him:

> Therefore, ask yourself: is there a greater need? Is there greater pain and suffering than that which will be inflicted upon the woman in our case if she gives birth to such a creature whose very being is one of pain and suffering and his death is certain within a few years, and the parents' eyes will witness [the child's agonies] without any capacity to alleviate it? And added to that is the pain and suffering of the infant . . . Hence, if there were a *halakhic* case to permit abortion because of great need and because of pain and suffering, this would seem to be the classic case in which to permit. Moreover, it does not matter what type of pain and suffering is endured, physical or emotional, as emotional pain and suffering is, to a large extent, much greater than physical pain and suffering.

---

[115] All Grossnass references and quotations are from A. Grossnass, *Lev Aryeh*, London, 1973, volume II, number 32.

[116] See above, chapter 3, pp. 90–91.

[117] Grossnass seems to be of the view that the viability of one born with a fatal disease ought to be considered compromised.

Waldenberg proceeds to offer a justification for his permission to abort as late as the seventh month. He acknowledges that Bacharach, in fact, had never made any differentiation between what is permissible before or after the fortieth day or before or after the passage of three months; as far as Bacharach was concerned, the abortion prohibition is always in place.[118] This reality, however, does not deter Waldenberg. "An instance as serious as that which is before us has never arisen in the memory of *halakhic* literature until now," he avers. Hence, to support an abortion so late in the pregnancy, Waldenberg turns to Al-Chakam for *halakhic* backing. From Al-Chakam's tentative statement that grounds exist to abort when "there is a family defect and disgrace and desecration of God's name if the fetus remains and is not aborted," Waldenberg concludes that "great need" is not invoked only for a bodily need of the mother, but includes an emotional need as well.

Parenthetically, it is noteworthy that, as Sinclair observes, Waldenberg's choice of Al-Chakam's *teshuvah* concerning a *mamzer* fetus was made deliberately in order to convey an important parallel: the case of the *mamzer* fetus is analogous to that of the fetus with potential deformities insofar as, in both instances, the chief impact of the fetal condition will be felt after birth, and will present no direct medical threat to the mother.[119] Waldenberg's implication is plain: while permission for abortion usually focuses exclusively on the physical and emotional impact upon the mother herself, this is not the only possible motivation. In the case of the *mamzer* fetus, Al-Chakam's concern centered on "family defect, disgrace and the desecration of God's name." In the same way, Waldenberg intimates, abortion ought to be contemplated for the fetus with Tay-Sachs disease, because of critical considerations that, in themselves, do not portend imminent physical jeopardy for the mother.

As to the issue of timing, the fact that Al-Chakam made his observations in the case of a pregnancy that was in its fifth month, leads Waldenberg to conclude that one can "permit [abortion], because of this [great need], even beyond three months of pregnancy." This conclusion is somewhat surprising given that Al-Chakam had limited himself to observations about the case before him and, in fact, had refused to rule in this manner. Waldenberg, then, uses Al-Chakam's statements as a foundation for a ruling that Al-Chakam explicitly declined to make.

---

[118] Waldenberg previously had relied on an errant understanding of Bacharach. See above, p. 158, n. 94.
[119] Sinclair, "Legal Doctrine and Moral Principle," p. 24.

Perhaps by way of deflecting criticism of this extension, Waldenberg reiterates that the case before him is one of the utmost gravity, far more
wrenching than the instance before Al-Chakam and that he, therefore,
seeks to construct his position on the appropriate time limits of the abortion, "not just [on the basis of] *binyan av* or *gezeirah shavah*, but even more
so from *kal ve-chomer*."[120]

Waldenberg again offers a strenuous refutation of the notion that an
abortion performed to alleviate maternal anguish could possibly constitute the "spilling of blood," before reiterating that an abortion in
the circumstances before him would be acceptable until seven months.
Waldenberg's repetition allows him to suggest that "it might be good
if it were possible for a female doctor to perform the abortion, since
in this way another element would be added that would tend toward
leniency in this matter." The reason that this would be a greater spur toward leniency is that Bacharach and Yaʻavetz had held that the abortion
prohibition was rooted in opposition to the "wanton spilling of seed,"
and women, according to the majority of *poskim*, are not commanded
concerning such spilling.[121] Hence, reasons Waldenberg, for a woman
doctor to perform the abortion would be less *halakhically* objectionable
than for her male counterpart.

It is surely not hyperbole to describe Waldenberg's Tay-Sachs disease
teshuvah as daring. Given the weight of rabbinic opinion, which, in the
previous two decades, had taken a forceful position against abortion in
cases of potential deformity, Waldenberg's stance is audacious. He appears, moreover, to be so sure that the consequences of Tay-Sachs disease
present unique horrors that he is prepared to allow for abortion effectively until the fetus becomes viable. There is no recorded *halakhic* precedent for this. Previously, whenever permission was granted to transcend
the abortion ban – for example, in the circumstance of a direct threat
to the mother's life – such permission generally was applied throughout
the pregnancy, until the onset of labor. Before Waldenberg's *teshuvah*, the
seven-month stage had never represented any type of determined turning
point.[122] Nor had Yaʻavetz's concept of "great need" been stretched quite

---

[120] These are three Talmudic hermeneutical principles. *Binyan av* is the tool of conceptual analogy:
    interpretation based on induction. *Gezeirah shavah* is the tool of linguistic or verbal analogy. *Kal
    ve-chomer* is the tool of *a fortiori* inference: drawing a comparison between two cases, one lenient
    and the other stringent. In this instance, Waldenberg is suggesting that if the law is a particular
    way in the milder case, how much the more so must it be this way in the more serious case.
[121] See above, chapter 3, p. 77.
[122] Rabbi Kassel Abelson, in a paper accepted as the majority opinion of Conservative Judaism's
    Committee on Jewish Law and Standards, explains Waldenberg's extension of abortion per-
    mission till the seventh month as being rooted in practical considerations: "The seventh month

as far as Waldenberg extends it. Waldenberg includes such issues as the mental distress of both parents and the pain and suffering of the infant in his evaluation of "great need," despite the fact that "great need" had not hitherto included such considerations. Plainly, Waldenberg regards the fetus with Tay-Sachs disease as presenting challenges that are sufficiently unparalleled to warrant making exceptions to the conventional *halakhic* boundaries in order to accommodate these unique circumstances. Furthermore, in arriving at his response, Waldenberg employs *halakhic* texts that, in actuality, provide him with little better than tenuous support. In a number of ways, therefore, this *teshuvah* goes beyond the usual evolutionary approach of the *halakhah* and breaks unanticipated ground.

It is hardly unusual for those who forge new approaches to become the subject of direct criticism, and disapproval of Waldenberg's position was soon expressed, despite the fact that reproof is relatively rare within the responsa literature. Given, however, the existence of two opposing viewpoints – one holding that aborting any fetus with potential deformities falls in the category of bloodshed, and the other holding that, at least in the case of a fetus with Tay-Sachs disease, such an act could be justified as a "great need" – the stage was set for a vigorous interchange. Hence, the fact that Waldenberg's position came to be disputed is perhaps less remarkable than the arguments that ultimately were adopted to combat his views.

It was Feinstein who led the opposition to Waldenberg's stance. Written in 1977, Feinstein's ruling on abortion did not emerge in response to any specific question, but rather, as became evident in the course of his writings, in response to Waldenberg.[123] Feinstein addresses his *teshuvah* to his son-in-law, Rabbi Moshe David Tendler, an expert in *halakhah* and bioethics in his own right. The title that Feinstein gave his piece immediately telegraphed his intended direction: "Concerning the abortion of a fetus, [in order] to clarify that it is prohibited even for maternal pain."

Feinstein begins his *teshuvah* by recapitulating that abortion is forbidden to Jews as an extension of the fact that it is prohibited to non-Jews. Feinstein, however, goes further: the reason that the non-Jew is

is allowed in this case, though most abortions would be permissible only in the first trimester, because doctors do not do amniocentesis until the end of the fourth month of pregnancy, when sufficient fluid is available. Most tests of the amniotic fluid then take three or four weeks to complete. Rabbi Waldenberg evidently permits sufficient time for the information to be gathered, a decision to be made by the parents, and the abortion to be performed"; K. Abelson, "Prenatal Testing and Abortion," in *Proceedings of the Committee on Jewish Law and Standards of the Conservative Movement 1980–1985*, New York, The Rabbinical Assembly, 1988, pp. 8–9.

[123] All Feinstein references and quotations are from M. Feinstein, *Iggerot Mosheh*, New York, 1961 and on, *Choshen Mishpat*, volume II, number 69.

prohibited from aborting is because of the prohibition of murder. In fact, avers Feinstein, under most circumstances a non-Jew, like a Jew, is required to ignore any prohibition in the name of *pikuach nefesh*. This is not, however, true when it comes to abortion. In the case of abortion, the ruling applied to the non-Jew against the killing of a fetus derives from the Noahide law against murder, as this is the only applicable injunction of the seven Noahide commandments, and a non-Jew is not bound by anything other than the Noahide laws. It follows, then, that if the killing of the fetus were subsumed under the provisions of murder, setting aside a prohibition on fetal destruction in the name of *pikuach nefesh* would be tantamount to murdering in order to save a life. Since taking one life to save another is unthinkable – "who is to say that your blood is redder than his?" – one must conclude that a non-Jew may not abort even to save the life of the mother. A Jew would be required to set aside the prohibition and save the mother, but only because the laws of *rodef* apply to a Jew. If the fetus were not behaving as a *rodef*, the legal outcome for Jew and non-Jew would be little different. Hence, Feinstein conveys, if the prohibition on Jewish abortion stems from the prohibition on non-Jewish abortion, then the prohibition on Jewish abortion must likewise be rooted in the prohibition of murder. Just as Unterman had done, Feinstein elects to classify abortion in a more extreme way than had been made explicit within any pre-modern stance.

Feinstein finds textual support for his position that a Jew is prevented from killing a fetus because of the prohibition of murder in the *Tosafot* to *Sanhedrin*.[124] While his reading of the *Tosafot* to *Sanhedrin* has been debated, a far greater challenge to Feinstein is how to deal with the *Tosafot* to *Niddah*, which records that, in the case of a Jew, "*mutar lehorgo*" (it is permitted to kill it [the fetus]). Feinstein, however, does not find the *Tosafot* to *Niddah* problematic at all. "It is simple and obvious," he writes, "that it is a scribal error..." Rather than reading "*mutar lehorgo*," opines Feinstein, the text should read "*patur hahorgo*" (one who kills it [the fetus] is not liable to execution). In order to justify this emendation, Feinstein advances some credible arguments: the *Tosafot* to *Niddah*, he observes, in part reads, "because of *pikuach nefesh* we transgress the *Shabbat* for [the fetus'] sake, even though it is permitted to kill it, as in the case of a *goses be-yedei adam*, when one who kills him is not liable..." The analogy to the *goses be-yedei adam* is instructional, argues Feinstein. After all, Feinstein maintains, notwithstanding other attempts to make sense

---

[124] The various *Tosafot* selections can be found above, chapter 3, pp. 62ff.

of this sentence,[125] the *goses be-yedei adam* analogy is only intelligible if
the intention in the case of the fetus, just as for the *goses*, is that one
who kills him is not liable.[126] Moreover, asks Feinstein, how is one to
explain the approval for transgressing *Shabbat* if one is "permitted to kill"
the fetus? If there is indeed permission to kill the fetus, then this would
imply that transgression of *Shabbat* is a voluntary matter: one might
decide to kill the fetus, or one might decide to transgress the *Shabbat* and
save the fetus. But transgression of the *Shabbat* is not voluntary, writes
Feinstein: "Any desecration of *Shabbat* that is permitted in order to save
somebody is obligatory and not voluntary." Hence, Feinstein holds, from
this perspective too, the *Tosafot* to *Niddah* can only be comprehended
logically if the sentence reads "*patur hahorgo*" (one who kills it [the fetus] is
not liable to execution) implying that, while transgression of the *Shabbat*
is obligatory, failure to transgress the *Shabbat* would not incur capital
punishment.

Feinstein, then, does not see any inconsistency among the various
Tosafot texts: the *Tosafists* were of one mind that there is an extant prohibition on fetal destruction that is grounded in the prohibition of murder. Moreover, Maimonides, Feinstein states, also had no doubt that
"the killing of a fetus is actual murder." Maimonides' *rodef* argument,
Feinstein holds, shows that the prohibition on killing the fetus is "like
actual murder," and that, therefore, it would be prohibited to kill the
fetus without a positive duty to save one being pursued. Indeed, so persuaded is Feinstein of the rectitude of Maimonides' position in this regard
that he goes to great lengths to defend the Rambam. Washofsky provides
a succinct summary of the defense strategies offered by Feinstein:

He [Feinstein] dismisses as "worthless" the suggestion that Rambam could possibly be wrong in his explanation of the warrant for abortion. Maimonides, after
all, was a great scholar, and to claim that he was imprecise in his interpretation of
Sanhedrin 72b is to show "contempt for all the rulings of Rambam throughout his
Code." To support Rambam's reading of the *sugya*, Feinstein proffers a formal
rule of decision-making: we are not entitled to reject the rulings of the Rambam
merely because we find them difficult. Who among us, after all, is worthy to
disagree with him? His great contemporaries, men such as Avraham b. David of
Posquierres who *are* worthy to express disagreement, do not object to this ruling.
And if some of the very latest authorities (*acharonei haʾacharonim*) do object, we have

[125] See above, chapter 3, p. 64.
[126] Understood this way, the *Tosafot* to *Niddah* would read as an exact parallel: "[B]ecause of *pikuach*
nefesh we transgress the *Shabbat* for [the fetus'] sake, even though one who kills him is not liable,
as in the case of a *goses be-yedei adam* when one who kills him is not liable . . ."

but to remember that Haim Soloveitchik, the greatest of all recent sages (*maran dedorot haàharonim shelifaneinu*), has sufficiently explained Rambam's position.[127]

By invoking Soloveitchik, it is clear that Feinstein is interested in defending not only Maimonides' position but, more particularly, the most stringent interpretation of that position. What is most interesting, however, is Feinstein's determination to elicit conformity with the Rambam. As Washofsky demonstrates, Feinstein's technique, while theoretically acceptable, represents an attempt at *halakhic* compulsion that is open to vigorous debate.[128] There are, after all, *halakhic* scholars of renown who are quite prepared to disagree with Maimonides on this issue, and who rule against him on any number of matters, based on their own assessment of the Talmudic evidence. Their freedom in this regard was never taken to represent any type of monolithic rejection of Maimonides' Code as a whole. Furthermore, through the centuries, the sages showed no tendency to cleave dutifully to any one viewpoint. As Washofsky observes, "[i]t is this independence, and not adherence to the views of one particular authority, that has characterized the abortion debate in the *halakhic* literature."[129]

Strenuous support for Maimonides' position is, then, at the core of Feinstein's approach. However, Feinstein by no means ignores Rashi. In fact, he sees no contradiction whatsoever between the views of Rashi and Maimonides. Like Meltzer before him, Feinstein is of the view that, in a situation of *extremis*, both mother and fetus ought properly to be seen as *rodfim* to one another.[130] Given this outlook, Rashi's understanding – that the fetus is not a *nefesh* – is necessary, Feinstein contends, in order to ascertain the superior status of the mother vis-à-vis the fetus and to permit the killing of the fetus as a *rodef* to a *nefesh*. Hence, Feinstein concludes, the *Tosafot*, Maimonides, and Rashi all agree that, as concerns the killing of a fetus, there is a prohibition of murder involved, a prohibition that finds its original roots in the *lo tirtzach* (you shall not murder – Exodus 20:13) provision of the Ten Commandments. Therefore, Feinstein infers, the killing of a fetus is completely prohibited, even for the sake of *pikuach nefesh*, with the exception that one must save the life of the mother "so that she does not die in childbirth." An abortion "for any need of the mother" short of saving her life certainly is not permitted.

Nonetheless, contends Feinstein, the provisions of *pikuach nefesh* dictate the transgression of *Shabbat*, or other commandments, even in cases of

---

[127] Washofsky, "Abortion and the Halakhic Conversation," p. 52.   [128] *Ibid.*, pp. 53–54.
[129] *Ibid.*, p. 54.   [130] See above, chapter 4, p. 105.

"remote doubt" that a life can be saved. But this is not the standard to be applied when considering whether a mother's life needs to be defended by means of abortion. Given that the life of the fetus is at stake, avers Feinstein, the doctors have to be "close to certain" that the mother will die if they take no action, before an abortion would be permitted. The reason for this is that in order for an abortion to be acceptable, the doctors are permitted to kill the fetus only on the basis that the fetus is behaving as a *rodef*. Hence, unless the doctors are certain that it is actually "pursuing" its mother, no grounds would exist to kill it. Feinstein immediately proceeds from this conclusion to the following observation:

It is clear, moreover, that there is, according to this, no difference between newborns. Even in the case of those newborns who, in the view of the doctors, are of the type who will not live for many years, like those children who are born with a disease called Tay-Sachs – even if it is known by means of fetal testing, which has just now become possible, that the newborn will be in this category – [abortion is] prohibited. Since there is no danger to the mother, and the fetus is not a *rodef*, one may not permit [an abortion] even though the pain will be very great, and the mother and father will suffer from this. And for this reason, I have said to Torah-observant doctors that they should not perform this test [Tay-Sachs screening], for there will be no benefit from it, since they will be forbidden to abort the fetus, and it will only cause pain to the father and to the mother, and they might also go to a non-Jewish doctor, not observant of Torah, to abort [the fetus], and will thereby transgress [the negative commandment of] "do not place a stumbling-block before the blind."

Feinstein's absolute opposition to the abortion of a fetus with Tay-Sachs disease at any point during pregnancy, let alone up to the seventh month, could hardly be plainer.

Feinstein, however, goes further. He next turns his attention to a critique of the writings of Bacharach, Maharit, Al-Chakam, and Yaʿavetz, among others. In the case of Bacharach, Feinstein, while satisfied with Bacharach's conclusion, is disturbed by the differentiation that Bacharach posited between a fetus before and after the onset of labor.[131] Bacharach had held that it is only with the onset of labor, when the fetus becomes a "separate body," that killing it would be considered a transgression. Despite the fact that Bacharach had grounded his view in more than one text, Feinstein sees Bacharach's distinction as being influenced heavily by the *Tosafot* to *Niddah* that Feinstein already had declared to be erroneous. The distinction between fetal standing before labor and after the onset of labor is a differentiation that Feinstein does not accept.

---

[131] See above, chapter 3, pp. 74–75.

Hence, he is content that, at least in practical terms, Bacharach derives no implications from it.

A far more difficult conundrum for Feinstein is that presented by the two seemingly contradictory responsa of Maharit.[132] Feinstein, however, is certain that a contradiction of this magnitude could not possibly exist in the writings of Maharit. His strategy for resolving this problem is, therefore, to accept Maharit's *teshuvah* number 97 at face value, while mounting a series of challenges to the more permissive *teshuvah* number 99. It is not possible, Feinstein contends, that Maharit would have thought that there is not the "faintest suggestion" of homicide when a Jew takes the life of a fetus. Moreover, how is it conceivable that Maharit "did not recall Maimonides, who permits abortion – in the case of a woman in life-threatening difficulty during childbirth – only because it is a *rodef*, and the *Tosafot*, who forbid abortion on the grounds that it is prohibited to gentiles"? All of this demonstrates, Feinstein declares, that "this *teshuvah* [number 99] is to be ignored, for it is undoubtedly a forgery, compiled by an errant disciple and falsely ascribed to him [Maharit]." Furthermore, even were both *teshuvot* genuine, it would be incumbent upon us to follow the more conservative approach of Maharit that forbids abortion. This strategy, however, is not necessary, Feinstein continues, for there is further evidence of the forgery. As previously noted, despite the fact that he had searched, Unterman had been unable to locate the responsum of Rashba, described in *teshuvah* number 99, that portrayed the way in which Nachmanides had rendered assistance to a gentile woman to abort.[133] The reason for this, Feinstein avers, is that there is no such Rashba *teshuvah*. Rather, this alleged *teshuvah* is also a product of the forger, who wrote it "to fabricate and to mislead." Since Feinstein is, however, aware of the fact that others had treated the Rashba *teshuvah* as if it were authentic, he adds that even if it were a "true" responsum, one ought, nevertheless, to follow the lead of Unterman in regarding Rashba's precedent as being intended for the first forty days of gestation only.[134]

Feinstein, then, is clearly of the view that Maharit's *teshuvah* number 99 requires no response whatsoever, but may be dismissed summarily as being counterfeit. Feinstein does not give a great deal more credence to the *teshuvah* of Al-Chakam. In the case of Al-Chakam, however, the problem that Feinstein discerns is neither one of scribal error nor forgery, but rather an instance of incomplete scholarship. Feinstein, perturbed

---

[132] See above, chapter 3, pp. 68ff.   [133] See above, p. 141.   [134] See above, p. 142.

by Al-Chakam's partial citation of the words of *Chavvot Ya'ir*, his failure to mention the conclusions of *Tosafot Chullin* and Maimonides, and his discussion of Maharit's *teshuvah* number 99 without detailing *teshuvah* number 97, ventures that Al-Chakam had not had access to the requisite books to allow for a full response. Hence, Feinstein advises, "one ought not to rely on his words at all."

Before turning his attention to Ya'avetz, Feinstein makes observations about the *teshuvot* of Weinberg, Grodzinsky, and Unterman, arguing against permissive features in the writings of each one. For example, Feinstein forcefully rejects Weinberg's claim that "the majority of the *Rishonim* differ with Maimonides" so that "it is possible that [one ought] to permit" even if the mother is not in immediate danger. This is an empty and untrue contention, Feinstein holds, because even those who rely on Rashi hold that the killing of a fetus is a Toraitic prohibition, based in the laws of murder. Grodzinsky's position that Maimonides intended that the *rodef* principle be applied only when the fetus has become a "separate body," is similarly rebuffed by Feinstein. "This is not correct at all," states Feinstein, as Maimonides gave no hint of making any such differentiation between fetuses. Even Unterman, with whom Feinstein generally concurs on this issue, was, in Feinstein's view, imprecise when he described a forced abortion – like that requested of the doctor in the First World War[135] – as an "appurtenance of the spilling of blood." It is murder pure and simple, opines Feinstein, albeit not of the type that would warrant capital punishment. Finally, Feinstein repels any notion that Ya'avetz's prominent permissive *teshuvah* could be taken seriously. Ya'avetz's logic, which allows for the killing of a *mamzer* fetus based in the laws of the death penalty, is "worthless," states Feinstein, "even though written by a man as great as Ya'avetz." Feinstein proceeds to cast doubt upon Ya'avetz's entire reasoning process and arrives at the declaration that "one may not rely on this *teshuvah*."

One by one, Feinstein attempts to dismantle the arguments of those who would allow for abortion under any circumstances other than an undeniable threat posed by the fetus to the life of the mother. It is not until the final paragraph, however, that Feinstein reveals a pressing motivation for his approach:

I have written all this because of the great outbreak of licentious behavior, in that the governments of many countries have allowed the killing of fetuses, among them political leaders of the State of Israel, and countless fetuses have

---

[135] See above, chapter 4, p. 119.

already been killed. Hence, at this time, there is a need to make a fence for the Torah, and not to undermine this most serious prohibition against murder. I was, therefore, horrified to see the *teshuvah* of a learned man in *Eretz Yisrael* ... who permits the abortion of a Tay-Sachs fetus, even beyond three months. He proposed that the nature of [the ban on] fetal destruction, in the eyes of many *poskim*, was rabbinic, and even if it were biblical, that it was instituted as a fence, but that there is not the slightest hint of murder (*ibbud nefashot*) involved. From Maharit, he cited *teshuvah* number 99 that permits [abortion], but did not mention that in number 97 [Maharit] forbids. On the contrary, he wrote that even in *teshuvah* number 97 [Maharit] permits. Moreover, based on the language "and even with a legitimate fetus, there is reason to be permissive where there is 'great need'," he wrote that *Sheèilat Yaàvetz* permits [abortion], even though he [Yaàvetz] explicitly prohibited. It is clear and simple that the language "there is reason to be permissive," conveys that there are many more reasons to prohibit [abortion], as Yaàvetz concluded. And, concerning the *teshuvah* in *Rav Paàlim* [Al-Chakam], on the basis of which he [the learned man] saw fit to rule that one is permitted to abort in the case of Tay-Sachs until the seventh month, this time-period is incomprehensible, and [I] have not found it at all. It is clear and simple, as I wrote, that in the *halakhah*, which is made clear by the *Rishonim*, the *mefarshim*, and the *poskim*, abortion is prohibited as it is considered actual murder, whether the fetus is pure or illegitimate, whether they are regular fetuses or those known to be afflicted with Tay-Sachs – it is strictly prohibited; and do not err and rely on the *teshuvot* of that learned man.

It becomes obvious in the course of this closing paragraph that a fundamental cause impelling Feinstein's *halakhic* writings on this matter is his deep concern over the proliferation of abortion brought about by legal liberalization. Moreover, when Feinstein declares, "there is a need to make a fence...," it becomes plain that he cannot countenance that the *halakhah*, in even the smallest measure, would lend a hand to such murderous "licentiousness." Hence, although Feinstein never mentions his name, his offensive against Waldenberg's position is perhaps as unbridled as it is because Feinstein refuses to tolerate the notion that *halakhic* sages could be perceived as contributing in any way to the pervasive culture of permissiveness. In the words of Sinclair, "Feinstein's own remarks are a sufficient indication of this strong concern for the decline in moral standards following in the wake of liberal abortion legislation, and it is, therefore, more than likely that it is this concern which is the operative factor in his analysis of the law."[136]

Feinstein's remarkable *teshuvah* did not pass without a reply. In his fifth foray into the abortion arena, Waldenberg retorts in a direct and

[136] D. B. Sinclair, *Tradition and the Biological Revolution*, Edinburgh, Edinburgh University Press, 1989, Appendix A, p. 96.

detailed fashion to Feinstein's analysis.[137] Waldenberg begins by disputing Feinstein's claim that the *Tosafists* were of one mind in considering the prohibition on fetal destruction to be grounded in the biblical prohibition of murder. There is an ongoing difference of opinion among the rabbis, writes Waldenberg, as to whether the prohibition is biblical or rabbinic. Perhaps even more importantly, Waldenberg cites several examples to show that there is absolutely no concurrence regarding the reason behind the prohibition – scholars throughout the centuries had provided a range of rationales.

Waldenberg next turns his attention to Feinstein's claim that the *Tosafot* to *Niddah* contains a critical scribal error that mistakenly appears to permit fetal destruction. Here, Waldenberg "sharply rebukes Feinstein for this tactic, in language rarely heard in *halakhic* argument."[138] In Waldenberg's words:

> With all respect, no sir. This is not the way. We live by the words of the great sages of the generations, each of whom has toiled in his own way to clarify and to reconcile the intent of the words of *Tosafot Niddah*. And not one of them ever thought to take the easy way out (*haderekh hapeshutah beyoter*) and say there is a scribal error in the *Tosafot*, that in place of *mutar* it ought to read *asur*.

Rejecting Feinstein's solution, Waldenberg points out that various authorities have grappled with and explained the *Tosafot* to *Niddah* in differing ways. Some took the view that this *Tosafot* was evidence that the prohibition was not Torah-based. However, none had ever even hinted at the notion that erroneous transcription was involved. Waldenberg, moreover, denies that permission to override the *Shabbat* in order to save a fetus suggests that one is not allowed to take the life of the fetus. Following Nachmanides, he avers that such overriding is accepted for the sake of the fetus' future potential and not because of its current status.

Waldenberg proceeds to counter Feinstein by expressing astonishment at Feinstein's perspective on Maimonides. In Waldenberg's view, Feinstein's position that Maimonides' use of the *rodef* category was founded in the prohibition on murder and allowed for the killing of the fetus only when there was an absolute certainty that the mother would die on account of the fetus, completely disregards the *halakhic* history to the contrary. Articulating his disbelief that Feinstein could have either "ignored" or "not noticed" the positions of numerous *poskim*, among

---

[137] References and quotations concerning this Waldenberg *teshuvah* are from *Tzitz Eliezer*, Jerusalem, 1985, volume XIV, number 100.
[138] Washofsky, "Abortion and the Halakhic Conversation," p. 54.

them some who "lived close to the period of the *Rishonim*," Waldenberg asks how Feinstein simply overlooks all those who took the opposite
point of view. Citing many texts from the tradition, among them that of
Zimra,[139] Waldenberg extensively illustrates that many authorities who
sought to be faithful to Maimonides did not perceive Maimonides as
holding feticide to be murder, explained Maimonides' use of the *rodef*
provision in a variety of ways, and, at times, regarded the fetus' lack of
nefesh status as the fundamental foundation that allowed for abortion.

Turning from Feinstein's handling of Maimonides to his approach to
the two *teshuvot* of Maharit, Waldenberg does not attempt to conceal his
incredulity:

> And what does Feinstein do with the words of Maharit? He again takes the easy
> way out (*haderekh hapeshutah be-yoter*), and writes that one simply may not rely on
> this *teshuvah* [number 99] at all, since it is obvious that it is a forged *teshuvah* from
> some errant student, and he [the student] wrote it in his [Maharit's] name.
>
> And I cry: Amazement! Amazement! How can one excise a whole *teshuvah* of
> Maharit on the strength of such a fanciful supposition? This would be so even
> were there no evidence to counter his assertion; yet that evidence exists.

Demonstration of the validity of both responsa, Waldenberg asserts,
comes from the fact that Rabbi Chaim Benveniste, the well-known and
highly respected student of Maharit,[140] cited both *teshuvot* in his glosses
to the *Shulchan Arukh*, and did not see them as contradictory. Moreover,
Waldenberg points out, just as Benveniste had arrived at a satisfactory
reconciliation of the two responsa without resorting to a forgery explanation, so Waldenberg himself had explained within his volume IX *teshuvah*
how the two pieces "complete each other."[141] This leads Waldenberg to
observe, "[a]nd Feinstein never saw the things I wrote on this in volume
IX ... and therefore he gratuitously suspected that I did not recall what
Maharit prohibits in *teshuvah* 97."

Waldenberg proceeds to marvel at the way in which Feinstein substan-
tiated his forgery allegation, a substantiation that necessitated positing
that Rashba's *teshuvah*, concerning Nachmanides' assistance to a gentile
woman, did not exist. The *teshuvah* – *Teshuvot HaRashba* 1:120 – most
certainly exists, Waldenberg declares, but both Feinstein and Unterman
misunderstood Maharit's use of it. Feinstein and Unterman were confused because Rashba's *teshuvah* actually refers to Nachmanides' provision of paid medical assistance to a gentile woman in childbirth, but

---

[139] See above, chapter 3, p. 67.   [140] See above, chapter 3, p. 72, n. 63.
[141] See above, pp. 160ff.

not to abortion. It was Maharit, explains Waldenberg, not Rashba, who made the connection to abortion. It was Maharit who extrapolated from Rashba's report to aver that not only is abortion not to be considered as homicide for a Jew, it is not to be considered as homicide for a gentile either.[142] Waldenberg is plainly in no doubt that Rashba's *teshuvah* is no more fictional than is either of Maharit's. Summarizing his outlook on Maharit, Waldenberg reaffirms that Maharit saw no trace of murder involved in the killing of a fetus and permitted abortion for the sake of the mother's healing, even if no imminent danger to the mother was anticipated.

Turning to a defense of Al-Chakam, Waldenberg writes that Feinstein has wronged this learned and pious sage. It is possible, Waldenberg posits, that Feinstein's attitude to Al-Chakam stems from never actually having seen Al-Chakam's *teshuvah*. For it is plain in the *teshuvah* that, contrary to Feinstein's assertion, Al-Chakam does cite both *teshuvot* of Maharit, but prefers to rely on *teshuvah* number 99, the *teshuvah* that permits abortion for the need of the mother. There is not the slightest hint, Waldenberg avows, that Al-Chakam lacked books, and Feinstein, therefore, had no cogent justification for dismissing Al-Chakam.[143]

Finally, Waldenberg deals with Feinstein's interpretation of the position of Ya'avetz. While Waldenberg expresses his own difficulty with Ya'avetz's logic permitting the destruction of a fetus destined to be a *mamzer*, this has no bearing on his acceptance of Ya'avetz's approach to an untainted fetus. Waldenberg makes a strong case that Feinstein's contention that "it is clear and simple that [Ya'avetz's] language [to the effect that] 'there is [a] reason to be permissive,' conveys that there are many more reasons to prohibit abortion," is simply not borne out by the sources. Citing an array of *teshuvot*, Waldenberg opposes Feinstein's dismissal of Ya'avetz by showing the extent to which the "permissive reason" was broadly invoked. All of this leads Waldenberg to the unwavering conclusion that, Feinstein's objections notwithstanding, a fetus with Tay-Sachs disease may indeed be aborted until the seventh month of pregnancy. Waldenberg again emphasizes that because Jews are imbued with a particular sense of holiness, they should never treat abortion lightly, but neither should cases of "great need" ever be ignored.

---

[142] See above, chapter 3, p. 70.
[143] Sinclair ("Legal Doctrine and Moral Principle," p. 27), supporting Waldenberg's view, makes the additional observation that "In any case, Yosef Hayyim's library was both extensive and wide-ranging and something of a legend among Baghdadi Jews."

Waldenberg however, was by no means alone in reacting to the unusual features of Feinstein's *teshuvah*. In fact, Feldman, clearly troubled by Feinstein's *teshuvah*, hinted at the possibility that Feinstein himself was not the author of the *teshuvah* published in his name.[144] Feldman reflects that "[t]he ruling, and, more important, the reasoning and the development of the argument, even making its point by imputing scribal errors to accepted rabbinic texts," are "all so uncharacteristic of the writings of Rabbi Feinstein..."[145] This opinion led Feldman to report that "a doctoral thesis analyzing the responsum concluded that if Feinstein is indeed its author, he was writing more in the mode of admonitory sermon than legal disquisition."[146] That doctoral thesis, however, written by Sinclair, was not nearly so explicit. Sinclair's most direct statement on the matter holds that:

It is unusual for a halakhic dispute to be resolved by declaring inconvenient sources to be forgeries, and the employment of such tactics raises doubts as to the legal integrity of the argument as a whole. (In any case, Feinstein's own remarks are a sufficient indication of this strong concern for the decline in moral standards following in the wake of liberal abortion legislation, and it is therefore more than likely that it is this concern which is the operative factor in his analysis of the law.)[147]

At the very least, then, Feldman and Sinclair harbor deep methodological concerns about Feinstein's *teshuvah*.[148] It was, however, Feinstein's conclusion, rather than his methodology, which seems more to have troubled Jakobovits. Writing in a 1976 article, Jakobovits wonders why those who take Feinstein's position ignore "the more permissive verdicts given by other rabbis," such as Weinberg, Yisraeli, and Grossnass.[149]

One more Tay-Sachs *teshuvah* appeared as the controversy began to subside. In the early 1980s, Freehof was asked about the reaction of "traditional law" to someone refusing to participate in a Tay-Sachs counseling program.[150] In the course of answering the question, he makes the following observation about the abortion of a fetus afflicted with

---

[144] Feldman, *Birth Control*, p. 346.
[145] Of course, even if this *teshuvah* were "uncharacteristic of the writings" of Feinstein, his 1973 *teshuvah* (see above, p. 165) provided corroboration that if the 1977 *teshuvah* was not penned by him, it was certainly not at odds with his position.
[146] Feldman, *Birth Control*, p. 346.   [147] Sinclair, *Tradition and the Biological Revolution*, p. 96.
[148] For more on Sinclair's reservations, see below, chapter 7, pp. 244–245.
[149] I. Jakobovits, "Tay-Sachs Disease and the Jewish Community," *Proceedings of the Association of Orthodox Jewish Scientists*, volumes 3–4, 1976: 16–17.
[150] "The Tay-Sachs Program," in S. Freehof, *Today's Reform Responsa*, Cincinnati, The Hebrew Union College Press, 1990, pp. 47–51.

Tay-Sachs disease: "When we consider, in the situation involved in our present discussion, the anguish that would come to parents if a fetus afflicted with Tay-Sachs would be born and die very soon thereafter, it would surely be a true benefit to the parents if…the fetus were destroyed by abortion."[151] While Freehof writes generally here about the "anguish" of "parents," he clarifies exactly what he means by this at the end of the *teshuvah*. In the case of Tay-Sachs disease, he contends, the law "would permit abortion if it is clearly for the mother's benefit." Freehof, then, continues to hold that abortion can only be countenanced if it is designed to address acute maternal suffering, but not for the sake of the fetus alone. Freehof's permissive response is one more piece of evidence that the vigorous Tay-Sachs interchange had sharpened and deepened the philosophical divide on the question of abortion in the case of fetal abnormalities.

THE POST-TAY-SACHS LANDSCAPE

With the Tay-Sachs debate concluded, Waldenberg, in yet one more abortion *teshuvah*, responded to an additional inquiry from Professor Meir, this time on the subject of whether it is permitted to abort a fetus that is afflicted with Down's syndrome.[152] Unlike Tay-Sachs disease, Down's syndrome is not a fatal condition, there is no excruciating physical suffering, and, while it does result in physical and intellectual deficiencies, individuals afflicted with Down's syndrome can live lives that are filled with human relationship and love.[153] Thus, for those *poskim* who are prepared to consider abortion in cases of fetal abnormalities, the question of aborting a fetus afflicted with Down's syndrome can be an even more anguished one than that for Tay-Sachs disease. This is clearly true for Waldenberg. While he is prepared to allow for the abortion of a fetus afflicted with Down's syndrome, based on the same textual foundations that he used in the case of Tay-Sachs disease, Waldenberg is careful to stress that, in this instance, he is not providing any type of general opinion. Rather, the decision whether an abortion may or may not proceed can only be made by a suitably ordained rabbi. Waldenberg

---

[151] *Ibid.*, p. 49.
[152] References and quotations concerning this Waldenberg *teshuvah* are from *Tzitz Eliezer*, Jerusalem, 1985, volume XIV, number 101.
[153] B. Kelly (medical ed.), *Family Health and Medical Guide*, Dallas, Word Publishing, 1996, p. 650, defines Down's syndrome as "[a] genetic disorder characterized by some degree of mental retardation and by various physical malformations, such as slanted eyes and a broad face."

describes Down's syndrome as being a condition that is "very undesirable" with invidious physical and mental consequences that can lead to a shortened life. Moreover, he regards it as an affliction "serious enough in many instances to cause destruction to the mental condition of the woman and her husband together," or to bring about mild or serious illness, or to interfere with normal relations between a husband and wife.

Conversely, Waldenberg is also cognizant that the prospect of Down's syndrome does not necessarily imbue a sense of hopelessness in every family. He cites the case of a couple who preferred that their fetus not be tested and were prepared for the possible consequences, as well as the case of a family that lovingly raised children affected by Down's syndrome, to emphasize that a decision in the case of a fetus with Down's syndrome cannot ignore family circumstances. Hence, only a competent rabbi, who is willing to weigh the *halakhic*, familial, and health considerations before him, is able to decide whether an abortion is appropriate in a particular instance of Down's syndrome.

Waldenberg's Down's syndrome *teshuvah* is far more tentative than his *teshuvah* on Tay-Sachs disease. In the case of Tay-Sachs disease, too, Waldenberg left it up to the individual rabbi to rule whether an abortion is warranted. However, his vigorous support for the legitimacy of abortion in cases of Tay-Sachs disease – all the way to the seventh month of pregnancy – provides a strong indication to the local rabbi that he would do well to rule in a lenient direction. In the case of Down's syndrome, though, Waldenberg simply affirms that the textual heritage would allow for an abortion to proceed and calls upon the local rabbi to determine whether the actual situation before him merits the invocation of the *halakhic* permission. Thus, his response accommodates abortion, but with none of the decisiveness evident for Tay-Sachs disease. Nevertheless, just as in his Tay-Sachs *teshuvah*, Waldenberg bases his reply on a range of familial concerns, including, but not limited to, the mother's mental well-being. For example, Waldenberg mentions issues like family deterioration which, though extremely testing, may not threaten the mother's mental stability. Once again, it is clear that Waldenberg understands the "great need" of the mother in a rather broad sense.

Rabbis who tended toward leniency, like Waldenberg, took one of two different approaches in weighing the interests of individuals beyond the mother. There were some, like Weinberg, who based their inclination to permit abortions in cases of fetal abnormalities upon the age-old *halakhic* argument that the well-being of the mother needed to be protected. According to this view, in order to safeguard the mental health of a woman who cannot cope with the bearing or the raising of an abnormal child, abortions should be allowed. Such abortions, though, would only be countenanced in those circumstances that involve an undeniable mental health threat to the mother. The second approach, discernible in the responsa of Yisraeli and Waldenberg, went further. It took the well-being of the fetus, and the prospects for its future pain and suffering, as possibly constituting a sufficiently important independent warrant for abortion, even if the mother were not *in extremis*. This latter view clearly opened the door to considering abortions in a far broader range of situations than would otherwise be conceivable.

Rabbi Walter Jacob, the successor to Freehof as the preeminent author of responsa for the American Reform community, used both approaches. In 1985, Jacob was asked about the timing of abortion.[154] In the course of a response that offers rulings on a variety of abortion issues,[155] Jacob writes, "[S]uch problems, as those caused by Tay-Sachs and other degenerative or permanent conditions which seriously endanger the life of the child and potentially the mental health of the mother, are indications for permitting an abortion."[156] The word "potentially" is significant in this sentence. If, after all, the "indications for permitting an abortion" include a "potential" endangerment to the mother's mental health, it would seem difficult to deny that such a potential is usually present in cases of fetal defects. Effectively, therefore, Jacob is prepared to allow abortions for a range of "degenerative or permanent conditions which seriously endanger the life of the child," no matter what the mother's actual mental state might be. It is not possible, from Jacob's words in this *teshuvah*, to discern how he might respond to fetal circumstances that are not life threatening, such as Down's syndrome. Nor does Jacob articulate exactly what he means by "endangering." After all, it is true that Tay-Sachs disease endangers the life of the child, but it usually does so after the transition of several years. Other genetic conditions endanger life, but only after several decades.[157] Would Jacob include these conditions as sufficiently endangering to permit abortion? This uncertainty notwithstanding, it seems that, like Waldenberg, Jacob's criterion for this type of abortion would permit the termination of pregnancy based on

[154] "When Is Abortion Permitted?," in W. Jacob, *Contemporary American Reform Responsa*, New York, 1987, # 16, pp. 23–27.
[155] For further discussion of this *teshuvah* see below, p. 204.
[156] W. Jacob, "When Is Abortion Permitted?," p. 27.
[157] Huntington's disease is an example of this phenomenon. For further discussion of this issue, see below, pp. 188–189.

fetal considerations, even if the mother's mental health is not substantially jeopardized.

Jacob, though, responds a little differently in a subsequent 1988 *teshuvah* about the abortion of an anencephalic fetus.[158] Here Jacob rules that "[a]n anencephalic fetus may be aborted under certain circumstances. The principal consideration, however, should be the condition of the mother and any danger, psychological or physical, which this fetus may pose."[159] In this *teshuvah*, unlike that of 1985, Jacob proposes that the "principal consideration" in contemplating an abortion should be maternal "danger." It is not hard to understand why Jacob's focus shifts towards the mother in this instance. As he states, "the anencephalic infant cannot survive for long."[160] Hence, since the swift demise of the fetus is sure, there is virtually no "life of the child" to be "endangered," and so maternal considerations logically come to the fore. From Jacob's previous *teshuvah*, however, it may still be safely assumed that where the fetus, once born, is expected to have some time to live, Jacob would permit abortion based on the anticipated nature of that life, even if the mother is not in demonstrable "danger." There is, then, something of a divergence on this point between the positions of Freehof and Jacob.

Yet another *teshuvah* written under Reform auspices reiterated the requirement that the mother be *in extremis* in order to justify an abortion. In 1995, the responsa committee of the Reform movement's rabbinic body, the Central Conference of American Rabbis, was asked whether a handicapped fetus might be aborted as a result of concerns that its prospective life "would impose an undue hardship on... other children who would be burdened by caring for this child in the future." The questioner continued: "The distinction is that the abortion would not be done to spare the mother suffering, but rather to spare the anguish of other family members."[161] After tracing the textual history, the responsa committee concluded:

Fetal life, though of lesser status than that of the mother, remains human life in potential, and is consequently of great significance. It can only be sacrificed for the most profound of reasons. Speculation and worry about the future are natural aspects of living, but do not themselves constitute a threat to the health

---

[158] "The Abortion of an Anencephalic Fetus," in W. Jacob, *Questions and Reform Jewish Answers: New American Reform Responsa*, New York, 1992, # 155, p. 253. An anencephalic fetus is one suffering from a congenital absence of most of the brain and spinal cord.

[159] *Ibid.*   [160] *Ibid.*

[161] W. G. Plaut and M. Washofsky (eds.), *Teshuvot for the Nineties: Reform Judaism's Answers for Today's Dilemmas*, New York, 1997, p. 171.

of the mother sufficient to justify the termination of unborn life. Hence, Judaism could not give its assent to an abortion under these circumstances. If serious maternal anguish were the result of genuine fears over a defined handicap, then abortion could be contemplated, but certainly not for the sake of 'hardship' or 'quality of life' issues for other family members. It is the degree to which the mother is suffering 'great pain' which remains determinative; the consideration of the anguish of others within the family is not pertinent to the question of an abortion.[162]

This statement reaffirms that maternal suffering is the pivotal issue. The potential torment that might be experienced by others as the result of the birth of an abnormal fetus cannot, according to this source, be determinative of the appropriateness of an abortion. This stance conforms well with the position articulated by Freehof.

However, a similar position to that taken by Jacob was expressed within two papers that became authoritative *halakhic* positions of Conservative Judaism, and therefore carried considerable influence.[163] The first, written by Rabbi Kassel Abelson, deals specifically with the issue of prenatal testing for fetal abnormalities, and concludes as follows:

There is clear precedent in the tradition, as it has developed to our day, to permit abortion of a fetus to save a mother's life, to safeguard her health, or even for "a very thin reason," such as to spare her physical pain or mental anguish. Some recent authorities also consider the well-being of other children, and the future of the fetus itself as reasons to permit abortion. All agree that there *must be a reason* to justify the destruction of the potential person the fetus will become after birth.

Where there is reason to believe that the fetus may be defective, it is advisable for the mother to go to her obstetrician and undergo amniocentesis and/or other prenatal tests. If the tests indicate that the child will be born with major defects which would preclude a normal life, and which make the mother and the family anxious about the future, it is permitted to abort the fetus.[164]

Abelson's ruling clearly considers the mental anguish of the mother, but places much greater emphasis on concerns over fetal defects that might interfere with "normal life." Abelson's viewpoint is, in fact, far more sweeping than that of Waldenberg, because it is not limited to

[162] *Ibid.*, p. 176.
[163] Orthodox *teshuvot* respond to individual cases and may or may not come to be precedents for later deliberations. Reform *teshuvot* are advisory in nature, and their rulings are not binding on the questioner or anybody else. Conservative *halakhic* papers, however, once they have been adopted by a majority of the Conservative movement's Committee on Jewish Law and Standards, come to represent the expected normative *halakhic* behavior for Conservative Jews. Hence, in theory, their practical impact ought to be substantial.
[164] Abelson, "Prenatal Testing and Abortion," p. 9.

the Tay-Sachs or Down's syndrome cases, but permits abortion for any "major defects" that might be portended. The rider that he attaches to his permission that these defects must also "make the mother and the family anxious about the future" describes a condition that is well short of a threat to the mother's mental health; which family, after all, when confronted with such defects, would not be "anxious about the future?" Indeed, it is precisely this anxiety that leads to the contemplation of abortion in the first place. However, "anxiety" or "concerns" might well be thought of as being in a different category from "mental anguish." Abelson, therefore, effectively follows Waldenberg's lead in allowing for abortions that are based upon concerns for the future of the fetus, whether the mother is mentally *in extremis* or not.

The second paper, written by Rabbi Robert Gordis, similarly holds that "[t]here is warrant in rabbinic responsa for permitting abortion if the mother is deeply concerned about the health of her unborn child."[165] Gordis includes the "pregnant woman's worry" over abnormalities as a "sufficient ground for an abortion because of the debilitating effects psychologically or otherwise on her well-being."[166] Weinberg, of course, had contemplated abortions for fetal abnormalities only in the context of maternal "pain" or "great need," and Freehof had described the appropriate criterion as being that of "mental anguish." While these are all rather vague terms, it is worth contemplating whether the maternal "deep concern" or "worry" articulated by Gordis constitutes the same standard as that enunciated by Weinberg or Freehof. Gordis, perhaps sensing that he needed more robust grounds for his permissive response, avows, "[u]nder any of these circumstances, few would be disposed to oppose abortions designed to prevent a major traumatic episode from being converted into a lifetime tragedy."[167] It is unclear in this statement whether Gordis is more concerned about the mother, the fetus, or both. Whatever the case, though, it is probable that all the lenient respondents would agree with Gordis' assessment that a "major traumatic episode" that could lead to a lifetime of mental "tragedy" might warrant an abortion. But this sentence does not address the circumstance in which the mother who is considering an abortion does not regard herself as being in the midst of a "major traumatic episode." Perhaps the mother does not deem her own plight to be deeply traumatic, but has come to the conclusion that, on balance, it is undesirable for the fetus to be born with the

---

[165] R. Gordis, "Abortion: Major Wrong or Basic Right?," in *Proceedings of the Committee on Jewish Law and Standards of the Conservative Movement 1980–1985*, New York, 1988, p. 24.
[166] *Ibid.*   [167] *Ibid.*

limitations that are anticipated. It seems likely that Gordis would regard this as an acceptable maternal "worry," and would, therefore, permit abortions in cases of fetal abnormalities for any amount of maternal discomfort.

A third Conservative position, offered by Feldman, utilizes the more exacting approach to maternal suffering. While Feldman correctly observes that there is often little real distinction between concerns for maternal well-being and that of the fetus, he nevertheless maintains that maternal "mental anguish" is the "normative" *halakhic* concern:

[A]bortion for fetal rather than maternal indications would not ordinarily be sanctioned by Jewish law. True, rabbinic opinion permitting abortion for fetal reasons alone is not altogether lacking, but the normative rabbinic view is to permit it for maternal indications only. Yet, the one can blend into the other, as fetal risk can mean mental anguish on the part of the mother, so that the fetal indication becomes a maternal one. The woman's welfare is thus the key to warrant abortion.[168]

While Feldman is of the view that frequently "fetal risk" will lead directly to maternal "mental anguish" he seems to differ somewhat from Waldenberg's position, as well as that of Abelson and Gordis, in contending that the "woman's welfare" is "key." If this is so, then it seems unlikely that Feldman would consent to an abortion when the mother expresses concerns for the fetus' future limitations but shows no signs that her own general welfare would be dramatically compromised if the pregnancy were to proceed.

Feldman's viewpoint, however, did not prevail within Conservative Judaism. In a "Statement on the Permissibility of Abortion" – a paragraph designed to summarize the collective stance of the aforementioned papers – Rabbis Ben Zion Bokser and Abelson write: "The Rabbinical Assembly Committee on Jewish Law and Standards takes the view that an abortion is justifiable if a continuation of pregnancy might cause the mother severe physical or psychological harm, or when the fetus is judged by competent medical opinion as severely defective."[169] The precise definition of what might constitute "severe" harm goes undefined in this statement; presumably it is to be left to the local rabbi to define

---

[168] D. M., Feldman, "Abortion: The Jewish View," in *Proceedings of the Committee on Jewish Law and Standards of the Conservative Movement 1980–1985*, New York, 1988, p. 16.

[169] B. Bokser, and K. Abelson, "A Statement on the Permissibility of Abortion," in *Proceedings of the Committee on Jewish Law and Standards of the Conservative Movement 1980–1985*, New York, 1988, p. 37.

"severe" within the context of individual cases. Plainly, though, the official *halakhic* voice of Conservative Judaism held that an abortion could be permitted based on fetal indications alone, regardless of the mother's condition.

However, Rabbi Elliot Dorff, a prominent ethicist within the Conservative movement, expressed serious qualms about this conclusion:

> Although I personally agree with this last approach, there are problems with it. Aside from the fact that it would represent an innovation in the law, it raises the extremely difficult issue of determining what constitutes a sufficient defect to warrant abortion. The "easy" cases are those in which the fetus has minimal brain tissue (e.g., an encephaly) or a degenerative disease like Tay-Sachs that will lead to the baby's death within a few years of birth at most. What about Huntington's chorea, though, where the degeneration will not usually begin until age thirty-five or forty? I believe that abortion is not justified in that case, since the person will live an extended period of time without suffering from any of the disease's debilitating effects – indeed, enough time to have children of his or her own and even participate in much of their rearing – and since there is reasonable hope that a cure may be developed in that time. But then where do we draw the line? Twenty-five years? Fifteen years? Ten years? And what constitutes a defect justifying abortion in the first place? Mental retardation? If so, how much? Blindness or deafness? We quickly slide into the danger of defining qualifications for a master race, with the corollary depreciation of disabled people.[170]

Despite Dorff's personal affinity for the approach taken by his Conservative colleagues and by Waldenberg, he nevertheless candidly contends that this strategy is undeniably "an innovation in the law." While he does not suggest that this makes such an approach *halakhically* untenable, he clearly denotes it as a response that is discontinuous with the *halakhic* past. This fact, in itself, might not so much have perturbed Dorff, had it not been accompanied by what he clearly regards as a pivotal challenge: the question of where to draw the line on the issue of "severity." While Tay-Sachs disease, in Dorff's estimation, represents an "easy case," other – less immediately debilitating – conditions pose vexing quandaries as to whether abortions should be permitted or not. This reality is exacerbated, Dorff asserts, given the fact that the very attempt to define this type of boundary leads to the categorization of certain disabilities as being humanly acceptable and others as unacceptable, with all the implications that accompany such specific expectations of wholeness for our humanity generally.

---

[170] E. N. Dorff, *Matters of Life and Death: A Jewish Approach to Modern Medical Ethics*, Philadelphia, The Jewish Publication Society, 1998, p. 131.

In Dorff's view, though, the "difficulty of making these decisions does not mean that we can or should shrink from them."[171] Quite the contrary, as Dorff sees it, Judaism has always taken the attitude that we ought not simply to let nature take its course, but should make responsible determinations as "partners of God." If, then, making such decisions is indeed our difficult duty, we should not make them, Dorff avers, based on the projected outcome for the fetus, for this is likely to lead to invidious inferences concerning the relative worth of disabled human beings. Rather, in "clouded" instances, it is perhaps most sage to determine whether or not an abortion is appropriate based on the "mother's mental reaction to the defect."[172] In other words, as far as Dorff is concerned, we should cleave closer to the traditional lenient criterion, and reject what he sees as the "innovative" path. While Dorff regards judgments based on the mother's mental state as the "wisest" on offer, he is nevertheless conscious of their deficiencies:

For some mothers, raising a mentally retarded child, while not pleasant, is manageable; for others it is beyond their psychological competence. This, of course, means that only the people who are psychologically strongest and most stable would have the responsibility for raising such children, and that is unfair. Moreover, if most families abort "defective" children, one wonders about the degree to which society in the long run will tolerate imperfections and provide for people who have them. Thus the very sensitivity of society to the sanctity of life is at stake.[173]

Notwithstanding these difficulties, Dorff advocates the creation of guidelines for deciding about abortions in cases of fetal abnormality, guidelines that are based upon the mother's "mental reaction," not the future of the fetus. Thus, Dorff's position is closer to that of Rabbis Weinberg and Freehof than to that of Rabbis Yisraeli, Waldenberg, or Jacob, or to the official outlook of Conservative Judaism.

CONSENSUS BECOMES APPARENT

From the perspective of the history of *halakhah*, it can readily be seen that, in the space of less than half a century, the challenge of abortion in cases of fetal abnormalities had fueled a legal discussion that yielded an unprecedented *halakhic* focus on abortion. While discrete answers to individual questions continued to form the foundation of the responsa process, this unparalleled *halakhic* interchange on the suitability of abortion

---

[171] *Ibid.*   [172] *Ibid.*   [173] *Ibid.*, pp. 131–132.

began to define the parameters and boundaries of acceptable *halakhic* discourse on the subject. Indeed, it became feasible to speak of emergent *halakhic* consensus on abortion in a way that would have been unthinkable in any prior period. Washofsky has defined this notion of a "*halakhic* consensus" within the Orthodox world as follows:

> A "consensus" position exists in *halakhah* when, despite the availability of other plausible interpretations of the sources, it is the view of the law held by a preponderance of orthodox authorities. A consensus ruling will often appear in *halakhic* literature as "the" *halakhah* on a given issue. If dissenting views are mentioned, they are presented as divergent, less "correct", not to be relied upon as authoritative statements of the law.[174]

It is clear, however, from the responsa that, while Washofsky was referring to the Orthodox world, consensus positions on abortion were not necessarily congruent with any particular ideological grouping. In fact, it seems most accurate to assert that not one, but two, distinct *halakhic* consensuses arose in the latter part of the twentieth century. In both the Orthodox and the non-Orthodox realms, these mounting consensuses acted effectively to submerge, though not to eliminate, some of the more diverse views that hitherto had been evident.

The more stringent consensus position was exclusively the preserve of Orthodox Jews, but not all Orthodox scholars subscribed to it. The "consensus" view among most Orthodox scholars had come to oppose abortions for fetal maladies. Waldenberg and Yisraeli had placed themselves outside this group by explicitly allowing for such abortions. Consequently, while summaries of traditional Jewish law on abortion often report on the views of Waldenberg, Yisraeli, and Grossnass, they do so only *en route* to their conclusion that Jewish law forbids abortion of a fetus with Tay-Sachs disease.[175] Authors representing this consensus tend, therefore, variously to describe Waldenberg as "aware that the vast majority of rabbinic decisors are in disagreement [with him]," as "the only recent authority to differ," or as "highly controversial"; it is always made clear that he is outside the more stringent consensus.[176] These authors

---

[174] Washofsky, "Abortion and the Halakhic Conversation," p. 40.
[175] For example, A. S. Abraham, *Nishmat Avraham*, Jerusalem, 1987, *Choshen Mishpat*, 425, p. 230.
[176] This consensus view, which, neither inaccurately nor unfairly, consigns Waldenberg to the status of minority opinion, can be found in numerous places: see Jakobovits, "Jewish Views on Abortion," pp. 109–115; Bleich J. D., *Judaism and Healing: Halakhic Perspectives*, New York, Ktav Publishing House Incorporated, 1981, pp. 96–103; Rosner, *Modern Medicine and Jewish Ethics*, pp. 139–160; F. Rosner and M. D. Tendler, *Practical Medical Halachah* (3rd edition), Hoboken, Ktav Publishing House Incorporated, 1990, pp. 33–34; J. D. Bleich, *Bioethical Dilemmas: A Jewish Perspective*, Hoboken, Ktav Publishing House Incorporated, 1998, p. 271.

never suggest that Waldenberg's or Yisraeli's *halakhic* technique is faulty; it is simply made plain that their conclusions put them beyond that outlook which, in the 1970s and 1980s, came to represent the dominant *halakhic* response from within much of Orthodoxy. Feinstein, then, hardly needed to be concerned about those who had criticized his methodology and conclusions, for it was around his position that a forceful consensus was coalescing.

This emerging consensus also concurred with the view, so well put by Unterman and strengthened by Feinstein, that non-therapeutic abortion should be regarded as a sub-category of murder. Thus, Jakobovits obviously takes Unterman's language to be normative when he asserts that "the killing of an embryo, while technically not murder due to a 'scriptural decree,' yet constitutes an 'appurtenance of murder...'"[177] Rosner, likewise, readily affirms that "[t]he destruction of the unborn fetus, although legally not considered murder, can be considered to constitute 'moral murder,'"[178] and Bleich chooses his words carefully when he reports without quibble that "[m]any authorities regard the destruction of the fetus as a form of non-capital homicide..."[179] The ease with which such formulations were adopted ought not, however, to hide their revolutionary nature. For there can be little doubt that these depictions would have been seen as exaggerated, if not wholly inaccurate, by a number of scholars who lived as recently as the first half of the twentieth century and certainly by many from centuries past. This is not in any way to suggest that the views of these authors of a more stringent consensus ought to be seen as incompatible with the tradition; they were clearly consistent with the approach of Maimonides and those who followed in his footsteps. It is merely to posit that, before the 1950s, such encapsulations would not have been regarded as the best way to epitomize the collective body of Jewish sources. While elevating a certain selection of the traditional materials, these writings suggest that the sources they emphasize represent the essence of the textual past – a claim that, were it to be made explicitly, would be difficult to justify.

It is noteworthy that in the Orthodox world the *halakhic* trend appeared to operate as a counterbalancing force to prevailing cultural tendencies. In the nineteenth century, when general abortion laws were more restrictive, there seemed to be a preponderance of more lenient *poskim*; yet in the second half of the twentieth century, when legal liberalization

---

[177] Jakobovits, "Jewish Views on Abortion," p. 123.
[178] Rosner, *Modern Medicine and Jewish Ethics*, p. 152.   [179] Bleich, *Bioethical Dilemmas*, p. 271.

became the societal theme, the predominant Orthodox *halakhic* response became decidedly more restrictive.

The second consensus position was dominated by non-Orthodox figures, but included some Orthodox scholars as well. Here, an altogether different view had come to the fore: because none of these respondents concurred with the stricter consensus that forbade abortions in cases of fetal defects, it can certainly be said that the more lenient consensus was no less cohesive than its more stringent counterpart. Unlike the more stringent consensus, however, this second consensus exhibited unanimity in its openness to abortions for a wide variety of fetal abnormalities. All the authorities who subscribed to this consensus agreed that if the mother were faced with a severe threat to her mental well-being, abortion of a disabled fetus would be warranted. These respondents did not make it appear as if their view represented the only possible reading of the *halakhic* texts; they simply depicted the approach they preferred as being the best reading of the historic *halakhic* alternatives.

Some of these authorities went beyond the lenient consensus view and permitted abortions based on fetal prognoses alone. Those who did so perhaps exhibited no less an innovative approach to abortion rulings than their more stringent counterparts who had designated abortion for other than life-saving purposes as "murder." After all, before the twentieth century, there were few precedents for *poskim* providing their consent to abortions for any reason save that of great maternal need. Again, this is not in any way to suggest that the views of these authorities who went further than the lenient consensus ought to be seen as incompatible with the tradition. It is merely to point out that they elevated parts of the tradition that, until the twentieth century arrived with its dramatic technological and social developments, had been more marginal.

Modernity, then, had finally had its impact upon Jewish abortion law. A century and a half after modernity's massive societal upheaval began to gather steam, its impact upon abortion *halakhah* had become palpable. Indeed, in some measure it is fair to contend that these two separate consensuses – each with its own extremes – were direct outgrowths of the loss of the independent, autonomous Jewish communal life that had been a predominant feature of the Jewish world until the nineteenth century. The autonomous Jewish community of the past had produced a *halakhic* inclination towards finding the middle ground, born out of the need for a law that was applicable to all Jews. With the dissolution of that communal structure, and with the passage of time, modernity undermined those conciliatory tendencies. As the contemporary jurist Rabbi Menachem Elon put it:

Still another consequence of the abrogation of Jewish juridical autonomy at the end of the eighteenth century was that the halakhic authorities were no longer called upon to adopt enactments or make legal rulings for the community as an entity, but only for particular groups of individuals; consequently, even had there been no split between religious and secular Jews, halakhic decisions would have lost much of their community-wide significance. The legal rulings of an organized autonomous juridical authority on matters such as communal administration, taxes, public order, etc. necessarily reflect the exercise of responsibility for the continued well-being of the entire community, as an entity, for which the authority acts. On the other hand, without such autonomy, no matter how many individuals accept the decision as binding, the decision is addressed to them as a group of individuals and not as a total Jewish community. Certainly, when the decision-maker is aware that his ruling is directed to only part of the community, broader considerations of the interests of the total community play less of a part in his decisions.[180]

The clear implication of Elon's words is that *poskim* in previous ages usually issued rulings that were tempered by considerations of the needs and concerns of all members of the Jewish community: the strict, the lenient, and even the unobservant. This phenomenon came to an end in modernity. In the modern world, when only a certain segment of the community hearkens to a particular *posek*'s ruling, it is natural for the *posek* to orient rulings towards the interests of that group. Hence, it comes as no surprise that as Jews who accepted the rulings of Orthodox *poskim* tended to embrace a stricter practice rather than leniency, the rulings of twentieth-century Orthodox *poskim* came to reflect this stringency.[181] Conversely, those who cleaved to the positions of non-Orthodox rabbis usually favored leniency, and the non-Orthodox authorities tended more in this direction. While there are exceptions to these generalizations, the impact of these trends on the shaping of abortion law, both in the Orthodox and the non-Orthodox worlds, ought not to be underestimated.

In the second half of the twentieth century, then, two extraordinary developments occurred in the Jewish response to abortion. First, "Jewish positions" on abortion began to crystallize. These "positions" were the

---

[180] Elon, *Jewish Law*, volume IV, p. 1587, n. 23.
[181] See also J. Katz, *Shabbes Goy: A Study in Halakhic Flexibility*, Philadelphia, The Jewish Publication Society, 1989, pp. 239–240. Katz argues that the traditional trend stems from a grave concern – brought about by modernity – that a lenient ruling will create a "breach" in "the wall of religion."

expression of two nascent consensuses that had emerged from deliberations over the painful and difficult realities of fetal abnormality. Thus,
a millennial history of multiple independent voices gave way to more
collectively held "views" on abortion. Second, the more stringent strand
of the *halakhic* past came to be seen as the "authentic" Jewish outlook on
abortion in much of the Orthodox world, even as the more lenient tendency of the tradition was amplified in most of the non-Orthodox world.
This is not to suggest that Jewish views on abortion became polarized,
but simply that both a more lenient and a more stringent position were
distilled from the material that hitherto had existed in an undifferentiated
fashion.

NEW CHALLENGES

While the plight of the defective fetus had initiated changes in the *halakhic*
landscape, the coherence of these new "Jewish positions" was tested by
other late-twentieth-century abortion challenges. By the 1980s, the vast
majority of Jews lived in places where abortions could be obtained for
any reason whatsoever, without threat of legal consequences.[182] Indeed,
the overwhelming percentage of abortions during this time was carried
out for reasons other than a profound threat[183] to the health of the
mother or the fetus. It is hardly surprising, then, that across the Jewish
spectrum, questions began to arise concerning the acceptability of abortion under a range of different circumstances. No longer focused on the
numerically marginal issue of fetal abnormality, the *halakhic* discussion
broadened to address diverse abortion issues, some prompted by medical advances, some stimulated by changed communal attitudes. Three
areas of discussion demonstrate that sometimes – unlike the issue of fetal
abnormalities, where the consensus to which one subscribed resulted in
quite different practical conclusions – adherence to different consensuses
led to identical recommendations for action.

[182] America and Israel had the world's largest Jewish populations, and between them they comprised
more than three-quarters of the world's Jews. From 1973 onward, the Supreme Court decision
in *Roe* v. *Wade* (see above, p. 135) made abortion a constitutional right in America. The legal
situation in Israel will be described below (see chapter 6). The Israeli legal parameters, however,
did not prevent women from obtaining abortions of their choosing.
[183] While, to be sure, any unwanted pregnancy has potentially serious consequences such as emotional trauma or depression, these are conditions that, if the mother is willing, are normally
susceptible to treatment. Hence, while they certainly constitute a threat to the health of the
mother, they need not be "profound" in the sense of leading to irreversible physical or mental
damage.

The first such issue is the difficult conundrum that has become known as "pregnancy reduction." One of the outcomes of the reproductive technology advances in the last quarter of the twentieth century resulted in women being treated with fertility drugs or undergoing *in vitro* fertilization sometimes becoming pregnant with multiple fetuses.[184] This was potentially life-threatening for the women involved. More usually, it resulted in the demise, or premature birth – with attendant problems and risks – of some or all of the fetuses. To prevent these results, physicians often recommended reducing the number of fetuses in the womb at an early stage of pregnancy, by means of selective abortion. It is clear, of course, from a *halakhic* perspective, that if the mother's life is at risk, then some or all of the fetuses should be destroyed in order to save her. It is, however, a far more difficult matter when the mother's life is not in danger, such that the fetuses cannot be designated as *rodfim* to her, yet the consequences of not intervening will be that the fetuses will die. In this circumstance, the significant *halakhic* question becomes, given that the fetuses are all in the identical non-*nefesh* category, and that they are in reality all *rodfim* to each other, does there exist *halakhic* justification for selective abortion, to kill some in order to save others, or does the law dictate taking no action, even if the outcome is that all will die?

Rabbi Shlomo Zalman Auerbach, a noted expert in the area, provided one of the first answers to this question.[185] Without explaining his reasoning, *Nishmat Avraham* portrays Auerbach's response to pregnancy reduction as tending towards permitting (*"daáto noteh lehatir"*) the killing of some of the fetuses to save those remaining. It is hardly surprising that those rabbis who adhered to the more lenient consensus view described above would concur with Auerbach's conclusion in this regard. Thus, in his sixth *teshuvah* related to abortion, within volume xx of *Tzitz Eliezer*, Waldenberg finds no difficulty in approving of pregnancy reduction.[186] Waldenberg was asked whether a woman who was pregnant with quadruplets could abort one fetus in order to save three, given that the doctors had advised her that without such a procedure all four would die. The question, which came from the woman's husband, further inquired of Waldenberg whether this was not a case in which the advice of the *Yerushalmi* that no selections be made – "even if all of them are [certain to be] killed they must not turn over one

[184] *Ibid.*, p. 269.   [185] Abraham, *Nishmat Avraham, Choshen Mishpat* 425:2, section 21, p. 234.
[186] References and quotations concerning this Waldenberg *teshuvah* are from *Tzitz Eliezer*, Jerusalem, 1963 and on, volume xx, number 2.

Jew"[187] – ought to be followed. In reply, Waldenberg contends that the
Yerushalmi was referring to instances when those at risk were within the
category of *nefashot*, and hence the principle of "be killed but do not
transgress"[188] applied. In other words, as *nefashot*, they were required to
give up their lives before agreeing to participate in a murderous process. Fetuses, however, Waldenberg avers, are clearly not *nefashot*, and,
hence the principle of "be killed but do not transgress" does not apply
to them. Moreover, Waldenberg reiterates, fetal destruction is not within
the boundaries of the "appurtenances of the spilling of blood," and consequently, the proposed pregnancy reduction most certainly would be
allowable. Even a non-Jewish doctor, Waldenberg rules, who normally
would be barred from fetal destruction, could perform this type of operation in order to save the remaining three fetuses.

Similarly, Rabbi Chaim David Halevy, in a *halakhic* opinion published
in *Assia*, does not hesitate to permit such procedures.[189] Both Halevy
and Waldenberg, it should be clarified, regard the abortion prohibition
as being rabbinic rather than Toraitic, both are of the view that the
fetus is not a *nefesh*, and both see no murder involved in fetal destruction.
It follows, therefore, that both regard the possibility of multiple fetuses
dying or being born in a severely impaired state as a far greater evil than
pregnancy reduction. Since, in their eyes, no element of murder would be
attached to such pregnancy reduction, these authorities readily approve
of such interventions in the name of allowing the remaining fetuses "to
be born healthy and whole."[190]

What, though, is the view of those rabbis whose response to abortion
conforms with the more stringent consensus that abortion, other than to
save the mother's life, involves some element of murder? How do they
approach the issue of pregnancy reduction? Rabbi Yitzhak Zilberstein
offers an example of an answer from one within the stricter consensus.[191]
Zilberstein, responding to a question on the permissibility of pregnancy
reduction, draws an analogy between pregnancy reduction and other
instances which require choices between equals, such as in the case of
the overloaded boat where the only way to save some passengers is by

[187] See above, chapter 3, p. 85.   [188] See above, chapter 4, p. 103.
[189] C. D. Halevy, "*Al Dilul Ubarim VeHaMa'amad HaHilkhati Shel Ubarim BeMivchanah*," in *Sefer Assia*, volume VIII, Jerusalem, 1995, pp. 3–6.
[190] *Ibid.*, p. 5.
[191] All Zilberstein references and quotations are from Y. Zilberstein, "*Dilul Ubarim: ShuT*," in *Sefer Assia*, volume VIII, Jerusalem, 1995, pp. 7–13.

throwing other passengers overboard. In this context, Zilberstein cites texts like *Panim Me̅irot*, which had ruled that it was acceptable to save the mother at the baby's expense when, after the baby had emerged, the alternative was the loss of both mother and baby.[192] From these sources, Zilberstein suggests that it indeed may be possible to offer textual foundation for the sacrificing of some lives in order to save others in situations like the boat example. This is, of course, a rather surprising and controversial position, and one that has little support within a tradition in which the usual response to such circumstances has been to give considerable weight to the counsel of the *Yerushalmi*.[193] Indeed, the editor of the journal in which Zilberstein's article appeared saw fit to append a footnote to Zilberstein's *teshuvah*, indicating that Auerbach had ruled that it is absolutely forbidden to kill one member of a group that is in jeopardy in order to save those remaining. Zilberstein's position on this point is, therefore, tenuous.

Zilberstein is, however, on much firmer ground when he maintains that even if this argument is not accepted, pregnancy reduction still is permissible by virtue of the fact that these multiple fetuses are non-viable. In other types of abortion, Zilberstein's view is that an abortion performed for reasons other than saving the mother's life – such as in the case of a fetus with Tay-Sachs disease – is tantamount to the spilling of blood. This is because these types of abortion represent the termination of a life without sufficient reason – a life that, if left undisturbed, could become viable. However, this is not so in the case of pregnancy reduction: left undisturbed these multiple fetuses have no chance at viability. Hence, Zilberstein contends, in the case of multiple fetuses, pregnancy reduction is "not killing" because these are non-viable beings in the first place. Zilberstein cites the *halakhic* provision that likens a fetus that is incapable of surviving for thirty days beyond birth to a stone, that is, an entity that is not animate.[194] "Even though now it is alive," writes Zilberstein, "it is clearly known that it will not live, and, therefore, there is no 'spilling of blood' prohibition involved in killing it." Indeed, opines Zilberstein, quite the reverse of viewing pregnancy reduction as taking life, it is only if intervention is allowed that life can be saved. Zilberstein's logic of non-viability, then, offers an approach that enables rabbis who are

---

[192] See above, chapter 3, p. 89.
[193] The advice of the *Yerushalmi* is that such selections are inappropriate. See above, chapter 3, p. 85.
[194] See *Shabbat* 135a, *Yevamot* 80a, and *Baba Batra* 20a.

within the more stringent consensus to condone pregnancy reduction.[195] There can be little doubt, then, that in the area of pregnancy reduction, whether a particular authority is within the more stringent consensus or outside it has bearing only on the methodology employed to arrive at the conclusion; near unanimity exists that the practice of pregnancy reduction is acceptable.[196]

The second issue upon which broad agreement emerged in the latter stages of the twentieth century is the matter of abortion to use the fetus for the well-being of others. It is possible, for example, that implantation of fetal tissue into those suffering from Parkinson's or Alzheimer's diseases may have significant therapeutic effect. This potential led to a 1995 question of the *Sefaradi* chief rabbi of Israel, Rabbi Eliyahu Bakshi-Doron. Bakshi-Doron was asked about a woman who wanted to become pregnant in order to use fetal tissue to help her father who was ailing with Parkinson's disease.[197] The two specific questions put to Bakshi-Doron were: is it permissible to become pregnant for purposes other than giving birth?; and is it permissible to abort in the name of a significant need, such as the fulfillment of the *mitzvah* of honoring father and mother?[198]

Beginning his answer with the second question, Bakshi-Doron immediately replies that there is a "serious prohibition" with the proposed abortion, and that it is impossible to fulfill the *mitzvah* of honoring one's father and mother through an act of transgression. It would be unthinkable, Bakshi-Doron points out, for a daughter to steal in order to feed her father. Bakshi-Doron proceeds to discuss abortion generally, and although his responses are generally restrictive, it is unclear from this *teshuvah* whether Bakshi-Doron adheres to the more stringent consensus view on abortion or not. Within this *teshuvah*, he does not connect abortion to the spilling of blood. He also refers to the possibility of abortion in circumstances other than a threat to the mother's life.

---

[195] Another rabbi who has written in the same vein as Zilberstein is Rabbi Joshua Ze'ev Zand. See J. Z. Zand, *Birkat Banim*, Jerusalem, 1994, chapter 12, section 41. Zand holds that pregnancy reduction can only be performed if none of the fetuses will survive without the procedure. If only one will survive, even in an impaired state, the procedure would not be permissible.

[196] There is further evidence of the strong support for pregnancy reduction: despite the fact that Bleich discerns a serious "conceptual problem" with the non-viability argument for those rabbis who are identified with the more stringent consensus, he goes to considerable lengths to resolve this conundrum in order to allow for pregnancy reduction. See Bleich, *Bioethical Dilemmas*, pp. 275–277.

[197] All Bakshi-Doron references and quotations are from E. Bakshi-Doron, "*Herayon LeShem Hashtalat Rikmot HaUbar LeTzorekh Ripui HaAv*," *Techumin*, volume 15, 1995: 311–316.

[198] It is important to note that this is a particularly germane question given that the rabbis classically understood "honoring" father and mother to imply taking care of their physical needs. See *Kiddushin* 31b.

Bakshi-Doron's conclusion on the initial question put to him is, however, unambiguous: becoming pregnant with a motivation other than
giving birth is not permitted. This is so for two reasons. First, pregnancy represents a danger to the woman, a danger that is *halakhically*
acceptable only for purposes of the fulfillment of the *mitzvot* associated
with child-bearing. In the instance under discussion, the planned abortion represents an additional danger to the woman beyond the primary
danger of pregnancy. Hence, the woman has no *halakhic* authorization,
Bakshi-Doron avers, to place herself in such danger even for a worthy
goal like improving her father's condition. It is true, Bakshi-Doron points
out, that the *halakhah* permits putting oneself in some amount of danger to save a life, as in the case of *in vivo* kidney donation. However, it
does not permit putting oneself in danger in order to save another from
tribulation.[199] The danger to the woman, therefore, would prohibit a
pregnancy leading to abortion as proposed.

The second reason that Bakshi-Doron advances to disallow such an
abortion is what he terms the *"kedushah"* (holiness) of pregnancy. Even
without the *halakhic* objections, Bakshi-Doron maintains, pregnancy in
human beings involves not just the production of a physical entity, but a
real partnership with God in the creation of a soul. As such, pregnancy
represents a holy endeavor, designed to foster parental devotion to a new
being and to the establishment of a deep bond between mother and child.
It is, and must be, far more than just a biological enterprise. Entering into
pregnancy with a goal less than the creation and embracing of a human
nefesh is an unacceptable frustration of the *kedushah* of pregnancy. That
kedushah arises from the totality of everything that inheres in bringing a
new human life into being, a totality that, in Bakshi-Doron's view, should
never be diminished.

Turning to a non-Orthodox perspective, it is noteworthy that Feldman
is in complete agreement with Bakshi-Doron on this issue:

The halakhic position is that it's clearly wrong to abort for this reason, and as
wrong to become pregnant in order to abort for this reason, but if abortion does
happen, the tissue may indeed serve the therapeutic needs of another.[200] While
there are situations in which one may place himself in some danger to save a

---

[199] Bakshi-Doron does not reveal how he would rule if the fetus were certainly able to provide some
life-saving substance. It is possible, however, to surmise from his next reason for forbidding this
type of abortion, that he may well be opposed even if the fetus could provide a life-saving gift.

[200] Rabbi Walter Jacob, writing from a Reform perspective, concurs with this view. Jacob responds to
the question, "[U]nder what circumstances, if any, would it be permissible to conduct medical
research involving an [already] aborted fetus?" He concludes that a scientist who is doing
research in Alzheimer's disease, which requires live brain tissue, would be acting "in keeping with

life, the creation of a life *only* as a means to an end (in a recent case, a mother conceived a child with the hope that she would *also* help a sibling) is a violation of medical ethics.[201]

It is, consequently, logical to infer that if those who concur with the more lenient consensus regard abortion for the medical welfare of another as a wrong, then those who see a connection between abortion and the spilling of blood will all the more reject this type of abortion. It follows that there is every reason to assume widespread *halakhic* accord in opposition to abortion for purposes of utilizing fetal tissue in the relief of illness.

The third issue, which has been the subject of not just accord but clear unanimity across the *halakhic* spectrum, is that of abortion for purposes of sex preselection. A careful reading of the texts reveals that the *halakhah* does not object to the aspiration to select the sex of one's children provided that it does not lead to potentially destructive societal imbalances between males and females.[202] Given, then, that the goal of sex preselection is largely unopposed within the tradition,[203] the *halakhic* reaction to sex preselection hinges on the means for arriving at the desired end. During the twentieth century, it became possible to employ amniocentesis or other testing methods to determine the sex of the developing fetus. Thus, a possible way to achieve the preferred sex is simply to test in order to ascertain the sex of the fetus and then to abort any fetus or fetuses of the unwanted sex. In the third world, where the cultural value of having a male child is high, the prevalence of such sex-selection abortions and other practices has already led to skewed gender ratios.[204] However, the Jewish attitude to abortions for the purpose of sex preselection is unambiguous. As Bleich expresses it, "[i]t must...be emphasized that Jewish teaching unequivocally rejects the option of terminating a pregnancy simply because the fetus is not of the desired sex... There is indeed some disagreement with regard to the grounds that would justify an abortion, but no authority would accept sex determination as legitimate cause for

Jewish tradition" if he were to use an aborted fetus for this purpose. See W. Jacob, *Contemporary American Reform Responsa*, New York, 1987, # 21.
[201] Feldman, *Birth Control*, p. 347.
[202] For a concise summary of the pertinent sources see Bleich, *Judaism and Healing*, pp. 110–115.
[203] For Jewish concerns about this goal, see D. L. Schiff, "Developing *Halakhic* Attitudes To Sex Preselection," in W. Jacob and M. Zemer (eds.), *The Fetus and Fertility in Jewish Law*, Pittsburgh, Rodef Shalom Press, 1995.
[204] Owen D. Jones, "Sex Selection: Regulating Technology Enabling the Predetermination of a Child's Gender," *Harvard Journal of Law and Technology*, volume 6, 1992: p. 11.

an abortion."[205] Bleich is surely correct: regardless of ideological per-spective, nobody responsive to the *halakhah* has deemed abortion for this purpose to be acceptable.[206]

Beyond these three areas of abortion for pregnancy reduction, fetal-tissue deployment and sex preselection, non-Orthodox authorities felt the need to address other matters that had become practical concerns. Thus, in both the Conservative and Reform movements, rabbis issued *halakhic* statements that responded to the dramatic rise in non-therapeutic abortions. In so doing, they clarified the range of circumstances in which those who adhered to the more lenient consensus envisioned abortions being acceptable. In 1970, for example, Rabbi Isaac Klein, one of the senior scholars of the Conservative rabbinate, advocated this position:

There is a distinction between the early and the later stages of pregnancy.

In the later stages we would permit abortion only when the birth of the fetus would be a direct threat to the life of the mother. This threat should be interpreted to include cases where continuation of the pregnancy would have such a debilitating effect, psychological or otherwise, on the mother as to constitute a hazard to her life, however remote such danger may be.

In the earlier stages we would allow therapeutic abortions wherever there is any threat to the health of the mother, directly or indirectly, physically or psychologically. Since such an interpretation is very flexible and therefore subject to abuse, the facts have to be established by reliable medical evidence.

We would therefore permit abortion in the case of thalidomide babies, cases of rape and the like, not because such a fetus has no right to life but because it constitutes a threat to the health of the mother. This is an area of controversy. Many authorities would disagree and limit abortion to cases where the threat to the life of the mother is direct.

We would not permit abortions that are prompted merely by the desire of the mother not to have another child.[207]

Klein proposes that Conservative Jews allow for abortions when the physical or psychological health of the mother, as judged by "reliable medical evidence," is threatened. Klein explicitly includes rape and

---

[205] Bleich, *Judaism and Healing*, p. 111.

[206] Abortion for sex preselection becomes a challenging issue when considering abortion with an eye to feminism. There is a feminist view, among others, which advocates that the *halakhah* should afford women considerable autonomy in the matter of abortion (for a full discussion, see below, chapter 7, pp. 251 ff.). This would presumably include abortions for purposes of sex preselection. In reality, however, sex-preselection abortions overwhelmingly destroy female fetuses, a matter of real concern for feminists. Hence, allowing for individual choice in this type of abortion may, in fact, undermine feminist objectives.

[207] I. Klein, "Abortion and Jewish Tradition," *Conservative Judaism*, volume 24, number 3, 1970.

pronounced fetal impairment in those categories that lead to considerable psychological damage to the mother. Conversely, Klein is emphatic
that abortions "prompted merely by desire" ought not to be countenanced.

Following Klein's lead, the *halakhic*-position papers that were accepted
as authoritative by Conservative Judaism in 1983 rejected abortions
where no severe health consequences were at issue. Thus, Feldman writes,
"[A]bortion for 'population control' is repugnant to the Jewish system.
Abortion for economic reasons is also not admissible. Taking precaution
by abortion or birth control against physical threat remains a mitzvah,
but never to forestall financial difficulty. Material considerations are improper in this connection."[208] Gordis concurs: "[A]bortion on demand
is a threat to a basic ethical principle which Judaism enunciated centuries [ago]...In sum, while the law does not categorically rule out
abortion since it is not 'murder,' the spirit of Judaism, reinforced by a
realistic understanding of human motivation, must look askance at any
blanket provision for abortion on demand."[209] These perspectives were
plainly what the Conservative Committee on Jewish Law and Standards
intended to convey when it declared: "The fetus is a life in the process of development, and the decision to abort it should never be taken
lightly."[210]

There is, moreover, little substantive difference between the rulings
of Conservative and Reform respondents in this area. Some confusion
exists on this point owing to the prominent role of the Reform movement in support of the American pro-choice cultural and political struggle. Thus, as early as the 1960s, Rabbi Israel Margolies, rabbi of Beth
Am congregation in New York City, while speaking to a national abortion conference, articulated Reform support for abortion becoming a
matter of choice. After quoting some lenient sources from the tradition,
Margolies constructs a forceful argument on behalf of abortion freedom
that is quite detached from the texts he cites:

Until a child is actually born into the world, it is literally part of its mother's
body, and belongs only to her and her mate. It does not belong to society at all,
nor has it been accepted into any faith. Its existence is entirely and exclusively
the business and concern of its parents, whether they are married or not. It is
men and women who alone must decide whether or not they wish their union

[208] Feldman, "Abortion: The Jewish View," p. 17.
[209] R. Gordis, "Abortion: Major Wrong or Basic Right?," pp. 25–26.
[210] Bokser and Abelson, "A Statement on the Permissibility of Abortion," p. 37.

to lead to the birth of a child, not the synagogue or church, and certainly not the state.[211]

Rabbi Balfour Brickner, a leading Reform figure in social action endeavors, strengthened the impression that Reform Judaism had few qualms about abortion in his congressional testimony in 1974[212] and 1980.[213] Rabbi Brickner testified that Jewish law does not consider abortion to be murder and that a fetus is not regarded by Jewish law as a "person" or as a "human being." Consequently, in Brickner's words, Judaism recognizes "the legality of abortion." While acknowledging the need for a "reverent and responsible attitude to the question of abortion," Brickner utilizes a textual principle to construct a Jewish argument for freedom of choice:

> We have always sought to preserve a sensitive regard for the sanctity of human life. It is precisely because of this regard for that sanctity that we see as most desirable the right of any couple to be free to produce only that number of children whom they felt they could feed and clothe and educate properly: only that number to whom they could devote themselves as real parents, as creative partners with God . . . It is that regard for the sanctity of human life which prompts us to support legislation enabling women to be free from the whims of biological roulette and free mostly from the oppressive crushing weight of anachronistic ideologies and theologies which, for reasons that escape my ken, continue to insist that in a world already groaning to death with overpopulation, with hate and with poverty, that there is still some noble merit or purpose to indiscriminate reproduction.[214]

Brickner was expressing a widespread sentiment among non-Orthodox Jews in presenting this type of argument. It should be noted, however, that his case is constructed with a particular purpose in mind: to convince American legislators that Judaism approves of American women having freedom of choice in the matter of abortion. While this proposition is itself controversial, it represents an entirely different enterprise from determining Reform Judaism's *halakhic* response to abortion. As other Reform Jewish leaders involved in the political struggle would observe about Brickner's testimony: "[I]s it not stretching the tradition to assert that it would support abortion on demand? Can Jewish tradition really sanction

[211] I. R. Margolies, "A Reform Rabbi's View," in R. E. Hall (ed.), *Abortion in a Changing World*, New York, Columbia University Press, 1970, volume 1, p. 33.

[212] B. Brickner, "Judaism and Abortion," in M. M. Kellner (ed.), *Contemporary Jewish Ethics*, New York, Hebrew Publishing Company, 1978, pp. 279–283.

[213] A. Vorspan, and D. Saperstein, *Tough Choices: Jewish Perspectives on Social Justice*, New York, Union of American Hebrew Congregations Press, 1992, pp. 216–217.

[214] Brickner, "Judaism and Abortion," pp. 282–283.

abortion on economic, psychological, or social grounds? Arguing for the right of free choice in the matter of abortion does not necessarily mean that the grave decision to abort a fetus is either ethical or wise."[215] Brickner, then, does not so much represent Reform Judaism's attitude to abortion, as Reform's attitude to the American abortion debate.

From a Jewish legal perspective, the actual closeness of the Conservative and Reform positions can be seen in the conclusion to the 1985 *teshuvah* authored by Jacob, dealing with the timing of abortion:

We feel that the pattern of tradition, until the most recent generation, has demonstrated a liberal approach to abortion and has definitely permitted it in case of any danger to the life of the mother. That danger may be physical or psychological. When this occurs at any time during the pregnancy, we would not hesitate to permit an abortion. This would also include cases of incest and rape if the mother wishes to have an abortion...

We agree with the traditional authorities that abortions should be approached cautiously throughout the life of the fetus...

It is clear from all of this that traditional authorities would be most lenient with abortions within the first forty days. After that time, there is a difference of opinion. Those who are within the broadest range of permissibility permit abortion at any time before birth, if there is a serious danger to the health of the mother or the child. We would be in agreement with that liberal stance. We do not encourage abortion, nor favor it for trivial reasons, or sanction it "on demand."[216]

Like Klein, Jacob includes abortions for incest and rape among those that might well cause significant psychological damage to the mother. The evidence is certainly convincing that, resembling their Conservative colleagues, Reform respondents were open to abortion in cases that presented serious health needs, but not otherwise. As the 1995 *teshuvah* of the Reform rabbinate's responsa committee summarized it: "[A]ll the Reform responsa concerning this subject are careful to couch their lenient rulings within the general traditional understanding of the importance of alleviating 'great pain' to the mother. None of them suggests that Judaism should countenance any other reason as a valid basis for abortion."[217] It is indeed striking that despite the public support of many non-Orthodox Jewish groups for laws that allowed for abortion on demand, Conservative and Reform *teshuvot* stood firmly against abortions proposed for financial or family-planning reasons.

[215] Vorspan and Saperstein, *Tough Choices*, p. 217.
[216] W. Jacob, "When Is Abortion Permitted?," p. 27.
[217] Plaut and Washofsky (eds.), *Teshuvot for the Nineties*, p. 171.

In the last half of the twentieth century, then, not only did it become meaningful to speak of "Jewish views" on questions of abortion, but those views came to include a convergence of thought on additional permutations of the abortion problem. Centuries of independent *teshuvot* that had been concerned mainly with what the traditional texts could bear, gave way in these decades to a period of greater homogeneity, within a surrounding culture that brooked no evasion. Broad *halakhic* agreement emerged on those issues for which the tradition's intersection with modernity offered the least ambiguity: the duty to abort in order to save a mother whose life is threatened by her fetus, the refusal to countenance abortions for any reason that did not constitute a "great need" for the mother or fetus, the permitting of pregnancy reduction, and the forbidding of abortion for fetal tissue initiatives or for sex preselection.

Beyond these areas of generalized assent were those topics for which the tradition yielded more than one cogent position. Thus, abortions performed for fetal abnormality, for genetic disease, for emotional needs of the mother, or when the mother's long-term health is at stake, all presented circumstances in which a divergence of views was expressed. Perhaps even more controversial than these practical concerns was the pivotal issue of whether feticide should be considered to be akin to murder in any way.

The *halakhic* response to abortion had exhibited contrary views in previous centuries as well. In the twentieth century, however, these dis-agreements became unusually stark. This reality is hardly surprising. *Halakhic* decisions, after all, were not being made in a vacuum. Unlike in previous centuries, *poskim* had additional concerns to factor into their rulings beyond how a given question might relate to the textual heritage. The significant transformations in legal and attitudinal approaches to abortion that had swept much of the world inevitably came to affect the thinking of *halakhic* decision-makers. Feinstein explicitly describes the profound influence of surrounding events upon his own perspective as an Orthodox respondent,[218] and a similar impact was surely experienced across the Jewish spectrum. True to its historic mandate, the *halakhah* at-tempted to be responsive to what the judges saw in the world about them, as well as in the texts before them. But what they saw in the world about them was so different from any previous epoch that it created an atmosphere in which the rabbis responded in sometimes dramatic, and increasingly divergent ways.

---

[218] See above, pp. 175–176.

In one place in particular, the milieu in which Jewish law functioned was unique, such that the interface of societal realities with the *halakhah* raised even more complex questions than the twentieth century had already offered: the State of Israel. After two thousand years of statelessness, Israel presented a host of unprecedented challenges for the appropriate functioning of Jewish law within an environment in which Jews exercised real temporal power. The significance and the effectiveness of the *halakhah* within this unparalleled context would offer important insights to the question of whether the *halakhic* approach to abortion could, in fact, be applied successfully to the day-to-day lives of the members of a modern mass society. In Israel, the practical impact of centuries of *halakhic* deliberations on abortion, together with the results of their confrontation with modernity, would come to be scrutinized and tested as never before.

CHAPTER 6

Confronting a new reality: legislation for a Jewish state

There is a compelling logic behind the widespread assumption that a Jewish state must surely be governed on the basis of Jewish law. Consequently, there are many who are surprised to discover that, with the exception of the laws of personal status, this is largely not the case for the State of Israel. While elements of *halakhah* do appear in many parts of the Israeli legal structure, they do not constitute the systemic underpinning of Israeli law. Despite the fact that this situation has come to be accepted as normative, it is, in fact, anomalous from a Jewish perspective. The *halakhah*, after all, was never supposed to be confined to so-called "religious" matters, but was envisaged as the appropriate source for the civic governance of any Jewish body politic. Hence, the creation of an Israeli legal enterprise that is separate and distinct from the classic Jewish legal wellsprings produces awkward implications for both systems.

The historical road that led to this situation was not smoothly paved. When the State of Israel came into existence in 1948, the law that had been in effect in the country until independence became the law of the fledgling Jewish nation. Thus, an extraordinary legislative mixture, derived from Moslem religious law, Ottoman civil procedure, and English Mandatory ordinances, once described as "a mosaic, destined perhaps to excite the eye of an archaeologist, but not able to serve as a firm basis for healthy and normal legal relations," became the law of the land.[1] Perhaps the principal reason why Jewish civil law could not supply the legislative foundation of the nascent state was that it was in no shape to do so. As previously discussed, the abrogation of Jewish juridical autonomy had effectively forestalled the responsive development of Jewish law through most of the nineteenth and twentieth centuries, the very period when other legal systems were adapting to prodigious societal and

---

[1] M. Silberg, as quoted in Elon, *Jewish Law*, volume IV, p. 1612.

technological changes.[2] This substantial deficit in adapting to the conditions of modernity could have been successfully addressed had there been sufficient time and opportunity to focus on the task. But there was not. As the religious Zionist leader Rabbi Meir Bar-Ilan observed:

> Had we been more fortunate, the leaders, rabbis, and scholars of observant Jewry would many years ago have prepared a code of law for the State of Israel for the time when we would be privileged to see it established. But because we lacked faith, the State of Israel caught us suddenly unaware, without our having adequately prepared a civil and criminal legal system for it. We cannot, therefore, criticize those legislators for using Mandatory law as their guideline and setting up courts accordingly. What they can be criticized for, however, is that they did not declare that that system was only a temporary expedient for an emergency situation.[3]

Just as the rejuvenation of the Hebrew language and its reapplication to daily life nourished the distinct national identity of the Jewish state, an even more profound contribution to the national culture could have been made through the reinvigoration of traditional Jewish legal structures and their application to a modern context. Thus, an extraordinary opportunity to revitalize the legal ethos of the Jewish people and to reconnect with it in a practical sense was lost. This historic chance to fuse together the textual and spiritual heritage of the Jewish people with the real life of the Jewish nation was an unrepeatable moment. "This failure," wrote Menachem Elon, "proved to be one of the gravest errors in the history of the religious-national movement."[4]

The outcome of this failure was that, in the early decades of the existence of the state, Jewish law was not the default starting-place for legislative initiatives, and in those instances where it did become a part of the Israeli legal structure, its incorporation was piecemeal. Notwithstanding this reality, Elon, who has written definitively on this subject, has shown that this non-systematic approach did lead to the assimilation of Jewish legal principals with some frequency.[5] Moreover, in 1980, a substantive change occurred when the Knesset adopted the Foundations of Law Act. The Foundations of Law Act formally "severed the Israeli legal system from the binding force of English common law and equity, and ... created a binding link with Jewish law, to which it gave official status as a complementary legal source, making Jewish law a part of Israeli positive law."[6] However, as dramatic as this sounds, the effect of the Act

---

[2] See above, chapter 4, p. 95.
[3] M. Bar-Ilan, as quoted in Elon, *Jewish Law*, volume IV, p. 1606, n. 82.
[4] Elon, *Jewish Law*, volume IV, p. 1605.   [5] *Ibid.*, chapter 42.   [6] *Ibid.*, p. 1828.

was less than revolutionary. Jurists, after all, do not necessarily interpret legislative acts uniformly, nor do they always do so in accord with the intent of the legislators. Thus, the Foundations of Law Act has regularly been construed narrowly, and recourse to the interpretative principles of American, English, or Continental law "is a daily occurrence as a matter of course."[7] While the reasons for this reality are not germane to the current discussion, its implication is this: although it is certainly possible for Jewish law to serve as a motivating source of Israeli legislation, there is no watertight requirement that its precepts must be given primacy in the consideration of Israeli legal enactments or deliberations.

It is against this background, then, that the unfolding history of abortion law in the State of Israel, and its relationship to Jewish law, should be considered. As in most Western countries,[8] abortion statutes in Israel underwent profound changes in the second half of the twentieth century. During the first three decades of the state's existence, Israeli abortion law encapsulated the conceptual approach of British Mandatory law, which was founded in the English Offence against the Person Act of 1861.[9] Though very rarely implemented, this Israeli law prohibited abortion under all circumstances and prescribed fourteen years of imprisonment for abortion providers and five years for women who underwent abortions. It was not long, though, before amelioration in the law's application surfaced. In 1952, the District Court of Haifa ruled that abortions were permissible for legitimate medical reasons, a position that was supported by the then Attorney General. Instructions were issued that charges should not be pressed in cases of abortions intended to protect the life or health of the mother. Despite the fact that in 1963 the legal standing of these instructions was called into question, leading to their revocation, the authorities continued to act as if they were in place. In 1966, penalties against women who had abortions were dropped, and the prison term for abortion providers was reduced to five years.[10]

It is worth noting that the "quasi-legal" arrangement that was in place from 1952 to at least 1963 could be viewed as having some faint similarities to the more liberal Jewish consensus on abortion. For more than a decade, Israeli society maintained a conservative legal prohibition on abortion, while openly allowing those abortions that might have been acceptable according to a liberal understanding of the *halakhah* on abortion.

[7] *Ibid.*, p. 1897.   [8] See above, chapter 5, p. 133.
[9] R. Bachi, "Abortion in Israel," in R. E. Hall (ed.), *Abortion in a Changing World*, New York, Columbia University Press, 1970, volume 1, pp. 274–283.
[10] *Ibid.*

Abortion in Judaism

One other feature of this period also deserves mention: the "quasi-legal" abortions that were carried out were dependent on the approval of a committee of two physicians at the *Kupat Cholim*, the large national sick fund. While not under rabbinic supervision, this process of approval by physicians ostensibly offered assurance that only "appropriate" abortions would be authorized. This factor could be seen as an echo of the *halakhic* assumption that competent experts should adjudge the suitability of abortion in individual cases.

In actuality, however, abortion was by no means limited to this accepted "quasi-legal" arrangement. Any woman who was denied an abortion by the *Kupat Cholim* had "no difficulty in finding the help of a private practitioner."[11] By the late 1960s this trend led the Israeli statistician, Dr. Roberto Bachi, to conclude that "abortion appears today to be one of the most popular methods of family plannning used in Israel."[12]

It is important to clarify that for the first two decades of the state's existence, abortion was not an issue that garnered much public attention. The predominant religious ethos in the country was that of Orthodox Judaism, an Orthodoxy that was moving toward the stringent consensus on abortion. From a sociological perspective, Israel, as a young nation with a small population, stressed the demographic importance of childbearing, rooted in the Torah's mandate to "be fruitful and multiply." Furthermore, in a post-Holocaust environment, within a society in which security was an ever-present concern, children had come to represent survival, stability, and the promise for a more assured future. Hence, bringing more children into the world became a declared national priority.[13] This public posture, combined with the relative ease with which illegal abortions could be obtained, meant that there was little impetus for modifying the abortion status quo.

In the early 1970s, however, this status quo began to be challenged, not so much out of concern over potential fetal abnormalities, as in response to two new currents in Israeli society. First, the impact of the Black Panthers – a protest group that drew widespread attention to the economic disparities between Israelis of Afro-Asian and those of European backgrounds – led to studies that revealed a significant correlation between large families and economic deprivation. One outcome of this awareness was the understanding that a heavy emphasis on

[11] *Ibid.*, p. 276.   [12] *Ibid.*, p. 281.
[13] Y. Yishai, "Abortion in Israel: Social Demand and Political Responses," in Y. Azmon and D. Izraeli (eds.), *Women in Israel*, Studies in Israeli Society 6, New Brunswick, Transaction, 1993, pp. 290–292.

childbearing was not without cost, and that, in extreme cases, abortion might offer a "last resort" option to stave off potential family disasters.[14] The second new trend in Israeli society was the emergence of the Israeli feminist movement. In line with other feminist organizations abroad, the Israeli feminist movement saw abortion as a critical feminist issue and petitioned the Knesset for legislation that would legalize abortion on demand.[15] The Black Panthers and the feminist movement, together with international trends, succeeded in placing the issue of abortion squarely on the Israeli public agenda.

Once abortion had been raised to the level of public debate, it was not long before members of the Knesset became involved. In 1972 the Minister of Health appointed a public committee to study the issue of abortion, and the committee submitted its report in 1973. It recommended the legalization of abortion, restricted solely to qualified doctors in authorized medical centers. It proceeded to stipulate five conditions under which abortion should be allowed, given the approval of suitable experts:

[W]hen a woman's physical or emotional health is endangered; when pregnancy endangers her life; when it results from rape or incest; when there is fear for the unborn child's physical or mental health, and … when there is a possibility of serious disruption of the life of the woman or other members of her family – such as would be the case in large families.[16]

As a result of this report, two private members' bills were submitted to the Knesset in January 1975. One bill sought to permit abortions for seven distinct circumstances, the five enunciated by the committee, as well as abortions sought for cases of pregnancy out of wedlock and abortions for all women under the age of seventeen or over the age of forty-five. The second bill essentially called for abortion on demand during the first twelve weeks of pregnancy. Neither proposed bill advocated including any type of professional panel to vet the appropriateness of individual abortions. The second bill was soon rejected in deliberations of the Public Services Committee. The first bill, however, was agreed to with one addition: the Public Services Committee opted to include the requirement of a two-member abortion approval panel composed of a gynecologist and any one of: a physician in general practice, a social worker, or a public health nurse.[17]

It was in this form that the bill came before the Knesset for a first hearing in February 1976. Despite the contention of the chair of the Public

[14] *Ibid.*, pp. 293–294. [15] *Ibid.*, p. 294. [16] *Ibid.*, p. 296. [17] *Ibid.*, pp. 297–298.

Services Committee that the bill was not designed to encourage abortions, the religious parties thought that it threatened to achieve precisely
that outcome, and expressed their vigorous opposition in no uncertain
terms. The Knesset passed the measure back to a joint committee for
further work. At this stage, those groups fighting the bill became particularly vociferous. Writing at the time, the legal scholar Professor Ze'ev Falk
described consideration of the abortion law amendment as "one of the
most controversial pieces of Israeli legislation," resulting in "hot debates
and public demonstrations."[18] Though staunch resistance was by no
means limited to the religious, many Orthodox groups were particularly
outspoken:

> Objection was elicited mainly by religious circles, who employed violent means
> in order to terminate the process of legislation, which was well under way. The
> chair person of the committee was accused of being the incarnation of Hitler;
> in addition, street demonstrations were held and manifestos were distributed
> against the "bill of murder." The protest against the bill was not confined to
> small religious zealot groups but was joined by figures such as the chief Rabbis
> of Israel who demanded that it be abolished altogether.[19]

Opposition to the bill also emanated from gynecological professional
groups, ostensibly out of concern for women's health issues. But, unlike
the religious groups, the gynecologists were persuaded to support the
bill after some adjustments were made, principal among them being the
expansion of abortion approval committees from two to three members:
a gynecologist, a doctor in general practice, and a social worker.[20]

   In January 1977, eleven months after the amendment to the abortion
law first came to the Knesset, the bill received the Knesset's assent.
In a late change, designed to assuage religious dissent, the bill that the
Knesset finally approved omitted reference to abortion for reasons of limiting the size of large families. Otherwise, with only minor alterations,
the bill that was enacted reflected the Public Services Committee recommendations. Thus, Section 5 of the Penal Law Amendment (Interruption
of Pregnancy) Law 1977 provides:

> 5. (a) The committee [deciding on abortions] may, after obtaining the woman's
> informed consent, approve the interruption of pregnancy if it considers it justi-
> fied on one of the following grounds:
> 1. the woman is under marriage age, or has completed her fortieth year;
> 2. the pregnancy is due to relations prohibited by the criminal law or incestuous
>   relations, or extramarital relations;

---

[18] Z. Falk, "The New Abortion Law of Israel," *Israel Law Review*, volume 13, number 1, 1978: 103.
[19] Yishai, "Abortion in Israel," p. 298.   [20] *Ibid*.

3. the child is likely to have a physical or mental defect;
4. continuance of the pregnancy is likely to endanger the woman's life or cause her physical or mental harm;
5. continuance of the pregnancy is likely to cause grave harm to the woman or her children owing to difficult family or social circumstances in which she finds herself or which prevail in her environment.[21]

"Informed consent" was to be obtained by the three-member approval committee by explaining to the woman concerned "the physical and mental risks involved" in the interruption of pregnancy. The law further required that the approval committee could not refuse an abortion before giving the woman an opportunity to appear and state her reasons for desiring an abortion. In addition, the woman was obligated to provide her consent to the abortion in writing, and the approval committee's decision, together with the grounds justifying termination, were also to be recorded in written form.[22] The approval committee's conclusion was not subject to review or appeal, but a woman who had been refused an abortion by one committee was allowed to bring her case before another approval committee or committees. The Israeli Supreme Court ruled that the law did not allow husbands or other third parties to make representation to an abortion approval committee.[23]

The passage of the 1977 amendment was not, however, the final legislative step in the saga. Section 5(a)(5) of the Act, the so-called "Social Clause," permitting abortion in various personal, familial, and environmental circumstances, continued to be the cause of intense discontent on the part of the religious parties. The Rebbe of Gur, Rabbi Simcha Bunim Alter, a member of the Council of Torah Sages, succinctly articulated the attitude of this constituency when he wrote in *Hamodia*, the newspaper of the *Agudat Yisrael* party: "If the law is not amended [to prohibit these abortions], Agudat Yisrael cannot be a partner to the murder of fetuses and for Agudat Yisrael to remain in the coalition would be tantamount to partnership in the murder of fetuses."[24] It is clear that, in making this declaration, the Rebbe of Gur aligned *Agudat Yisrael* with the stringent consensus that had already declared abortion, other than to save the life of the mother, to be equivalent to an act of murder. What is perplexing – from

---

[21] Falk, "New Abortion Law of Israel," p. 109.   [21] *Ibid.*, 110.
[23] N. Morag-Levine, "Imported Problem Definitions, Legal Culture and the Local Dynamics of Israeli Abortion Politics," in F. Cass, *Israel, the Dynamics of Change and Continuity*, London, 1999, p. 230.
[24] Rebbe of Gur, as quoted in *Ha'Aretz*, November 15, 1979, cited in M. Zemer, *Evolving Halakhah: A Progressive Approach to Traditional Jewish Law*, Woodstock, Jewish Lights Publishing, 1999, p. 335.

a *halakhic* perspective – is why *Agudat Yisrael* restricted its opposition solely to the Social Clause:

> The Rebbe of Gur and his colleagues on the Council of Torah Sages never demonstrated that there was something amiss only with the "social" clause of the abortions law and that it is halakhically permissible to participate in a coalition that permits abortions in the circumstances enumerated by other sections of the law, such as pregnancy in women who are below the age of consent (seventeen), past forty, or unmarried.
>
> Why, in these cases, was membership in the coalition not a matter of being accessories to feticide?[25]

Notwithstanding this palpable inconsistency, it is plain that the religious parties were determined to eliminate any possibility of "Social Clause abortions," which they regarded as being essentially groundless.

Their lobbying efforts against the clause were finally successful in 1980 when coalition politics within the conservative Likud-led government resulted in the elimination of the Social Clause as a reason for abortion.[26] In reality, though, this change had little practical effect. The numbers of abortions being approved dipped, but then quickly returned to their previous levels, owing to the fact that abortion approval committees simply interpreted abortions sought for "social" reasons as coming under the heading of a mental or physical risk to the mother and approved them in this way. This development highlights the extent of autonomy enjoyed by the approval committees under the law. This autonomy, moreover, is unlikely to be shaken: a 1990 Knesset attempt to regulate the functioning of the more liberally oriented private-hospital approval committees failed in the face of widespread opposition.[27] Thus, notwithstanding the liberalization of the law, the previously established Israeli tradition of balancing a more conservatively expressed law with a more liberal application of the law continued to operate.

The Israeli abortion statute that emerged from the amendment process was a construction that placed Israel's enactment in the middle of the spectrum of international abortion laws. A 1997 global review ranked Israel in a group of about twenty countries that all allowed abortion on similar grounds; almost eighty countries had more restrictive standards than this group, while approximately fifty countries had more liberal standards.[28] It is important to note that almost all of the nations to

[25] Zemer M., *Evolving Halakhah*, p. 337.
[26] Morag-Levine, "Imported Problem Definitions," p. 230.   [27] *Ibid.*, pp. 238–239.
[28] A. Rahman, L. Katzive, and S. Henshaw, "A Global Review of Laws on Induced Abortion, 1985–1997," *International Family Planning Perspectives*, volume 24, number 2, 1998: 56–64. One

which Israel normally looked for its legal models – the United States, Great Britain, and the countries of Western Europe – had more liberal legislation than Israel.

How is it that Israel came to adopt a more centrist abortion law than so many other Western democracies? Professor Noga Morag-Levine, a political scientist, offers some insights. In her estimation, the amendment agreed to by the Knesset

is more in harmony with the traditional Jewish approach than the more absolute prohibition it replaced. The Israeli statute combines principled disapproval of abortion with exemptions under specified circumstances, a solution much in keeping with rabbinical case by case decisions on abortion. While Israeli law substituted the secular authority of the committees for the rabbinical, it retained the norms and logic of the traditional religious process.

The primary difference between the 1977 law and Jewish tradition lay in its inclusion of socio-economic conditions among the specified exemptions. The difficulty of reconciling socio-economic exemptions with religious formulations of maternal health led to ultimately successful ultra-orthodox agitation against the Social Clause.[29]

"Formal state law," Professor Morag-Levine later affirms, "accords with pertinent Jewish religious tenets…"[30] This perception suggests that the amended abortion law, unlike the strict prohibition it replaced, was fashioned with the "norms and logic of the traditional religious process" as a central concern. Indeed, there can be little doubt that this is so, given that two *halakhic* opinions are appended to the report of the 1973–74 public committee that fashioned the groundwork for the bill[31] and given the legislative tendency to look to Jewish law in circumstances where this was possible. Setting aside the provision permitting abortions for women under seventeen and over forty years of age, Israel's abortion amendment – as revised in 1980 – provides an approximate legislative reflection of the *halakhic* grounds sufficient to allow for an abortion to be permitted, viewed from a lenient perspective.

hundred and fifty-two nations with populations of more than one million people were included in the review. Nations were divided into five categories: (1) nations that permitted abortions only to save the life of the mother; (2) nations that permitted abortions to save the mother's life, or in the interests of her physical health; (3) nations that permitted abortions for life, physical health, or mental health; (4) nations that permitted abortions for life, physical and mental health, and on socioeconomic grounds; and (5) nations that permitted abortions without restriction as to reason. Israel was assigned to category three, the middle category.

[29] Morag-Levine, "Imported Problem Definitions," p. 231.   [30] *Ibid.*, p. 241.

[31] Committee for the Investigation of Abortion Prohibitions, "Commission Report: Appendices 4 and 5 – *Halakhic* Opinions," *Public Health*, volume 17, number 4, 1974: 495–502.

There is, however, an irony here. If the bill was fashioned in part with the idea of bringing Israeli abortion law better into "harmony with the traditional Jewish approach than the more absolute prohibition it replaced," then why did the Orthodox religious parties object so vehemently to this attempt to embody *halakhic* notions in legislation? How could a proposed enactment aimed at making the law of Israel comply more closely with traditional principles evoke bitter protests and accusations of Hitler-like malevolence? The answer is to be found in the divide alluded to previously between the more lenient and the more stringent consensuses. As has been seen, the stringent consensus – which, while not congruent with Orthodox Judaism, certainly included the Israeli Orthodox political parties and the majority of their adherents – regarded abortions carried out for any reason other than to save the life of the mother as tantamount to murder.[32] Consequently, when presented with a choice, the Israeli Orthodox political parties found the original prohibitory Israeli law and its application to be a far better fit with their understanding of the *halakhah* than any of the proposed amendments. When Professor Morag-Levine writes of the amended law embodying a greater "harmony with the traditional Jewish approach," she is correct only insofar as the traditional Jewish approach is viewed through the prism of the liberal consensus. The fierce denunciation of the abortion amendment on the part of the Orthodox political parties stemmed from the reality that the conservative consensus actually found greater "harmony" with the pre-1977 law and saw the amendment as moving away from traditional Judaism.

If, then, the amendment could not have hoped to please the majority of Orthodox Israelis, why did the Knesset not opt to accede to the will of the other vitally concerned constituency, the feminist movement, that wanted to make abortion-on-demand an individual right for all women? After all, the United States had already moved in precisely that direction, providing women with relative freedom to decide about the appropriateness of having an abortion.[33] Israel's amended abortion law, by contrast, was highly interventionist, dictating the circumstances under which abortion would be acceptable and then subjecting women to the scrutiny of a committee charged with ascertaining whether the proposed abortion met the legal criteria or not. Indeed, there can be no doubt that the Israeli law placed complicated restrictions on women's freedom and, hence, presented a much more difficult challenge in its application.

[32] See above, chapter 5, pp. 190–192.   [33] See *Roe* v. *Wade*, 410 US 113 (1973).

Why endure such struggles? If the law were going to be liberalized in a manner that the Orthodox would find unacceptable in any case, why not follow the American model by simply avoiding the list of sanctioned circumstances and the approval-committee gatekeepers altogether?

In all likelihood, one of the central reasons why the abortion-on-demand path did not garner widespread support in Israel was "due to tensions between the rights-based focus of the imported feminist agenda and the national collectivist values that many Israeli women continue to hold."[34] Put differently, the responsiveness of American society to an individual-rights-based argument for abortion was more than balanced in Israel by a range of perceived cooperative needs, not the least being a continued demographic concern that echoed across the political spectrum. As Professor Morag-Levine expresses it:

> The American focus on rights, whether of the fetus or the woman, was thus countered in Israel with arguments couched in the language of national rather than individual well being. The marginality of rights to definitions of abortion problems in Israel is in part explained by continuing deference to the state as an embodiment of nationally defined collective values.[35]

Abortion-on-demand did not galvanize the enthusiasm of many Israelis because, to some degree, it was perceived as being contrary to national values and needs, and the majority did not question the importance of raising national goals above individual privileges. According to this perspective, the amended Israeli abortion law was fashioned not only with an eye to Jewish sources, but with an appreciation that abortion-on-demand was not in consonance with the widespread perception of what was most conducive to the national interest.

Though this reality is, in large part, due to the particular conditions of Israeli society, it is possible that Jewish law may have exerted some small influence here as well. For Jewish law, based as it is in a series of *mitzvot*, is primarily oriented towards instilling responsibilities to God and society, rather than to carving out areas of individual privilege. Duties, it is fair to assert, are far more important to the Jewish legal system than rights. Consequently, in a society in which Jewish law can be said to have a voice, the impetus towards fulfilling mandates that uphold broader joint objectives is a more natural fit.

While this "national interest" reason certainly illuminates why a centrist path was initially palatable to the Israeli electorate, it does not explain how that path was comfortably maintained in practice. It is one thing,

---

[34] Morag-Levine, "Imported Problem Definitions," p. 236.   [35] *Ibid.*, p. 237.

after all, to agree to a national law for the sake of communal interests that seem remote from one's personal situation; it is an altogether different matter, within the context of a free democracy, to be denied an abortion that one personally feels is essential. Had the law operated as worded, it ought to have led to large numbers of denied abortions and to numerous prosecutions for performing illegal abortions.[36] As written, it would have been reasonable to expect that the law would have resulted in disgruntled families, imprisoned physicians, and fulminating discontent.

But no such outcome ever eventuated. Since the abortion-law amendment in 1980, while political parties of a left-leaning persuasion have persistently called for the restoration of the "Social Clause," no groundswell of public unhappiness has led to any movement towards further liberalization of the law.[37] There are two clear reasons why the public never became sufficiently disillusioned with the law to pressure politicians to make changes. Both have to do with the law's application. The first relates to the remarkably high approval rate generated by the committees operating in public and private hospitals around the country. The statistics for the years 1992 to 1996 show the approval rate for abortion applications running between 90 and 95 percent in each year. In actual figures, the total number of legal abortions carried out was sixteen to seventeen thousand per year, representing a rate of thirteen to fifteen abortions per one thousand women aged fifteen to forty-four every year.[38]

Why, it must be asked, was the approval rate so high? Was it because only those women who conformed to a strict reading of the legislation were applying for abortions, and it was therefore easy to approve almost all applications? It is highly unlikely that this was the case. After all, a strict reading of the legislation would have disallowed all abortions that did not portend health implications for the mother. Comparing Israel's abortion rate to that of the United States, a much lower abortion rate per thousand women would have been anticipated had such a strict reading been utilized.[39] Hence, as set out above, the generally accepted explanation

---

[36] The law specifically provided that a woman who underwent an illegal abortion would not be subject to any criminal penalty. However, the person carrying out the procedure would be "liable to imprisonment for a term of five years or a fine of fifty thousand pounds." See Falk, "New Abortion Law of Israel," 109–110.

[37] Morag-Levine, "Imported Problem Definitions," p. 236.

[38] *Israel Yearbook and Almanac 1998*, Jerusalem, Israel Business, Research and Technical Translation / Documentation Limited, 1999.

[39] According to the United States Centers for Disease Control, national abortion rates in the United States fell from a 1990 high in the mid twenties per thousand women aged fifteen to

for the very high approval rate is that the committees interpreted the law in a most lenient way, expanding the definition of maternal "health" to permit a wide range of abortions that the framers of the legislation intended to disallow when the "Social Clause" was removed.

There was, then, little cause for widespread public agitation about the restrictive nature of the committees; largely the committees did their work in a most lenient fashion. Further explanation, however, is still required. For, notwithstanding the high rate of approval, the committees still did reject 5 to 10 percent of the abortion requests that came before them. Moreover, this figure does not begin to take into account those women – probably considerable in number – who either had no desire to appear before a committee or simply came to the conclusion, correctly or not, that the committee would reject their requests, and so decided not to apply. Added together, these two groups should have represented a sizable pool of women prevented from having abortions, leading to a great deal of familial anguish. Why did this group not protest vociferously? To answer this question, it is necessary to turn to the second major reason why the public did not become more exercised about the abortion law.

This second reason can be located in the long-standing phenomenon of illegal abortion. According to the 1987 estimate of the Minister of Health, illegal abortions, normally carried out by physicians, were being performed at twice the rate of legal abortions in Israel.[40] While there is disagreement as to whether this is an overestimation or an underestimation of the true rate of illegal abortion, a consensus has coalesced around the view that there are at least as many illegal abortions as legal abortions in Israel, and probably far more.

It is worth noting that when totaled, the overall number of legal and illegal abortions carried out in Israel since the founding of the state may approach one million. For Israel, whose population at the close of the twentieth century was around five and a half million, abortion has had a substantial impact on its potential population numbers. For the Jewish people, moreover, which has not succeeded in replacing the enormous

forty-four, to twenty per thousand in 1996. See "Abortion Surveillance – United States, 1997" at http://www.cdc.gov. Though the United States has some restrictions on abortion, abortions are obtainable with comparative ease. It is inconceivable that Israel could attain an abortion rate that is approximately three-quarters of that of the United States had the law been read and applied in a strict fashion.

[40] Minister Shoshana Arbelli-Almosnino, replying to a Knesset question on July 14, 1987, as cited in M. Kaufman, *The Woman in Jewish Law and Tradition*, Northvale, Jason Aronson Incorporated, 1993, p. 172 and p. 282, n. 84.

population losses of the Nazi Holocaust, abortion has certainly been a limiting factor in potential population gains.

It is, then, fair to assert that, in keeping with the historic Israeli response to abortion laws, the 1980 law has been both applied and not applied in a most lenient fashion. Nor should this reality be perceived as a matter that has simply escaped the attention of the legal community. Indeed, on one of the two occasions that abortion issues have come before the Israeli Supreme Court, Justice Ben-Ito "acknowledged the precariousness of the legal structures underpinning the abortion status quo when she described the pertinent law as a delicate compromise aimed at determining not whether but how abortions would be performed and cautioned against judicial interference in this fragile equilibrium."[41] In other words, despite the fact that the 1977 law specifically prohibited abortion, albeit with delineated exceptions, Justice Ben-Ito seemed to perceive the legislation as being an abortion-enabling statute. Justice Ben-Ito's caution against "judicial interference," moreover, constitutes an acknowledgment that judicial intervention might well have become necessary, were it not for the desire to maintain the status quo. Hence, a striking dichotomy exists in Israel between a relatively exacting law on the one hand and the knowing acceptance of frequent transgressions of the statute on the other.

Professor Morag-Levine offers a succinct description of this unusual state of affairs:

> In contrast to American concerns with dyadic divisions between constitutional and unconstitutional moves, Israel's abortion arena has unfolded along a spectrum marked by much more subtle gradations in legality. Israeli legal rights, whether those of the fetus or the woman, have been marginal to an abortion management process only marginally constrained by its legal shell. Instead, both sides, out of mutual fear of backlash, appear committed to compromise premised upon the circumvention of law.[42]

Indeed, not only does the illegal behavior represent a largely uncontested "circumvention of the law," but Professor Morag-Levine cogently asserts that the approval-committee structure effectively "constitutes an institutional bypass within the law,"[43] providing official permission for the letter of the law to be breached. Thus, it is reasonable to assert that the Israeli abortion law is certainly not the only, and probably not the most powerful, determining source of authority in the "abortion management

[41] *Plonit* v. *Ploni*, Civil Appeal 413/80, p. 60, pp. 85–86, as cited in Morag-Levine, "Imported Problem Definitions," p. 240.
[42] Morag-Levine, "Imported Problem Definitions," p. 240.   [43] *Ibid.*, p. 241.

process." Societal realities proceed according to the dictates of what doctors and those for whom they care deem to be appropriate, substantially
untrammeled by the confines of the law.

Such "illegalism" or "extra-legalism" is not unique to Israel. In some
measure, it exists everywhere. However, a variety of researchers have
discerned that this response may be particularly apparent where there is
a sense of dual loyalty to two alternative legal cultures.[44] The unspoken
logic appears to hold that respect for both of the legal cultures involved
can be preserved effectively by carefully negotiating the tensions between
"formal symbolic messages and actual practices."[45] Thus, Israeli abortion "illegalism" represents a fine example of a delicate attempt on the
part of the body politic to preserve a Jewish legal culture – albeit a lenient
version – in the formal structure of the law, while allowing for a secular
legal ethic to prevail in practice. Seen this way, illegal behavior, within
acceptable limits, becomes a reasonable price to pay to ensure that both
systems can be respected, without forcing one to yield to the other.

What message, though, does all of this convey about the *halakhic* approach to abortion? Those who contend that there is no connection
whatsoever between Israeli abortion law and the *halakhic* treatment of
abortion would answer that realities in Israel are not at all informative
when evaluating the impact of the *halakhah*. Those, however, who accept
the viewpoint that the current Israeli abortion law is indeed a plausible
rendering of the lenient *halakhic* consensus are presented with a considerable challenge. For if the law is an approximate representation of
a lenient *halakhic* position, then Israeli abortion realities at the close of
the twentieth century lead to a rather disconcerting conclusion: even a
lenient *halakhic* consensus position on abortion seems to be essentially unworkable in practice. After all, as has been seen, upholding such a legal
position – without threatening considerable societal discontent – requires
a far-reaching elasticity in interpreting the law, as well as a preparedness
for the law to be circumvented with impunity where necessary.

Hence, while maintaining a law with *halakhic* features may well have
symbolic significance, it can hardly be argued that the law is well adapted
to the task of regulating social realities. This is not to suggest that the
amended abortion law is futile; it certainly articulates a clear set of values
that provides an important educational message, which might well have

---

[44] *Ibid.* Professor Morag-Levine cites studies from Korea, Brazil, and varying parts of Europe,
which show correlations between the existence of competing legal structures and tolerance of
illegal or extra-legal conduct.
[45] *Ibid.*, p. 242.

an impact on the process of making decisions on abortion. This possibility should not be taken lightly. Professor Mary Ann Glendon, a law professor at Harvard University, argues that the law, particularly in this area, can have a critical role in shaping societal attitudes over time:

> Law itself often assists in the formation of a consensus, influencing the way people interpret the world around them as well as by communicating that certain values have a privileged place in society. We need only think here of the roles that the equality principle and the enactment of civil rights legislation played in shaping our moral attitudes about racial discrimination.[46]

The educational function of the law in helping to influence society's viewpoint cannot be underestimated. However, while Professor Glendon is correct in this regard, it is difficult to discern any significant educational impact from the first decades of the law's functioning in Israel. In terms of creating an environment that is likely to shape "right and good"[47] behavior, arguably a central role of the *halakhah*, the law as it stands appears to be lacking in effectiveness. This results in a difficult conundrum. If, in the view of Israeli society, it is "right and good" essentially to allow for abortion on demand, then the lenient *halakhic* position, insofar as it is reflected in the law, is restrictive and obsolete. If, conversely, the current law is in fact a viable expression of what is "right and good," then its demands seem too restrictive for Israeli society to accept. Either way, while the *halakhic* position offers informative ethical insights, it seems to be wanting in terms of its responsiveness to practical realities.

Does this inevitably imply that *halakhah* is essentially irrelevant when it comes to the framing of a usable law for the Jewish state? Is it a necessary conclusion that any law designed to address the realities of abortion, as opposed to symbolism, must begin with a dismissal of *halakhic* nostalgia? The answer depends on one's view of *halakhah*. It is common to view the *halakhic* enterprise primarily as a textual matter, wherein once the textually "correct" answer – be it lenient or strict – has been determined, that answer becomes the *halakhic* response, notwithstanding its impact upon real circumstances. The frequent outcome of this approach is that a majority of Jews in any pluralist Jewish society decides to disregard numerous *halakhic* textual determinations. Some find this disregarding to be of no great concern. After all, they contend, the *halakhah* is *vox Dei*, not *vox populi*, so that the attitude of any majority or minority grouping

[46] M. A. Glendon, *Abortion and Divorce in Western Law*, Cambridge, MA, Harvard University Press, 1987, p. 59.
[47] Deuteronomy 6:18.

cannot be pivotal in the formulation of the law. This perception of the *halakhah* as an attempt to embody God's will is compelling. For the *halakhah* is indeed structured so as to fashion human behavior, to elevate human conduct above the temptation of our base instincts; it would be hard pressed to do this if some majority group were allowed to utilize its own instincts to form *halakhah*. According to this understanding, the *halakhah* acts as a legal stimulus to Jews, designed to elevate behavior toward the best possible human encapsulation of the Divine intent, no matter what practical consequences for compliance or effectiveness might ensue.

So long as a particular *halakhic* ruling is broadly respected as being ethically worthy – whether it is widely observed or not – there can be little quibble with this *halakhic* model. The problem for this model arises not when the law goes unobserved, but when its widespread application as written threatens some measure of societal revolt. If the enactment of a *halakhic* principle into a legal statute becomes unworkable not simply from an unwillingness to observe it but from a profound and widespread dissent from the law's correctness, can the "textual model" continue to be deemed a sufficiently responsive view of the *halakhah*? In Israel, if the *halakhah* provides a textual response that ignores societal realities, then Israelis are likely to seek a "realistic" response from the secular legal system. It follows that while there may be a desire to create laws based in *halakhah*, these laws inevitably will result in tolerated illegal behaviors, so long as the *halakhic* response is solely textually based. Such laws, grounded in the text, will express a *halakhic* aspiration that the majority of people are unprepared to keep, while the tolerated illegal behaviors will reflect the consensus view of what is deemed sensible. Hence, maintaining laws that are founded in this type of textual *halakhah* will require openness to their circumvention, because few will regard these laws as being reasonable in a practical sense.

Standing in contradistinction to this vision is Elon's above analogy between the process of revitalizing the Hebrew language, and the situation of Jewish law.[48] Imagine, Elon's analogy posits, if modern Hebrew had never come into existence, but instead Israeli law required the use of biblical Hebrew in official communications. Since biblical Hebrew cannot hope to offer a huge range of technical terminology that is critical for current discourse, "illegalism" would be the inevitable response: people would either resort to a foreign language to find the necessary terminology, or invent their own terms. In either case, the legal requirement

[48] Elon, *Jewish Law*, volume IV, p. 1941.

to use biblical Hebrew, while symbolically attractive, would almost of necessity be circumvented. Furthermore, a great deal of the language of interaction that is most critical in the day-to-day world would have no roots in Jewish sources whatsoever.

As is well known, however, the revitalization of Hebrew took an altogether different path. While the core of modern Hebrew is certainly drawn from ancient wellsprings, it was decided early in the revivifying process to create new Hebrew words – fashioned from old Hebrew roots – to give a truly Hebrew voice to the technological language of modernity. Instead of simply pronouncing foreign terms with a Hebrew accent, Hebrew words were crafted, often creatively built from ancient precedents, to address the linguistic requirements of a new epoch. Whereas other languages had been able to rely on an evolutionary process to produce the required modern terms, the unprecedented resurrection of Hebrew as the spoken language of a nation required a skillful manufacturing of words in order to make modern Hebrew a usable and self-sufficient language. In large measure, this has been a successful endeavor. Hebrew has developed in a Hebraic, rather than a foreign direction, and it has stimulated closer ties to the Hebrew-Jewish past in those who speak it.

Elon raises the question whether the *halakhah* can become a usable and self-sufficient law, just as Hebrew has become a usable and self-sufficient language. Elon believes that this goal is not only possible, it is critical:

Continuous creativity founded upon the past is characteristic of all Jewish culture ... The example of the Hebrew language provides reason for hope that Jewish law will be integrated into the legal system of the Jewish state and that the legal system of the State will thus take its place in the historical record of Jewish creativity.[49]

According to this model, *halakhah* is a larger enterprise than just the coherent application of textual mandates to the realities of a given Jewish community. If *halakhah* is to operate as the true legal foundation for the Jewish nation, it will only be effective if it is incorporated systematically into the legal structure of the nation and if Jewish creativity drives Jewish law to flourish in new directions from out of the seeds of the past. This model would anticipate the continued incorporation of the vast majority of *halakhic* provisions in their historic form, but when certain laws require adaptation in order to stimulate ethical behavior, a dynamic evolutionary process – rooted in traditional principles – would be initiated.

[49] *Ibid.*

How does all of this illuminate the status of *halakhah* and abortion law in Israel? It highlights the reality that there exists a variety of reactions to Israel's abortion law. One view – widely held by those who adhere to the stricter consensus on abortion – holds that the 1977 law is a travesty and should, ideally, be replaced with a law that allows for abortion only in cases of legitimate threat to the life of the mother. A second, more skeptical, view asserts that Israel's abortion law does not bear sufficient similarities even to a lenient-consensus *halakhic* view to arrive at any conclusions about how the application of a law founded in *halakhah* might operate in practice. A third view contends that the law is actually a reasonable attempt to enshrine *halakhic* principles in contemporary Israeli legislation, and that the evident legal circumventions required to preserve the law's viability demonstrate that the provisions of the *halakhah* are not suited to the demands of a pluralist Jewish environment. A fourth view states that the law indeed expresses *halakhic* principles, and that this can have an important educational role in molding behavior. A fifth view maintains that while the law is a possible way to encapsulate a *halakhic* position in contemporary legal terms, a final verdict about the role of *halakhah* cannot yet be returned. Until such time as *halakhah* has become integral to the Israeli legal system in such a way that it can be fully responsive to the Israeli milieu, it will be impossible to judge the viability of discrete *halakhic* provisions based on episodic *halakhic* grafts. While all five views have their adherents, the fifth is perhaps the most provocative in prompting reflection about the potential for *halakhic* influence within the Israeli legal structure.

However, not only are there complex political problems associated with any attempt to make *halakhah* a more organic part of the Israeli legal system, but there are numerous philosophical obstacles as well. Rabbi Shalom Carmy, a scholar contemplating the theoretical possibility of legislating a *halakhic* approach to abortion, foresaw virtually insurmountable difficulties in such a project:

On several practical issues, we cannot count on a consensus of rabbinic decision. These areas involve primarily questions about the kind of danger to the mother that would justify abortion (e.g., is danger to a mother's sanity equivalent to a threat to her life?). It would be unreasonable to prohibit legally, on moral grounds, an act of abortion that would be permitted by a mainstream halakhic decisor. On the other hand, it is not always obvious what constitutes a lenient ruling within the mainstream of halakhic development: does a theoretical suggestion count as a mainstream ruling (e.g., Jacob Emden's startling suggestion about abortion for bastards)?; what if the *Posek* later changed his mind?

To formulate the desirable limits of legislation would thus require the services of rabbis who are not only competent to rule on these issues but also able to formulate the acceptable range of decision. That such cooperation need be relied upon is not the least Utopian aspect of the project.[50]

While, as has been seen, it is possible for "a consensus of rabbinic decision" to evolve,[51] Carmy points to a number of significant methodological obstacles in formulating *halakhically* authentic abortion legislation. Beyond the contentious problem of locating suitable rabbinic authorities for the task lies what is clearly the most formidable difficulty of all: formulating "the acceptable range of decision." If the *halakhah* is to respond coherently to real life circumstances, how will the variety of *halakhic* voices be coordinated to produce a result that is *halakhically* valid as well as relevant?

Attempts to delineate how the *halakhah* ought to be systematized to produce an "acceptable range of decision," have yielded several differing approaches. A number of these strategies are worthy of consideration, not only for what they teach about abortion, but for the light they shed on the understanding of those involved in the *halakhic* enterprise concerning the nature of the *halakhic* venture itself. Thus, Israel's attempt to grapple with abortion in a Jewish state has focused renewed attention on the critical and intriguing question of how the *halakhah* should best be encapsulated and further developed. It is, therefore, valuable to ponder the ways in which Jewish abortion law might conform optimally with the received textual tradition, and yet function effectively in this unprecedented Jewish era.

[50] S. Carmy, "Halakhah and Philosophical Approaches to Abortion," *Tradition*, volume 16, number 3, 1977: 151.
[51] See above, chapter 5, pp. 189ff.

CHAPTER 7

A halakhic *challenge: discerning Jewish abortion principles*

Among the few observations that may be made with certainty concerning Judaism and abortion is that, in its practical rulings, Jewish law has usually eschewed extreme positions. This outcome was not strategically planned in order to make Jewish views more palatable to external critics. Polarized positions on abortion are, after all, normative within contemporary society. There are outlooks that advocate that abortion should always be prohibited, even if it is to save the life of the mother.[1] Conversely, there are standpoints that express precisely the opposite: that a woman's decision to have an abortion ought to be accepted, no matter what her reason for desiring the procedure.[2] As the rabbis have demonstrated, however, the Jewish consensus views on abortion do not accord with either of these approaches.[3] Rather, normative *halakhic* positions have always held that some amount of abortion is required – in order to save the life of the mother – but have uniformly rejected abortions that cannot be justified either because of maternal need, or for a threat to the fetus, or perhaps to save another child. In reality, however, while this more centrist position has much to commend it, it has also proven to be

---

[1] The Catholic Church is the most prominent proponent of this position. Pope Pius XII succinctly expressed the unwavering view of the Church when he stated that every human being, even the infant in the mother's womb, is afforded the right to life from God. No authority or "indication for abortion" can take away that right. Thus, for example, to save the life of the mother is a most noble end, but the direct killing of the child as a means to this end is not licit: "The child, formed in the womb of the mother, is a gift from God, who confides it to the care of its parents"; Pope Pius XII, *Acta apostolicae sedis*, 43 (1951), pp. 838–839, as cited in Grisez, *Abortion*, p. 182.

[2] Feminist perspectives regularly articulate this view with great clarity. A concise example, from among many, holds that "While a fetus resides within her, a woman has the right to decide about her body and her life and to terminate a pregnancy for [disability] or any other reason"; M. Fine and A. Asch, "Shared Dreams: A Left Perspective on Disability Rights and Reproductive Rights," in M. Fine and A. Asch (eds.), *Women with Disabilities: Essays in Psychology, Culture and Politics*, Philadelphia, Temple University Press, 1988, p. 302.

[3] For a good discussion of Jewish approaches in contrast to the more polarized positions see M. Gold, *Does God Belong in the Bedroom?*, Philadelphia, The Jewish Publication Society, 1992, pp. 118–134.

somewhat unfocussed: more extreme stances have a clarity that it is difficult to maintain closer to midstream.

Indeed, the historic record has ably demonstrated that the *halakhic*
response to abortion is anything but sharp. The *halakhic* picture abounds
with complexities and nuances. Consequently, it is hardly surprising that
some have proposed the application of structural templates to Jewish
abortion deliberations in order to achieve greater consistency and coherence, as well as what they deem to be more appropriate outcomes.
Assuming that such principled methodologies may have some influence
on future *halakhic* directions and rulings, it is important to evaluate criti-
cally the insights provided by their strategies.

The first such approach is that of Rabbi Ratzon Arusi, who, in
the 1990s, served as the chief rabbi of Kiryat Ono and as a member
of the Israel Chief Rabbinate Council. Arusi draws a distinction between "*halakhah*," which he regards as a theoretical legal construct, and
"*halakhah le-maʾasei*," which he understands to be the practical application
of *halakhah* to actual situations.[4] In the area of *halakhah*, it is immediately clear that Arusi is intent on demonstrating that the cacophony of
halakhic voices could be tamed by examining the worthiness of a particular source in terms of its place within a *halakhic* hierarchy that he
perceives to be operative. According to Arusi, the rules by which this
hierarchy is governed, if applied correctly, are fully capable of eliminat-
ing equivocation and yielding authoritative answers to difficult problems.
Thus, in Arusi's estimation, the *halakhah* in a given area can be deemed to
have been correctly ascertained provided that there is adherence to five
rules. The first rule is that priority should be given to the examination of
Mishnaic and Talmudic sources that deal directly with the subject under
consideration – Arusi designates these as "primary" sources. The second
rule is that attention should be paid to the proper application of those
halakhic principles that are genuinely relevant to the solution of the problem. The third rule is that insight should be sought from "secondary"
sources, all the while taking great care that such sources are indeed germane to the issue at stake.[5] Arusi's fourth provision is that the rulings of a
posek should take precedence over the positions of a *parshan* (commentator), because the *posek* has an intent to create a *halakhic* ruling, something
that may not be true of the *parshan*. Finally, his fifth provision holds that

[4] R. Arusi, "*Halakhah VeHalakhah LeMaʾasei BeBitzuʾah Hapalah Melakhutit BeMishpat HaʾIvri*," *Dinei Yisrael*, volume 5, 1977: 119. *Halakhah le-maʾasei*, then, may, depending on the *posek* concerned, exhibit considerably more flexibility than the theoretical *halakhah*. See Arusi, p. 132.
[5] *Ibid*., p. 120.

rulings found in works of *halakhic* codification should be preferred over rulings found in *teshuvot*, since the former offer a more "pure" view of the *halakhah*, while the latter represent specific instances of *halakhah le-maàsei*.[6]

Arusi proceeds to illustrate how the system that he has elucidated in theory actually works in practice, by applying it to the abortion issue. Put briefly, Arusi holds that *Mishnah Ohalot* 7:6 is the sole relevant primary source on abortion, and that the plain implication of the text is that one is only permitted to sacrifice the fetus in order to save the life of the mother. In Arusi's view, it follows from this that the reason the fetus may not be killed is because such an act represents an appurtenance of the spilling of blood. Consequently, Arusi holds that Rashi's viewpoint could be understood as conveying that the fetus ceases to possess *nefesh* standing only in those instances when it is threatening its mother's life, but does not carry implications for *nefesh* standing at other times. Hence, there most certainly could be no permission to kill the fetus "just for the purpose of preventing the pain of the mother."[7] Arusi expresses astonishment at Sinclair's assertion that Unterman's description of abortion as the appurtenance of the spilling of blood involved "an element of a novel approach, [as] this type of idea was not encountered among the *Rishonim* and *Acharonim*, according to the best of our knowledge."[8] Not only is there nothing novel about it, asserts Arusi, but it was given at Sinai and reaffirmed by a long line of *poskim*, both *Rishonim* and *Acharonim*, who held that the law of the spilling of blood is at the root of the matter. In Arusi's estimation, then, the only primary text on abortion, *M. Ohalot* 7:6, clearly states that abortion is only permitted when the fetus poses a substantive and immediate danger to the life of the mother.

Arusi's second rule, requiring the proper application of those *halakhic* principles suitable to the matter under consideration, leads him in the same direction. Arusi first gives an example of a *halakhic* principle, which, he avers, is not well adapted to the "solution" of the abortion "question": the use, by some scholars, of the *ubar yerekh imo* concept is not helpful. According to Arusi, this principle was sometimes misused to demonstrate that the fetus, as a "limb" of its mother, might be readily sacrificed for the sake of the mother's well-being. However, the use of this principle is under dispute not only in the Talmud, but among the *poskim* as well.[9] Moreover, Arusi recalls, Ellinson already indicated that *ubar yerekh imo* has no bearing

[6] Arusi R., "*Derakhim BeCheker HaHalakhah UVeVeirurah*," *Techumin*, volume 2, 1981: 518–520.
[7] Arusi, "*Halakhah VeHalakhah LeMaàsei*," 122–124.
[8] Daniel Sinclair, as quoted in Arusi, "*Derakhim BeCheker HaHalakhah UVeVeirurah*," 520.
[9] Arusi, "*Halakhah VeHalakhah LeMaàsei*," 124–125.

on fetal status, and is limited to a few situations, none of them having the slightest association with abortion.[10] Conversely, Arusi maintains, the principle that "there is nothing that is permitted to a Jew but prohibited to a non-Jew" is both pertinent to and instructive within the abortion context. Arusi sees this principle as being pivotal to the abortion issue for a variety of reasons, perhaps the foremost being that the capital punishment meted out to a non-Jew for an act of feticide provides strong evidence that the "spilling of blood" is the core concern in abortion. This principle, in Arusi's view, was effectively made an inseparable part of the *halakhah* on abortion through the prohibition of the *Tosafists*.[11]

Arusi's third rule, that insight should be sought from germane "secondary" sources, also offers no contradiction to his established trend. By way of example, Arusi points to the two apparently conflicting sources in the *Arakhin Gemara*. One calls for a pregnant woman who is convicted of a capital crime to be executed without delay – seemingly implying that fetal interests are sufficiently subordinate that the fetus can be destroyed so as to prevent "dishonor" for the condemned mother. The other demands that the *Shabbat* be overridden in order to extract the fetus of a mother who has died – which suggests that the fetus has sufficient independent standing to warrant transgressing the *Shabbat* on its behalf.[12] Both of these sources, in Arusi's view, are "secondary" when it comes to the matter of abortion, because they do not address the subject directly. Furthermore, Arusi posits, not only are they secondary, but neither is truly germane to the abortion issue, the first because it is a special regulation peculiar to the provisions of punishment within Jewish law and the second because it deals with the future potential of the fetus, whereas abortion is concerned with the fetus' present disposition.[13] It is clear, then, that in Arusi's estimation, where secondary texts are used they must be treated with considerable caution in order to ensure that they are indeed fully applicable to the matter at hand.

Arusi's last two directives, that the rulings of a *posek* take precedence over the positions of a *parshan* and that legal statements found in works of *halakhic* codification are to be preferred over rulings found in *teshuvot*, are consistent with the outcome of his other rules. If a *posek* takes precedence

---

[10] See above, chapter 2, p. 32.   [11] Arusi, "*Halakhah VeHalakhah LeMaʿasei*," 125–128.

[12] See above, chapter 2, pp. 45ff.

[13] Arusi, "*Halakhah VeHalakhah LeMaʿasei*," 128–131. There is, of course, a strong position that holds that a knife could be brought on the *Shabbat* in order to remove a live fetus from the body of its dead mother. This was explained on the basis that, although a clear transgression of the *Shabbat* was involved, the transgression of one *Shabbat* was permitted because of the potential of the fetus to preserve many *Shabbatot* in the future. See above, chapter 2, p. 48.

over a *parshan*, then handling the problematic *halakhic* divergence between Rashi and Maimonides, which through the centuries had elicited
so many ingenious resolutions, turns out to be a relatively simple matter.
The Maimonidean outlook trumps that of Rashi because Maimonides is
a *posek* and Rashi is a *parshan*. Similarly, the Codes, for the most part, reiterate Maimonides' *rodef* stance, whereas positions that are more lenient
are to be found in the *teshuvot*. Hence, preferring *halakhic* codification to
teshuvot most certainly helps to extract clarity from disorder, a clarity that
is indeed capable of yielding "answers" to abortion questions.

Every application of Arusi's system, then, leads to the same conclusion: the true *halakhah*, stripped of what Arusi sees as imprecise distrac-
tions and inaccurate accretions, is capable of producing an unmistakable
halakhic position on abortion. This position, delineated by Arusi, deems
the more restrictive stance of the tradition to be the "true," core intent
of the *halakhic* heritage. It is an undeniably neat system for ordering the
untidiness created by a plurality of varying *halakhic* perspectives. Arusi's
approach, however, has been vulnerable to criticism. Shortly after the
publication of Arusi's first article, Moshe Drori, who, at the time, was
a member of the Institute for the Research of Jewish Law in Jerusalem,
wrote about the teleological nature of Arusi's endeavor:

It appears to the reader that after the author has crystallized his own position
as to the approach of the *halakhah* to a [given] problem, he "orders" the sources
in a manner that is convenient to him: those that follow the line that he has
chosen for himself are [designated as] primary [texts] or general principles, and
the rest, which are not compatible to his view, are [designated as] being only
secondary.[14]

Drori proceeds to contrast Arusi's approach to that of Sinclair, whose
work he praises, opining that Sinclair's "objectivity" is likely to produce
"better fruit."[15] Arusi's strategy is inferior, in Drori's estimation, because
it is an exercise in giving greater prominence to those sources favored
by Arusi, precisely because they provide what Arusi preordains to be the
"right" answer.

Arusi, however, has a response to this judgment of his system: he
points to Sinclair's own assessments of the *halakhic* material[16] and inquires
rhetorically about the fundamental techniques employed by Sinclair:

[14] M. Drori, *"HaHandassah HaGenetit: Iyun Rishoni BeHeibetim HaMishpati-im VeHaHilkhati-im,"*
Techumin, volume 1, 1980: 294, n. 81.

[15] See below, pp. 243–251, and D. B. Sinclair, *"HaYesod HaMishpati Shel Issur Hapalah BaMishpat*
HaIvri," *Shenaton HaMishpat HaIvri*, volume 5, 1978: 177ff.

[16] See below, pp. 243–251.

How then do we allow the assembly of *halakhic* material without examining its sources, and without taking a position on the nature of its sources, and, in the end, [we countenance] a determination between the positions without any reason? Is this what is called objectivity?! And why are the fruits [of this strategy] better? Only because he [Sinclair] tends towards the view of those who are lenient, even though he does not demonstrate [the validity of] this [view] from the power of Talmudic sources?![17]

Rejecting the idea that he had chosen his texts in order to support a particular position, Arusi counters his detractors by saying that Sinclair is, in fact, guilty of something worse: presenting texts without offering any principles by which to analyze them and then arbitrarily evaluating their worthiness based on a preexistent bias. Surely it is better, Arusi proposes, to employ agreed-upon tools of analysis by which to arrive at a conclusion, rather than to rely on subjective appraisals of the sources.

This defense, however, was not sufficient to deter further misgivings about Arusi's approach. Washofsky also points to real difficulties with Arusi's conceptualization. Washofsky writes that as far as Arusi is concerned:

The stringent position is the correct *halakhah* on abortion, therefore, because it accords with Arusi's formal rules of decision-making. Arusi contends that these rules can function as a universal key to *halakhic* correctness, identifying the "right" answer to every controversial question by distinguishing the proper sources for decision. The problem, however, is that there is little evidence that *halakhic* authorities other than Arusi himself would accept this system as an objective standard of *halakhic* truth. Indeed, each of Arusi's "rules" is vulnerable to critique.[18]

Washofsky proceeds to provide a detailed critique of Arusi's rules. Washofsky's three main objections can be summarized as follows. First, that Arusi's classification of texts as "primary" or "secondary" vis-à-vis a given subject is both foreign to the texts and forced upon them. Notwithstanding, for example, that Arusi sees the *Arakhin* 7a text as dealing with specific laws of punishment and, therefore, as not being pertinent to the abortion issue, a number of leading *poskim* did not read the text this way, but regarded it as being most relevant. Arusi's designation in this regard, Washofsky contends, is inescapably subjective. Second, preferring a *posek* to a *parshan* is not the accepted manner in which to evaluate *halakhic* positions. In actuality, *poskim* function as commentators as well, such that

[17] Arusi, "*Derakhim BeCheker HaHalakhah UVeVeirurah*," 521.
[18] Washofsky, "Abortion and the Halakhic Conversation," p. 57.

the only way to decide which view is to be favored is to make an intellectual selection based upon the "persuasiveness" of each individual's interpretation of the texts under discussion. Third, many *halakhic* experts hold that the decisions found in *teshuvot* are in fact preferable to those found in codes because *halakhah le-maʿasei* affords better legal insights than "theoretical learning."[19] Given these various objections, Washofsky concludes that attempts like those of Arusi to impose rigid rules upon the *halakhah* are, perforce, doomed ventures:

> Thus has it always been. For every Yosef Caro, who posits a set of rules for decision-making, there is a Moshe Isserles who offers a different set of rules, and there is a Shelomo Luria who rejects them both. Arusi's system is therefore a failure. For any system of decisory rules to "work", to yield the indisputably correct legal solution, the rules themselves must be above controversy. They must be accepted as "the rules of the game" by the preponderance of those who play it ... Yet no such perception is current among the rabbis. Indeed, Arusi is forced to spend a great deal of time critiquing all those eminent *posqim* – Trani, Bacharach, Waldenberg, Benzion Ouziel, Yehiel Yaʿakov Weinberg, Shaul Yisraeli – who do not analyze the abortion question according to the rules he finds obvious ... Arusi "finds" that the lenient *posqim* are objectively wrong, but in fact they are wrong only because he says so, because they fail to conform to his own version of proper legal procedure. He therefore cannot argue that he has identified the objective standard of *halakhic* correctness.[20]

Washofsky makes a strong point. From the viewpoint of simplicity and clarity, one might wish that it were otherwise. After all, even those who do not favor Arusi's conclusions on abortion would certainly find it immensely easier if unarguable rules could be applied that might determine with some certainty what the *halakhic* response ought to be to a given issue. But, as Washofsky has shown, the reality is that Waldenberg and Unterman, Yisraeli and Feinstein, Ouziel and Soloveitchik are far from agreeing with each other on the relative importance to be accorded the various *halakhic* sources and their interpretations, let alone agreeing with Arusi's structure.

Indeed, one could reasonably argue that if legal systems were intended to operate in the way that Arusi contends that the *halakhah* ought to function, the need for judges to utilize their judgment in order to evaluate a particular issue would be vastly reduced. The "true" *halakhic* response could be effectively discerned by the more or less automatic application of a set of "Arusi rules" on the part of skilled "judicial technicians,"

---

[19] *Ibid.*, pp. 57–59.   [20] *Ibid.*, p. 59.

without the need for unpredictable judges. Those who bemoan so-called "activist judges," judges whose rulings are seen to reshape the law in ways that allegedly were not intended by the framers of the law, would be well satisfied with Arusi's attempts to curb judicial independence. But most *poskim* are unlikely to derive contentment from the application of interpretative restrictions like those set forth by Arusi. For, despite the existence of a range of possible governing principles, the *halakhic* system has always been sufficiently open to allow for an unusual position like that of Yaȧvetz to be deemed as authoritative a response as that of Feinstein. While it is plain, therefore, that the *halakhah* does have generally accepted parameters of interpretation, these parameters cannot be drawn nearly so narrowly as Arusi portrays.

Even as Arusi is absolutely persuaded that the *halakhah* ought to provide unequivocal "answers" to abortion conundrums, it should be stressed that he applies this strategy not just in the field of *halakhah le-maȧsei*, but in the area of theoretical *halakhic* research as well. The Arusi rules are designed to yield conclusions as to the direction preferred by the *halakhah* generally, notwithstanding the manner in which a particular *posek* might rule in an individual circumstance.[21] It is hardly surprising that Arusi should be so concerned with finding the "correct" conclusion. As Washofsky has observed, since the *halakhah* is supposed to represent the distillation of God's will into human action, "how can the *halakhah* appear simultaneously to affirm both 'X' *and* 'not-X' as answers to the same question?"[22] It is possible, however, that Arusi's attempt to invoke *halakhic* order in the pursuit of definitive outcomes is based on a misconstruing of the *halakhic* endeavor: perhaps indeed the aim of the *halakhic* system is not so much to arrive at "solutions" to problems as it is to engage in a process of thoughtful consideration and response.

Indeed, the second approach to the functioning of the *halakhah* in the light of the abortion issue focuses precisely on the significance of *halakhah* as "conversation." Offered by Washofsky, this outlook draws heavily on an approach to jurisprudence called "law as practical reason."[23] Washofsky first rejects the model of "legal formalism," of which Arusi's structure is an example, as inapposite to the *halakhah*. Legal formalism, a conceptualization which "conveys a theory of judicial decision-making

---

[21] Arusi, "*Derakhim BeCheker HaHalakhah UVeVeirurah*," 522.

[22] Washofsky, "Abortion and the Halakhic Conversation," p. 60.

[23] *Ibid.*, pp. 67–77. Washofsky cites a number of proponents of this way of understanding the law. Among them are: Steven Burton, Vincent A. Wellman, Neil MacCormick, and John Ladd. See Washofsky, p. 87, n. 100.

according to rule, the use of deductive reasoning to yield correct answers to even the most difficult questions of law,"[24] is, according to Washofsky, not the way that any legal system operates in reality, and certainly not the *halakhah*. Washofsky also rejects the opposite end of the spectrum, the "Critical Legal Studies movement," as being a poor fit with the *halakhah*. The Critical Legal Studies perspective views the legal enterprise as suffused with subjectivity such that there is "no objective constraint upon judicial discretion."[25] A decisor, according to this stance, "can manipulate the texts so as to arrive at whatever answer is dictated by his or her value-preferences," with the result that the law ends up being "but politics by another name."[26] The Critical Legal Studies model fails to represent the *halakhah*, Washofsky suggests, because the *halakhah* in actuality does exert objective constraints: the fact that there are those understandings of the law which are considered to be "legitimate," and, hence, those which are "illegitimate," argues that the *halakhah* imposes boundaries upon judicial interpretation. To contend, then, that the formalist system of attaining one "right" answer does not comport well with the *halakhah* is most certainly not to maintain that all answers are feasible.

Rather, Washofsky posits the notion that *halakhah*, especially in a complex area like abortion, sets forward "more than one right answer," but by no means an unlimited number of acceptable responses. Moreover, Washofsky explains, within the "law as practical reason" conception, what constitutes an acceptable response is determined principally by its "reasonableness," or, in other words, by its success in describing a compelling "vision of how things ought to be." "Law as practical reason," then, does not attempt to disavow the subjective element involved in the legal process. It acknowledges that judges will, at times, arrive first at a tentative decision about the subject under consideration and then proceed to find the means. It views the judicial task as one which regularly is "a process of thinking which starts not from the premises but from a vague conception of the conclusion and which searches for principles or data that either support the conclusion or lead to intelligent choice among rival conclusions."[27] This "intelligent choice" will be made by selecting that conclusion which best supports the "relevant goals and purposes" of the system in question.[28]

Discerning good arguments or acceptable goals and purposes within any legal framework is, in Washofsky's estimation, a function of the

[24] *Ibid.*, p. 61. [25] *Ibid.*, p. 68. [26] *Ibid.* [27] *Ibid.*, p. 69. [28] *Ibid.*, pp. 69–70.

rhetorical success of the positions being advanced.[29] If one is able to persuade a particular "community of legal interpretation" that a given argument or goal is cogent and that it fulfills the aims of the system, that stance will attain validity, notwithstanding the fact that the author may have arrived at a conclusion before constructing the logic to get there. Washofsky offers an example from the abortion context:

> Yair Bacharach's prohibitive ruling is an instructive example of *halakhic* rhetoric, of practical reasoning employed in the service of justifying the desired conclusion. Bacharach, we will recall, begins by offering arguments which would permit an abortion for the repentant adulteress; then, after citing the "widespread custom" among Jews and Gentiles alike to prohibit abortion as a means of discouraging illicit sex, he refutes each one of these arguments, giving the law a stringent cast. His rhetorical strategy, I think, is clear: he sweeps the reader in his wake towards a lenient reading of the sources which clashes directly with the reader's moral sense, which in that day can be assumed to conform with the "widespread custom." Then, by showing how the sources can be understood so as to affirm the moral sense, he leaves the reader with the distinct impression that the prohibitive theory is the better of the two possible ways of reading the law. Given the indeterminacy of the precedents, Bacharach determines that the law must accord with that alternative reading that lies closer to the Torah's overriding purpose, to establish justice and holiness. His answer is both textually justifiable and chosen, over the other textually justifiable possibility, on the basis of criteria that are external to the texts but no less vital to the law as we know it must be.[30]

From Washofsky's perspective, then, the task is not to "prove" a particular case, but rather to offer persuasion that it is a case that fits the available texts and accords well with the values and priorities of the *halakhah*. Since there can be no such thing as objective legal validity, Washofsky contends, a given stance will be valid if substantial elements within the "legal community" can be satisfied that it is *halakhically* cogent and meritorious.

According to this model, it follows that in some fields there will be more than one viable, legitimate solution to a given conundrum. To be sure, in many *halakhic* areas the response to questions of considerable complexity will see judges arrive at one "right" answer; the available texts, precedents, and systemic values will usually preclude alternative responses. Nevertheless, uncomfortable though it may be for the formalists, for subjects like abortion a plurality of answers will prove to be feasible.

---

[29] Washofsky explains that his use of the term "rhetoric" "includes all the means by which a writer or speaker attempts to persuade an audience, to elicit its 'adherence' to the rightness of a proposition. In this sense, rhetoric is equivalent to argumentation itself"; *ibid.*, p. 70.

[30] *Ibid.*, pp. 71–72.

Moreover, Washofsky maintains, the very existence of a plurality of possible solutions to a particular question elevates the significance of the
judge's assessment, "when the texts could lead their readers toward more
than one conclusion, argument of necessity becomes goal-oriented. The
purely legal reasoning is directed toward ends which, though not demanded by the texts themselves, are informed by the *poseq*'s general
sensibilities, his deeply held convictions as to what God and the Torah
require of us."[31]

Hence, Washofsky's vision of *halakhic* functioning sees the *halakhah* as
a legal conversation in which multiple differing positions on an issue can
coexist and interact within a framework of mutually recognized legitimacy. In this conceptualization, the feature that makes one particular
response stand out as being superior within a "conversation" is the ability to convey a case that is convincing. In those *halakhic* conversations
that are "profoundly controversial," such as abortion, particular communities will arrive at their own conclusions from among the *halakhically*
possible options. The "conversational model" is preserved, provided that
those options that are *halakhically* possible – namely those that have been
endorsed by a recognized *posek* and chosen by a given *halakhic* community – can enjoy a "legitimate and serious claim to *halakhic* validity."[32]
Suggesting, for example, that the position of either Rashi or Maimonides
might be dispensed with by formalist techniques is artificially to end a
significant *halakhic* conversation. While a particular judge may persuade
a given community that one or other viewpoint is more acceptable at a
given juncture, the *halakhic* legitimacy of both views must be maintained
if the "conversational model" is to be sustained. The alternative is the
stifling or censoring of *halakhically* legitimate positions, a move that would
result in such positions becoming inappropriately inaccessible to future
generations. Washofsky argues that, especially for contentious issues, the
halakhah best fulfills its mandate to set forth the manner in which a Jew
should act not when it "arbitrarily denies options" in the name of a single solution, but when it sustains a plurality of reasonable and reasoned
positions:

Halakhah, like law, is best understood not as science but as an enterprise in
world construction . . . It is by ongoing argument, the refusal to be committed
to the existence of one exclusively correct answer to every question of law,
that Jewish law has preserved the vitality needed to accommodate the never-
ending changes and transformations of Jewish life . . . [We] should reject any

[31] *Ibid.*, pp. 72–73.   [32] *Ibid.*, p. 74.

and all attempts to impose "scientific" methods that would arbitrarily force an end to the *halakhic* conversation on abortion and other questions of legitimate controversy. For Jewish law has always worked best as an argument, the search for truth conditioned by the humble realization that "the" final truth may always escape us. *That* is *halakhah* at its best.[33]

One of the great advantages of the conversational model proposed by Washofsky is that it requires none of Arusi's rule making, or his elaborate rejection of incompatible positions, in the pursuit of some "final answer." It presents, furthermore, a most satisfactory accounting of the openness evident in the history of the *halakhic* response to abortion, at least until the middle of the twentieth century. Rejecting foreclosure by fiat, Washofsky's model embodies a clear commitment to safeguard those positions that have historically been considered *halakhically* possible and legitimate, as "live" options from which subsequent generations of *poskim* can make responsible selections.

It is important to observe that Washofsky's approach to practical abortion matters is entirely consistent with his preferred encapsulation of the *halakhah*. Indeed, it might well be said that Washofsky's commitment to choice appears to be at the heart of his intellectual methodology. Elsewhere, when writing about abortion, Washofsky gleans from the *halakhic* literature that "the morality of any particular decision for abortion must be judged on a case-by-case basis." In explaining this idea, Washofsky asserts that:

In the here and now of this situation, her religious tradition or her conscience will demand of a woman the conclusion that an abortion is morally justified, even though well-meaning observers, judges and legislators may disagree. The interests of morality are served and not frustrated when we allow her to make that decision. It is an odd form of morality that strips the individual of her power to choose a morally justifiable action. Yet that is precisely what happens when we operate under the misconception that morality is synonymous with the restriction of choice.[34]

From the outset, Washofsky had expressed his determination to show that "freedom of choice in abortion is a morally defensible doctrine,"[35] and the statement above represents the nub of his argument. Washofsky does not accept the proposition that all abortions are morally justifiable. He does maintain, though, that it would be a "distortion" of morality to refuse to permit those abortions that are morally justifiable.

[33] *Ibid.*, pp. 76–77.
[34] M. Washofsky, "Morality and Choice: A Response to Daniel Callahan," in B. S. Kogan (ed.), *A Time to Be Born and a Time to Die: The Ethics of Choice*, New York, Aldine de Gruyter, 1991, p. 76.
[35] *Ibid.*, p. 74.

The problem with Washofsky's approach is that he does not offer a defined way to ascertain whether a particular abortion is morally justifiable or not, beyond indicating that "danger" to the mother's life and some circumstances "including her physical health and emotional well-being" are "morally significant and may warrant the termination of pregnancy."[36] This claim, however, is open to challenge. Why, for example, should the state of the mother's emotional well-being be a "morally significant" justification for abortion? While Washofsky has arguments to support his position, there is deep disagreement on this very question in both Jewish and non-Jewish circles. It follows that if Washofsky, or some other arbiter, is unable to supply an account of what is morally justifiable that can be held to be generally acceptable within a given community, then what Washofsky is actually defending through his argument is the moral appropriateness of making a *subjective* decision about what is morally justifiable. Without some external standard of what is morally justifiable, Washofsky's argument allows a woman to make such a decision according to her own judgment of what is morally justifiable, free to ignore the "observers, judges and legislators" around about her. While Washofsky's argument may have appeal, many will express concern at the difficulty of avoiding the natural and understandable human tendency to rationalize one's desires as being morally appropriate under these circumstances.

Given that Washofsky does not hold to the view that any decision to abort made by a pregnant woman is *ipso facto* moral, his entreaty not to place moral restrictions on choice will inevitably lead to the performance of abortions that cannot in fact be morally justified. Apparently, though, this is a price that Washofsky is prepared to pay in the name of defending abortion choice. If the alternative is the artificial foreclosure of options that may, in certain circumstances, be morally justifiable, it is more important to Washofsky that full choice be available, even though it means that some may make choices that are morally wanting.

Whatever one might think of Washofsky's argument, it bears a similarity to his systemic model for the *halakhah*. As Washofsky envisages the *halakhah* "at its best," no *halakhically* feasible position should be excluded from potential use by a judge through the narrowing of the law via artificially imposed criteria. Whatever was once *halakhically* possible and legitimate ought to remain on the agenda so that a *posek* may utilize that option to make a persuasive case that the *halakhah* ought to be applied that way in a given situation. Just as no abortion option that could, in

---

[36] *Ibid.*, p. 76.

theory, be morally justified should be ruled out of consideration for a pregnant woman, so no "*halakhically* feasible" position should be ruled out of consideration for a *posek*. In both cases, Washofsky makes choice his doctrine.

The question, consequently, that must be asked is: if Arusi drew the parameters of acceptable *halakhic pesikah* too narrowly, does Washofsky depict them in a way that makes them look overly broad? Rabbi Joel Roth, an expert on *halakhic* process, cites the legal scholar P. J. Fitzgerald in drawing a useful distinction between what Fitzgerald calls "law in the first sense," and "law in the second sense." Simply put, a question of "law in the first sense" is one that the judge "is bound to answer in accordance with a rule of law – a question which the law itself has authoritatively answered." A question of "law in the second sense" is different: it is "a question as to what the law is."[37] Later, Roth uses these categories to make the following observation about different types of approaches to the *halakhah*:

In light of the tendency of legal systems, as they develop, to limit areas of judicial discretion in favor of matters of law in the first sense, it is not unanticipated that we find the same tendency operative in the halakhic system as well. Moreover the degree to which the recognized greats of the legal tradition acquiesce in this development, or fight against it, gives us an indication of what each conceived to be the best way of ensuring the viability of the system. To the degree that some advocate the retention of maximal and expanding realms of judicial discretion and theoretical flexibility within the *halakhah*, they indicate their conviction that its viability is ensured by openness and nonuniformity. If, on the other hand, others reject this view and favor the imposition of uniformity through the elevation of increasing numbers of questions to the realm of matters of law in the first sense, they are arguing for definitiveness as the best guarantor of the viability of the system. Since both positions, in their extreme forms, are problematic – the former because of the danger of legal chaos, and the latter because of the danger of the stultification of the system – one seeks to discover how the masters of the past have balanced these opposing forces.[38]

While Washofsky, then, harbors appropriate concerns that Arusi's conception could lead to "stultification of the system," his own conceptualization may well be vulnerable to the accusation that it tends toward legal unruliness. Indeed, as has been seen, the price that must be paid for the conversational model of *halakhah* is that no position that was at

---

[37] J. Roth, *The Halakhic Process: A Systemic Analysis*, New York, The Jewish Theological Seminary of America, 1986, pp. 49–50. The explanations given here are Professor Roth's quotations of P. J. Fitzgerald, *Salmond on Jurisprudence* (12th edition), London, Sweet and Maxwell, 1966, pp. 65–75.
[38] Roth, *The Halakhic Process*, pp. 93–94.

any time historically feasible within the *halakhah* can be definitively ruled out of *halakhic* contention, even if that position is deemed to be ethically inferior. Thus, even if the overwhelming majority of *poskim* were to view the killing of a Tay-Sachs fetus as not only forbidden, but as ethically indefensible, they would be unable to deactivate the approval of Tay-Sachs abortion made *halakhically* possible by Waldenberg. That approval would always be potentially part of the "conversation," waiting in the wings for its rhetorical reactivation in the hands of a skilled judge.

Proponents of the conversational model would most likely respond that this is as things ought to be and that the conversational model of the *halakhah* is, in fact, self-correcting. This is so because a position that is generally regarded as being ethically indefensible would gain no rhetorical traction and would, therefore, continue to be irrelevant to the practical thrust of the law. While this may be so, a central concern with the model remains: the conversational model does nothing to stimulate an evaluation of competing rulings based on their moral acceptability. Thus, for example, Waldenberg and Feinstein cannot both be offering positions that are equally morally worthy: either the killing of a fetus with Tay-Sachs disease at seven months is morally acceptable or it is repugnant. The conversational model, however, holds that, since both positions are *halakhically* feasible, so long as they can garner a supportive constituency, they cannot be explicitly designated as being "beyond the bounds," even if they are viewed as morally less than desirable. If, then, a central goal of the *halakhah* is the distillation of those behaviors that will lead to the greatest good and the most elevated holiness, the conversational model does little to provide direction in this search.

The conversational model, moreover, is not a wholly satisfactory encapsulation of the way that the *halakhah* has functioned historically. While the metaphor of the *halakhah* as conversation has much to recommend it, it is not altogether fitting to see the *halakhah* as a conversation that stands ready to give voice to any view that was once held to be legitimate. As Bleich expresses it:

With the redaction of the Mishnah, and later of the Gemara, binding decisions were promulgated with regard to many matters of *Halakhah* which served to establish normative practices in areas which previously had been marked by diversity born of dispute. This, of course, did not preclude subsequent disagreement with regard to other questions, which had not been expressly resolved.[39]

[39] J. D. Bleich, *With Perfect Faith: The Foundations of Jewish Belief*, New York, Ktav Publishing House Incorporated, 1983, pp. 3–4.

Hence, Washofsky's model may well be accurate in theory, for it is true that practices once rejected could conceivably be resurrected if a successful rhetorical argument were to gain the assent of a given *halakhic* community. Nevertheless, there is a very real sense in which even attempting such an endeavor would be deemed extraordinary, because the *halakhah* tends to arrive at resolution and then "move on."

Normally, this process of resolution is achieved through the accumulation of what Roth terms the "weight of precedent."[40] Roth makes the point that the codification of the *halakhah* marked "a watershed in the development of the halakhic process," since the codes became the "repositories" of the "weight of precedent." He notes that the amassing of codified material, particularly in the *Shulchan Arukh*, gave the "weight of precedent" more presumptive power than had hitherto been the case, such that, in most instances, judges came to take their direction from it. This having been stated, it should be noted that Roth readily affirms the right of the judge to make an independent decision that is appropriate to the circumstances before him, utilizing whichever sources are deemed suitable. This decision, moreover, may be completely contrary to the "weight of precedent": "In the final analysis, only the systemic principle '*ein lo la-dayyan ella mah she'einav ro'ot*' (a judge must be guided by what he sees)[41] stands as the ultimate judicial guide."[42] It is reasonable to conclude, then, that Washofsky's *halakhic* vision better accounts for the reality of judicial independence than does that of Arusi. Where Washofsky's model does not fare so well is in explaining the practical limits that, in reality, precedent often places upon a *halakhic* conversation, theoretical openness notwithstanding. Put differently, once a body of precedent has coalesced within the *halakhah*, it will come to have a presumptive power, such that independent voices will need to work far harder to gain a hearing. Washofsky's entreaty, therefore, to preserve *halakhic* choice may well be in order so long as abortion matters remain questions of "law in the second sense," but would lose relevance, were these matters, through increasing "weight of precedent," to be changed into questions of "law in the first sense."[43]

---

40 Roth, *The Halakhic Process*, p. 113.   41 This is a Talmudic principle found in *Baba Batra* 130b.

42 Roth, *The Halakhic Process*, p. 113.

43 It is important to note that Washofsky's model has a further weakness: it seems to presuppose a *halakhah* that lacks real temporal power. As has been seen, however, the existence of the State of Israel requires a broader response. In this sense, Washofsky's appeal for maximum *halakhic* flexibility appears more suited to a Diaspora environment, where the voluntary acceptance of *halakhic* rulings makes *halakhic* diversity and variability more tolerable than it does in a milieu where it is envisaged that the *halakhah* might serve as a foundation for actual temporal law.

Is there, then, an alternative approach to the path of Arusi and Washofsky? Sinclair offers a third possibility. Sinclair is convinced that, historically speaking, the *halakhah* on abortion has been shaped by a somewhat unusual "combination of legal doctrine and moral consi-derations."[44] The legal doctrine to which he refers is simple, consisting of two points: "the principle of fetal non-personhood and the absence of any well-defined legal category for prohibiting non-therapeutic abortion."[45] The "moral considerations," however, are more complex. The *Rishonim* and *Acharonim* inherited a *halakhah* that did not regard the fetus as a per-son. It follows from this that abortion was not considered to be homicide within Jewish law. According to Sinclair, however, this idea seemed "to offend against a very pervasive moral intuition prevalent in most Chris-tian countries to the effect that feticide is indeed associated with the destruction of life and not with any lesser type of offence."[46] Sinclair posits that much of the *halakhah* on abortion can be understood as the rabbis' attempt to resolve this tension between the prevailing standards of external morality and the extant *halakhah*, in order to "compensate for the apparent shortcomings of the classical doctrine of fetal non-personhood in Jewish law."[47] This is tantamount to conceding that the *halakhah* on abortion appeared, when compared with the standards of surrounding society, to be morally deficient and was in need of refinement.

According to Sinclair, this refining was first undertaken by the *Tosafists* when they declared that feticide is "not allowed," based upon the con-nection between *halakhah* and the Noahide laws.[48] In Sinclair's estima-tion, this connection is significant because, in the *halakhic* world-view, the Noahide laws "served as a blueprint for the moral framework of civilised societies in both Jewish and non-Jewish circles alike."[49] Coupling this view of the Noahide laws with Maimonides' position that the Noahide laws are rational in their nature, Sinclair concludes that the Noahide laws "may very well be regarded as a fundamental moral framework for society, the foundation of which lies in rational thought."[50] Given that this is so, it becomes clear that the Talmudic provision that "there is nothing permitted to an Israelite yet prohibited to a Noahide"[51] effec-tively ensures that Jews are bound by the provisions of this preexistent, fundamental corpus of Noahide morality, even if its provisions are not explicitly enjoined by the *halakhah*. Consequently, it is possible, explains

---

[44] Sinclair, "Legal Doctrine and Moral Principle," p. 18.   [45] *Ibid*.   [46] *Ibid*., p. 13.
[47] *Ibid*.   [48] See above, chapter 3, p. 62.
[49] Sinclair, "Legal Doctrine and Moral Principle," p. 15.   [50] *Ibid*.
[51] *Sanhedrin* 59a. See above, chapter 3, p. 62.

244 *Abortion in Judaism*

Sinclair, to understand the *Tosafists'* use of the terminology that feticide is "not allowed" – as opposed to the more usual *halakhic* term *assur* (prohibited) – in this way: "Implicit in the use of this phrase is the notion that without a criminal sanction, there can be no infraction of the criminal law and hence, the only possible source for putting non-therapeutic abortion beyond the pale of acceptable conduct is the moral mechanism of the Noahide code."[52]

From this analysis, Sinclair discerns the "moral considerations" that are critical to the construction of abortion *halakhah*:

The moral element is the Noahide law which places unjustified feticide in the category of acts which are "not allowed" on the basis of the fact that they offend against the foundations of the moral order. Now, it is certainly arguable that the distinction made here between law and morality is neither watertight nor is it made in general usage. It must, therefore, be emphasized that it is rooted in later halakhic literature on abortion in Jewish law rather than the primary definitions and first principles of jurisprudence and ethics... [T]he tension between the Biblical and Talmudic positions on fetal status and the awareness that they both seem to fall below the general moral standard is endemic to the *responsa* in this area, especially in the more recent period. The resulting rulings have on occasion made this tension explicit and have generally resolved it by turning, in effect, to general morality in order to bring the *halakhah* up to what is regarded as an acceptable moral standard. Indeed, there is at least one halakhic authority who makes this point quite explicitly, whilst others direct their responses to non-Jewish sources of morality and ethics.[53]

The authority, who Sinclair contends makes the point "explicitly," is Bacharach. It is important to recall that Bacharach had written, "Therefore, according to what we have shown, the law of the Torah would permit what you ask, were it not for the widespread practice among us, and among them, to seek to establish a fence to curb the immoral..."[54] In Sinclair's view this is a clear statement that the abortion prohibition, which Bacharach sought to justify with the "tentative argument" of the wanton spilling of male seed, was, as far as Bacharach was concerned, grounded in "conventional morality rather than halakhic doctrine."[55]

Sinclair proceeds to make the case that there are other examples in which "conventional morality" appears to be the preeminent concern of the *poskim*. Besides Bacharach, he cites Al-Chakam, Zweig, and Feinstein in this regard.[56] While Sinclair's reading of Al-Chakam raises

[52] Sinclair, "Legal Doctrine and Moral Principle," p. 18. [53] *Ibid*., pp. 18–19.
[54] See above, chapter 3, p. 78. [55] Sinclair, "Legal Doctrine and Moral Principle," p. 21.
[56] *Ibid*., pp. 22–30.

problems,[57] Zweig's concern about how Judaism would look in comparison to "jurists, physicians and the Church" if the *halakhah* were to take a permissive stance,[58] ably supports Sinclair's contention. Feinstein also lends credence to Sinclair's hypothesis, albeit from a different perspective, in his declaration, "I have written all this because of the great outbreak of licentious behavior, in that the governments of many countries have allowed the killing of fetuses . . . hence, at this time, there is a need to make a fence for the Torah."[59] It is primarily an external moral concern that seems to propel Feinstein's more restrictive *halakhic* approach. Indeed, Sinclair speculates whether some of the differences between Waldenberg and Feinstein may in fact be attributable to the diverse moral milieus in which they lived:

> In this respect, it is noteworthy that Feinstein's country of residence is the United States where abortion is a highly controversial issue and the subject of an ongoing public debate. The authentic moral position is often identified, in the mind of the general public, at any rate, with that of the strict forms of Christian doctrine in both Catholicism and Protestantism. Waldenberg, however, lives in Israel where the issue has a much lower public profile and where the moral highground is less well-defined, even in the mind of the public.[60]

While this point is conjectural, Sinclair's overall argument is persuasive: "Moral concerns with regard to the image of *halakhah* figure in the decision-making process in abortion cases and often manifest themselves in striking deviations from regular halakhic reasoning in *responsa* or specific cases in this area."[61]

This depiction of the unfolding development of abortion *halakhah* leads Sinclair to two noteworthy observations. The thread common to both is Sinclair's inference that specific ethical criteria – criteria that are external to "regular halakhic reasoning" – will form an indispensable part of the future of abortion *halakhah*. Sinclair's first observation is that the link that hitherto has existed in abortion *halakhah* between the non-*nefesh* standing of the fetus and concern over maternal welfare is in the process of being severed. As has been seen, until the latter part of the twentieth century, permission for abortion was almost always predicated either on the notion that the fetus was behaving as a *rodef* or on the idea that the non-personhood of the fetus, combined with maternal distress, allowed for abortion, following Rashi.[62] In either instance, feticide was only

---

[57] See above, chapter 4, pp. 114–116.   [58] See above, chapter 5, p. 148.
[59] See above, chapter 5, pp. 175–176.
[60] Sinclair, "Legal Doctrine and Moral Principle," p. 28.   [61] *Ibid*.
[62] See above, chapter 3, pp. 58–59.

countenanced because of some measure of maternal anguish. Even in the case of the *mamzer* fetus – in which those who permitted abortion did so, to some degree, because of the ignominious outcome of being born a *mamzer* – the suffering of the mother was seen as a vital component.[63]

However, contends Sinclair, this link can no longer be viewed as inviolate. Modern issues have stretched the nexus between fetal non-personhood and maternal suffering to the breaking point. In the matter of pregnancy reduction, if there is any maternal pain involved, it is "hardly the same order of suffering as that indicated in traditional sources on abortion in halakhic literature."[64] Moreover, the question of whether it is permissible to sacrifice the fetus to obtain fetal material for healing purposes also challenges this link. In contradistinction to many, Sinclair is not certain that the *halakhah* has fully resolved this issue, for even if there is a consensus against the "commodification" involved in using a fetus to provide fetal tissue in order to save someone other than the mother, what of those cases where the fetus is not wanted for "parts," but must die if a relative is to be saved?

For example, ought a mother to undergo a bone-marrow transplant to save her sister's life even if this might cause the death of her fetus? Is the prime consideration here the mental suffering of the mother as a result of knowing that she could have saved her sister's life but did not do so in order to preserve her fetus, or is it the determination that her sister's life overrides that of the unborn child, or a combination of both?[65]

This instance, too, Sinclair suggests, portends a disconnection of fetal non-personhood from a threat to the mother's well-being. Of course, this would not be the case if *poskim* were to rule that where there is no maternal suffering the pregnancy should proceed. If, however, *poskim* rule that the fetus, lacking *nefesh* status, ought to be sacrificed in the name of saving the full-*nefesh* sister, this would certainly appear to be a ruling based on fetal non-personhood, without substantive maternal danger. This leads Sinclair to a provocative conclusion:

Clearly, the advent of new technology is bringing a great deal of pressure to bear upon the traditional link between the doctrine of fetal non-personhood and maternal welfare. It is also evident that it is unlikely that the link will survive this pressure and the question of defining the parameters of the Biblical and Rabbinic principle that a fetus is not a legal person will require new answers for the first time in several centuries.[66]

---

[63] See above, chapter 3, pp. 8off.   [64] Sinclair, "Legal Doctrine and Moral Principle," p. 32.
[65] *Ibid.*   [66] *Ibid.*, p. 33.

If Sinclair is correct, and he may well be, then the task of "defining the parameters" of fetal non-personhood will, of necessity, be informed by a variety of ethical considerations, not previously a part of the "halakhic reasoning" in this area. No easy task, such a mission will involve a principled reappraisal of the standing of the fetus within the Jewish legal world-view.

Sinclair's second noteworthy observation is that "[a] concerted effort is required ... to develop a set of moral principles in the area of abortion to which *halakhists* may turn in order to test the conclusions of their doctrinal reasoning in a particular case."[67] Sinclair arrives at this conclusion after observing that many contemporary *halakhists* "tend to measure the moral appropriateness of their rulings in terms of Christianity alone."[68] Not only has this tendency been responsible for the strictness evident in the more stringent consensus view,[69] but it has produced, Sinclair posits, a *halakhic* picture that is arguably less Jewishly "authentic" because it is not grounded primarily in the "classical concept of the Noahide system." The original Jewish approach, according to Sinclair, was to ground abortion law in this most universal of codes, a code which had as its aim "the principle of the preservation of society and its defence against attacks on the bodies and property of its citizens."[70] Though Sinclair concedes that there is genuine difficulty in imbuing this principle with "specific content," he nevertheless contends that embarking on this project might well be "more profitable" than "merely taking on the dogmas of the dominant faith."[71]

Sinclair offers an illustration of the importance of establishing a set of moral principles to deal with the abortion issue. He suggests that proponents of "*halakhic* positivism" – allowing *poskim* to apply available *halakhic* precedents to abortion questions, unfettered by external considerations – ought to consider the rulings of Waldenberg. Those who applaud the "liberalism" of Waldenberg's ruling in the Tay-Sachs case[72] and regard Waldenberg's position as being "perfectly humane" might well contend that the application of moral principles to the *halakhah* is unnecessary and that *halakhic* positivism of the type offered by Waldenberg is perfectly adequate to deal with abortion matters. However, Sinclair notes, Waldenberg's *teshuvah*, in which he permits the abortion of a fetus afflicted with Down's syndrome, is significant.[73] There is, Sinclair cautions, "little to distinguish" the two cases "in terms of halakhic doctrine." Indeed,

---

[67] *Ibid.*, p. 34.   [68] *Ibid.*, p. 33.   [69] See above, chapter 5, pp. 189ff.
[70] Sinclair, "Legal Doctrine and Moral Principle," p. 33.   [71] *Ibid.*, p. 34.
[72] See above, chapter 5, pp. 166ff.   [73] See above, chapter 5, pp. 181–182.

Sinclair notes that while Waldenberg appeared more hesitant to permit the abortion of a fetus with Down's syndrome, Waldenberg stated that "[O]n the basis of my *responsa* on Tay-Sachs there are more than adequate grounds to use the same sources in order to permit the abortion of a Down's Syndrome fetus."[74] Sinclair questions whether it is just as "perfectly humane" to apply the same permissive stance to a fetus with Down's syndrome as to a fetus afflicted with Tay-Sachs disease.

If this is not enough to prompt a reconsideration of *halakhic* positivism, Sinclair echoes Dorff in pointing out that some genetic diseases that are detectable in fetuses hold the possibility of fatal consequences for the bearer only decades hence. Would it, he asks, be morally acceptable to those of a more permissive viewpoint if a *halakhic* positivist approach were to permit the abortion of these fetuses because of such a condition? Sinclair implies that even the more liberally minded might demur at this juncture and might welcome limitations on the scope of *halakhic* positivism. This leads him to conclude as follows:

> Tosafot's remark about there being no legal sanction on feticide but that "it is not allowed" in situations of a non-therapeutic nature then becomes highly relevant, and the Noahide principle of the preservation of the moral fabric of civilized society combines with pure legal doctrine in order to find a solution to the problem, which is both halakhically valid and morally sound.
>
> There can be little doubt that one of the greatest challenges of the 21ˢᵗ century to ... abortion *halakhah* in particular, will occur in the form of genetic technology ... Halakhists concerned with abortion must ensure that there is a suitable body of moral principles available for directing the application of their legal doctrine in this complex field of Jewish law.[75]

Sinclair again interprets the *Tosafists'* position to be that feticide is forbidden not for "pure" legal reasons, but because non-therapeutic feticide does not comport well with the universal Noahide vision of the moral standing of a civilized society. It is this Noahide vision, contends Sinclair, that should continue to act as a corrective to *halakhic* positivism today. The creation of specific moral principles that will apply this vision within Jewish abortion law is, therefore, an important contemporary priority.

Sinclair clearly offers a path between that of Arusi and Washofsky. He eschews both the automatic application of systemic rules espoused by Arusi, and the openness to any position that *halakhic* positivism might yield and that a given community might be persuaded to accept, as

---

[74] Sinclair's translation from *Tzitz Eliezer*, volume XIV, number 101.
[75] Sinclair, "Legal Doctrine and Moral Principle," p. 35.

proposed by Washofsky. Instead, Sinclair opts for an approach in which *poskim* would continue to have considerable latitude in their decision-making, limited not just by *halakhic* precedent, but by an expectation that they will operate within a specific set of moral principles.

Sinclair's central point, that since the time of the *Tosafot*, the *poskim* were concerned to ensure that the *halakhah* on abortion conformed to high moral standards, is convincing. Indeed, it accounts well for a number of the struggles encountered within abortion deliberations: the effort to find the correct balance between Rashi and Maimonides, the search for the justification behind the prohibition on abortion, and the circumstances under which the prohibition could be circumvented. These can be seen, at their core, as attempts to define the *halakhah* according to stricter or more lenient standards of what is deemed to be morally acceptable.

Furthermore, Sinclair's insight that permission for abortion no longer appears to depend upon a link between fetal non-personhood and maternal suffering may well denote a significant turning point in the development of abortion *halakhah*. Sinclair is of the view that this demands a rethinking of what actions the doctrine of fetal non-personhood – in cases where there is no threat to the mother's welfare – should permit. In actuality, as has been seen, the widespread permission for pregnancy reduction to save the maximum number of fetuses has already begun to create a response to this new reality, albeit without any disciplined rethinking.[76]

Indeed, it could well be argued that the broad consent accorded to pregnancy reduction is further evidence of how external moral concerns continue to play a significant role in abortion *halakhah*. After all, for those who subscribe to the more stringent consensus view of abortion, one might well have expected that, absent any significant danger to the mother, *halakhic* positivism would contend that pregnancy reduction ought to be dismissed as "tantamount to bloodshed." Indeed, not only might *halakhic* positivism lead to this conclusion, but the *halakhic* case most analogous to pregnancy reduction, that of the sinking boat,[77] also argues against making any selection. That authorities like Zilberstein and Bleich go as far as they do to construct arguments that are contrary to the thrust of *halakhic* positivism[78] hints powerfully that they are disturbed by the idea of embracing a *"shev ve-'al ta'aseh"* (take no intervening action) approach that will probably doom all the fetuses, when some could be

---

[76] See above, chapter 5, pp. 195–198.   [77] See above, chapter 4, pp. 104ff.
[78] See above, chapter 5, pp. 195–198.

saved. Indeed, when Bleich describes pregnancy reduction as an act of "rescue,"[79] he invokes a moral imperative to commit feticide in the name of saving fetal life, an imperative that is certainly not dictated by *halakhic* positivism.

Perhaps the problem with Sinclair's approach is not his description of the manner in which abortion *halakhah* has unfolded, but rather his prescription for the appropriate way ahead. To be sure, the development of a set of explicit moral principles grounded in the notion of the "preservation of society and its defence against attacks on the bodies and property of its citizens" is an attractive proposition. But this Noahide moral vision, which Sinclair wants to use to shape legal principles, is by Sinclair's own admission, beset by vagueness. Consider, for example, the way that Professor Louis Newman perceives the application of the Noahide principles within the contemporary abortion context:

> Relying upon a peculiar, forced reading of Genesis 9:6, the rabbis concluded that abortion is categorically prohibited as a matter of Noahide law. The rabbinic sources dealing with this interpretation do not delve into the rationale behind it, though most probably it rests on a concern to preserve all human life as something sacred. Indeed, it may be that the ancient rabbis were especially concerned to instill a respect for human life among non-Jews, whom they viewed as more prone to violence than Jews. The inclusion of feticide as a form of homicide, then, would reinforce both the social and theological bases of the prohibition against murder.
>
> Certainly this Noahide principle, if applied to modern society, would warrant a strongly "pro-life" position on abortion. Arguably, our society is characterized by a growing disrespect for human life that is reflected and perhaps even promoted by the high rate of abortion. Prohibiting, or at least restricting, abortion could promote greater appreciation that human life in all its forms is sacred and so not readily expendable. Others, of course, will disagree. The point here is only that this viewpoint, based on Noahide law, has a legitimate place within the public forum, not that it will necessarily be compelling.[80]

Plainly, Professor Newman views the application of the Noahide principle as a prohibitory mechanism in much the same way as the *Tosafot* originally envisaged it. Indeed, there is likely to be little practical difference between the position on abortion yielded by Newman's use of the "classical concept of the Noahide system" and that arrived at by those rabbis who "merely [take] on the dogmas of the dominant faith." Sinclair, however, clearly envisages a considerably broader understanding and

---

[79] Bleich, *Bioethical Dilemmas*, p. 27.
[80] L. E. Newman, *Past Imperatives: Studies in the History and Theory of Jewish Ethics*, Albany, State University of New York Press, 1998, pp. 211–212.

utilization of the Noahide concept than that offered by Newman. While Sinclair might derive some modicum of satisfaction from seeing *halakhic* decisions on abortion grounded in Jewish rather than non-Jewish sources, this is surely not his major goal. Rather, it is the creation of a more flexible and comprehensive moral structure for abortion *halakhah* that he envisages. It is not the specific application of the historic Noahide standard that he desires, so much as the ability to apply a set of moral principles crafted in the Noahide spirit of preserving "the moral fabric of civilized society."

The difficulty with this goal, however, is that filling it with any specific content may be a "utopian" endeavor. Even if general agreement could be reached on the *halakhic* validity of mandating the type of governing principles that Sinclair proposes – and this is dubious – the prospect of creating a series of precise moral statements that would comprise a broadly acceptable tool for *halakhic* decision-making is remote. Sinclair, in effect, ends up returning us to Carmy's difficulty in conceiving of any authoritative body that might be "able to formulate the acceptable range of decision."

Arusi, Washofsky, and Sinclair open up differing conceptual vistas for responding to the range of abortion conundrums. Each of their insightful positions has difficulties of a greater or lesser nature. Nevertheless, the fact that there exists a plurality of attempts at systematization demonstrates a noteworthy desire to refine and advance *halakhic* outlooks on abortion beyond the consensus viewpoints of the twentieth century. It shows, moreover, that there continues to be a strongly perceived need to reframe the *halakhic* picture in order to produce the most conducive *halakhic* response. However, the call for *halakhic* reframing has not only come from men with diverse *halakhic* visions. For the first time in *halakhic* history, voices that had never before been taken seriously in *halakhic* deliberations have begun to be heard.

WOMEN'S PERSPECTIVES

Like all the abortion texts of the past, each of the three approaches examined above represents the thoughts of a male. Given the inherent dissimilarities between men and women, as well as the reality that abortion has potential personal consequences for women in ways that it does not for men, it would hardly be surprising if women saw abortion and appropriate *halakhic* responses to abortion quite differently from men. However, while the authors of *halakhic* texts were possibly influenced to some extent by the women around them, *halakhic* texts on abortion have not overtly encapsulated women's perspectives. If women of centuries past took an approach to the *halakhah* on abortion that was in any way divergent from their male counterparts, their input has been irretrievably lost to us.

We will never know what might have occurred, but it is possible that the *halakhah* on abortion could have been either subtly or significantly altered had women been active in the formulation of legal responses. Indeed, this is precisely the point made by Professor Dena Davis, a teacher of law, in her contemplation of abortion within Judaism. Davis argues that the legal analogies selected by a particular *posek* are not inevitable ones, but are choices, such that "analogic argument is necessarily subjective."[81] In fact, Davis maintains, *halakhic* texts do not "interpret themselves." Hence, our interpretative assumptions and the decisions we make about the way that the textual material ought to be construed profoundly influence our conclusions about the lessons to be learned from the textual heritage. Davis' chief concern, however, is not limiting the subjective features of the *halakhic* structure, but demonstrating that determining which individuals may make decisions can have critical effects:

[T]here is a deeper, prior problem: *who* is allowed into the interpretative process and whose subjective experience is to count? . . . Just as in American law, feminist jurisprudence and critical race theory present the view that excluding women and people of color from casuistic scholarship has resulted in an ideological interpretation of law that reflects the bias of white males who flourish under the *status quo*, so I argue that in a culture as powerfully gender-oriented as Judaism, it is reasonable to assume that the body of law would be different had women been part of the interpretative process.[82]

Davis does not, however, limit her argument to the observation that "the body of law" would have been different had women been involved. She proceeds to critique the current *halakhic* rulings as being *ipso facto* compromised because they do not take women's perspectives into account: "Because men and women experience pregnancy, childbirth and child-rearing very differently, excluding women from the casuistic process – thereby excluding the unmediated use of their experience – necessarily results in a flawed process whose conclusions are called into question."[83] Not only, then, does Davis maintain that the absence of women's

[81] D. S. Davis, "Abortion in Jewish Thought: A Study in Casuistry," *Journal of the American Academy of Religion*, volume 60, number 2, 1992: 319.
[82] *Ibid.*, 320. [83] *Ibid.*, 323.

contributions lessens the breadth of *halakhic* insights, but it raises concerns about the cogency of what she regards as partial perspectives.

Davis' observations lead to speculation over what the potential impact of women's participation in the "interpretative process" might in fact be. There are glimpses of initial responses to this inquiry. In the last quarter of the twentieth century – for the first time in *halakhic* history – women's views on the shaping of the *halakhic* response to abortion began to be expressed and afforded public recognition. Though not yet involved in the issuing of actual rulings, women started to articulate diverse visions of how the *halakhah* on abortion ought to be conceptualized.

One of the earlier and more daring approaches was that proposed by Blu Greenberg, an Orthodox thinker, who takes a somewhat radical approach to abortion in her pivotal work, *On Women and Judaism*.[84] Noting a tension between her devotion to Orthodoxy and her concern for the social realities she encounters, Greenberg calls for a broadening of the *halakhic* "interpretation of therapeutic abortion."[85] She proposes that the *halakhic* response to abortion needs to be "framed as part of a theological whole," giving far greater weight in the process to various *halakhic* meta-principles in determining the appropriate *halakhic* outcome. Jewish legal deliberations, in other words, should not involve simply an application of textual precedent to current circumstances, but should include far broader considerations:

A Jew should ask and answer personal questions with wider reference to a religious code that has as its value-source God and community. This is the reverse of how abortion decisions often are made today.

It will take courage for the framers of Jewish law to rule that in certain instances abortion is the higher morality, in keeping with overall principles of *kavod ha-briot* (respect for all living things) and *tzelem elohim* (in the image of God) – principles that sometimes are lost in the myriad of laws developed to express those very priorities. For example, Jewish law, as we have seen, sanctions abortion in cases where the mother's health is at stake. In various responsa, rabbinic authorities have extended this notion to include her psychological health as well. Those responsa could support new ones, which would encompass such variables as physical strength, stress, even delay in child rearing for purposes of family planning. Further, the fact that in Jewish law love and marriage are positive values should allow room to deal with cases where a wife becomes pregnant before the couple has had a chance to develop a solid relationship.[86]

[84] B. Greenberg, *On Women and Judaism*, Philadelphia, The Jewish Publication Society of America, 1981.
[85] *Ibid.*, p. 150.   [86] *Ibid.*, pp. 151–152.

There can be little doubting the daring nature of this proposal. As an Orthodox woman, Greenberg not only demonstrates that she is outside the more stringent consensus on abortion, but outside the more lenient one as well. In suggesting the utilization of broad *halakhic* principles to enable the *halakhah* to be read in such a way as to countenance abortions when maternal stress or family-planning priorities are the central issues at stake, Greenberg comes close to calling for *halakhic* permission to abort pregnancies that portend any measure of distress to the mother.

Clearly aware of the likely response to such a notion, Greenberg offers the reassurance that "Halakhists should not be fearful of extending Jewish law to create a better meshing of personal needs with traditional dictates."[87] The *halakhic* response, she avers, will not be put in the position of needing to accede to every "claimant" – indeed, in adopting "a more realistic position," there will be a better chance that *halakhic* rulings "will be taken seriously" on those occasions when permission for abortion must be denied.[88] In Greenberg's view, her proposals will rescue the *halakhic* stance from becoming "simply a matter of opposition to abortion, with grudging exceptions granted in particular cases."[89] Rather, her approach will serve to stress the positive values contained within the *halakhic* system, including such concerns as having children, love, and care. Greenberg, then, is anxious to rehabilitate what she perceives to be a widespread disrespect for the *halakhah*. Consequently, she holds that a *halakhic* framework that places a "stress on proper ethical, social and sexual decision-making" is one that is most likely to be respected as a "moral force" for contemporary life.[90]

From the start, Greenberg states that she believes that abortion should be a "legal option," and that the Jewish tradition should be reexamined "to see where the more lenient interpretation of the law can support legalized abortion."[91] Having set herself this task, Greenberg goes about accomplishing it. She does so while conceding that "there are no traditional Jewish precedents for abortion on demand" and acknowledging that her strategy is "one way to maintain some integrity within the halakhic framework."[92] It is not, though, immediately clear why a "stress on proper ethical, social and sexual decision-making" should necessarily lead to the conclusion that lenient abortion rulings are required – other

---

[87] *Ibid.*, p. 152.   [88] *Ibid.*   [89] *Ibid.*, p. 153.   [90] *Ibid.*
[91] *Ibid.*, p. 148.   [92] *Ibid.*, p. 150.

than the fact that Greenberg wants things to be this way. Greenberg does not explain why proper ethical decision-making demands the elevation of the considerations that she proposes.

Greenberg's approach seems to be that the *halakhah* has always regarded the priority of the mother's life over that of the fetus as being the ethically correct alternative. In relative terms, it is a less significant damage to destroy life that has not reached *nefesh* status than that of a full *nefesh*. Consequently, it is appropriate, in Greenberg's view, to posit that maternal priority should "include serious regard for the quality of [her] life as well."[93] Greenberg, then, takes the opening provided by Rashi and extends it further than anybody had hitherto contemplated. In Greenberg's estimation, it is ethically defensible to assert that considerations of the mother's "quality of life" should outweigh those of continued fetal existence when such conditions as the mother's need to support her family, stabilize her marriage, or respond to the needs of other children, pertain.[94] Greenberg's strong reaction to unwanted pregnancy[95] impels her to call for a bold rethinking of the *halakhic* position on abortion. Indeed, Greenberg arrives at a conclusion about the appropriate circumstances for abortion that represents a considerable departure from the outlooks of virtually all the males who have issued rulings in the area.

A similar meta-*halakhic* approach, albeit more rigorously argued, is offered by the philosopher, Dr. Sandra Lubarsky. Lubarsky begins her analysis by pointing out the convergent nature of (male) rabbinic thought on abortion: "Though agreement among rabbis as to what constitutes *sufficient reason* for abortion falls short of unanimity, it does not fall short by much. In the greatest number of decisions made by members of both the 'lenient' and the 'stringent' schools, abortion has been permitted on medical grounds only."[96] This convergence, Lubarsky observes, is curious, given the lack of any specific *halakhic* prohibition of non-therapeutic abortion within the biblical and Talmudic sources. Lubarsky's explanation

---

[93] B. Greenberg, "Abortion: A Challenge to Halakhah," *Judaism*, volume 25, 1976: 204.

[94] *Ibid.*

[95] Greenberg writes with conviction that "the other facets of unwanted pregnancy are inescapable – fatigue and harassed parents, the shame of rape, the premature end of youth because of a foolish mistake, the degradation and danger of coat-hanger abortion, and, not the least, the overwhelming and exclusive claim that a child makes on a woman's life for many of her strongest years"; *ibid.*, p. 201.

[96] S. B. Lubarsky, "Judaism and the Justification of Abortion for Non-Medical Reasons," *Journal of Reform Judaism*, volume 31, number 4, 1984: 1.

of this reality is that the rabbis arrive at their abortion rulings through the use of a set of "extra-legal premises" which they employ because "they find themselves uncomfortable with the *legal* position on abortion and attempt to mitigate the influence of that position."[97] In other words, Lubarsky is of the view that the rabbis apply a set of values to the abortion issue that is not intrinsic to the original legal response, so as to make the law more congenial to their perspective on the subject. Lubarsky discerns evidence for these extra-legal premises in an instance of rabbinic disagreement: the very fact, Lubarsky maintains, that there is "no single interpretation" of Maimonides' *rodef* argument "suggests that interpretive decisions are based not on 'pertinent sources' but rather on preconceived ethical stances."[98]

Lubarsky proceeds to identify six non-legal assumptions which, she asserts, are widespread among *poskim*, though not all six are necessarily held by every Jewish authority:

1. With the exception of God, human life is valued over every other kind of life.
2. In almost all cases, an increase in human life amounts to an increase in value.
3. All humans are of equal worth from God's perspective.
4. God is unchanging, or, at least, God's essence is unchanging.
5. The mental or psychological aspect of human life is (somehow) less basic than the physical aspect.
6. Existing human life has precedence over potential human life.[99]

Without these assumptions, Lubarsky contends, Jewish abortion law would look more like its biblical and Talmudic foundations, supporting abortions for "both medically advised and other than medically advised reasons." According to Lubarsky, it is, therefore, the customary rabbinic understanding of these six assumptions that undermines the case for non-medically advised abortions.

Consequently, Lubarsky regards the critical evaluation of these six assumptions as an essential task. Taking the first three assumptions together, she offers an intriguing line of reasoning. Assumptions one and three lead to a world-view in which all human beings are distinct from and superior to all other beings – the ultimate form of anthropocentrism. Within this world-view, it makes sense to support assumption two, because – given that human life is superior to all other concerns – any loss of potential or actual human life requires justification. Put differently, the preservation of human life becomes a paramount issue, no matter what its cost to other life forms. In Lubarsky's estimation, however, the

---

[97] *Ibid.*, 2.   [98] *Ibid.*, 3.   [99] *Ibid.*, 5.

separation of the "human realm from the non-human realm is a distorted world view," with implications that are deeply problematic:

From an ecological perspective (which includes humanity), life itself is robbery, for the living depend on the dead to sustain them. Because life feeds on life, "the robber requires justification." Human life requires some sort of justification for the sacrifice it demands from other forms of life. The taking of any life, human or non-human, must be justified. Abortion, then, becomes an issue that cannot be considered apart from ecological issues.[100]

This ecological argument seems to imply that an abortion desired for any reason could have moral standing. Lubarsky appears to convey that only the fervent desire to have a child can justify the ecological "robbing" which that child represents. Without such desire, the interests of bringing that fetus into the world would need to be considered together with a host of other ecological concerns, and it is not at all clear that, when weighed in this way, the fetus would be deemed more worthy.

Lubarsky supplements her ecological argument with a further point about the relative value of different beings. Given that we acknowledge that both humans and non-humans have "some degree of intrinsic value," it does not follow, Lubarsky states, that they have equal value. Jewish tradition accepts this notion, Lubarsky points out, in the differentiation that it makes between God and humans, humans and animals, or a being that is a *nefesh* and one that has not attained *nefesh* status. What factor, Lubarsky inquires, separates one category from the other and allows us to make sense of such a hierarchy? Lubarsky contends that the answer to this question is to be found in the level of experience of each of these beings. The reason why a non-*nefesh* can be said to have a lesser standing than a *nefesh* is that the "fetus' experience lacks the richness, intentionality, and consciousness of a person's experience." It follows from this, Lubarsky states, that abortion may be reasonable in non-medical circumstances as it allows the mother's superior level of experience to find full expression: "Abortion may then be justified for other than medical reasons. Abortion may be judged to be beneficial to the mother's experience as a whole, including her intellectual, moral, emotional, and physical health and her sociological and ecological milieu."[101]

Lubarsky uses a similar strategy to deal with assumption four, the belief in the unchanging nature of God. It is incorrect, Lubarsky posits, to suggest that God's laws are unchanging such that they would,

---

[100] *Ibid.*, 8.   [101] *Ibid.*, 9.

for example, favor human procreation under any conditions. Rather, what is in fact unchanging is God's commitment to "elicit intensity of experience." Thus, to illustrate her point, when the human population was small, "intensity of experience" was best upheld by calling for procreation. However, when human beings became numerous, ensuring the "intensity of experience" for human beings might well argue against encouraging procreation. Hence, if "intensity of experience" is indeed God's desire for humans, it follows that there might be times when non-medical abortions might be called for so as to uphold the "intensity of experience" in the life of a given person or family. Understanding God to permit abortions of this type would actually show that God desires to be responsive in this way.[102]

Lubarsky, though, reserves her strongest comments for assumption five, the assumption that conveys the notion that mental or psychological issues are less important than physical ones. Lubarsky first notes that even on those occasions when mental issues are considered within the *halakhah* they are seen to be important only when they constitute a potential threat to maternal health, never in terms of their overall impact on a woman's intellectual life. Moreover, Lubarsky contends, those who shape abortion *halakhah* continue to posit that physical issues are more critical than mental ones and that acceptable mental criteria for abortion can only be defined narrowly. This, in Lubarsky's view, is simply demeaning to women:

> Not to take a woman's mental life, in all its aspects, seriously is to deny a woman what has been permitted to men: the assumption of interiority, and, thereby, of individuality. Not to accord significance to the mental aspects of her life – significance that at least equals and ought to surpass the physical aspects of her life – is not to accord her the freedom and creativity that is given to men. In this kind of Judaism, women bear children, not witness. So long as mentality is subservient to physicality in the discussion about abortion, or any issue concerning women, the tendency will be to perceive women as being less than fully human.[103]

In other words, to regard women's thoughtful choices as being of less moment than threats to maternal health is to place the preservation of women's physical well-being on a higher plane than the defense of women's self-determination as independent decision-makers. To do this, Lubarsky contends, is to pay primary attention to women as physical objects in a way that is wholly divergent from the manner in which male

---

[102] *Ibid.*, 10.   [103] *Ibid.*, 11.

"interiority" is respected. Going even further, Lubarsky suggests that the outcome of this inequality might lead to the dehumanization of women.

It is possible that Lubarsky overstates her case here. While restricting women's choices in this particularly pivotal area may be seen as undesirable by many, to contend that this will lead to a diminution of women's humanity may be exaggerated. Those legal systems that curtail women's abortion choices usually do so in order to protect another being, namely the fetus. Thus, while the diminution of women's "interiority" might be the perceived result of this protection, the intent of the law is to establish a reasonable balance between the woman's "interior" interests and the interests of the fetus. It would, therefore, clearly be offensive if women who were not pregnant did not have access to the same "freedom and creativity" as men. The fact, however, that pregnancy might lead to the limiting of some freedoms does not necessarily indicate a lessening of women's humanity. Rather it might signify that, while a woman is pregnant, her "interiority" does not enjoy the same independence as at other times, as the interests of the fetus must be considered alongside the needs of self. According to this line of reasoning, some amount of "individuality" is ceded in these circumstances, not because the individual concerned is a woman, but because the individual concerned is pregnant.

Lubarsky's final analysis brings her to assumption six, that existing human life has precedence over potential human life. While Lubarsky regards the *halakhic* distinction between actual life and potential life as a praiseworthy one, she contends that it would be a mistake always to value actual life more highly than potential life. Referring to the human capacity for self-sacrifice, Lubarsky writes that sacrifice "is an important corrective to the view that potential life is always less valuable than actual life."[104] Thus, self-sacrifice is an example of future potential outweighing present actuality. Seen this way, Lubarsky suggests, we should be open to the possibility that there are times when the "intrinsic value" of potential life will appropriately be regarded as more significant than existing life. From here, Lubarsky takes a significant additional step: the list of considerations that could be deemed to hold sufficient "potential value" to outstrip that of existing life encompasses more than just the nascent fetus. In Lubarsky's view, ample "potential value" may be found in a range of mental conceptions which, as yet, have no existent reality: "[T]hose cases include ... that potential which is completely unactualized (i.e. the

[104] *Ibid.*, 12.

value of potential fetuses) and that potential which is part of the future
life of those who are already persons, e.g., the existing mother's future,
the existing family's future, the future of the population at large, and
so forth."[105] Given Lubarsky's assertion that there are times when the
"possible" should be given greater weight than the "actual," her position
appears to be that there are instances when what the future might hold
for a woman's, a family's, or a population's future, could be of enough
moment to warrant abortion of the fetus. Lubarsky is actually calling
for a reasoned choice between two potential realities, a task that is considerably more complex than the classic one between an actual and a
potential being.

For each of the six assumptions, then, Lubarsky illuminates alternative
ways of thinking about these postulates that stress the centrality of experience and lead to a philosophical justification of abortion for non-medical
reasons. Indeed, the values decisions that are apposite to the type of world
in which we should aspire to live, Lubarsky posits, are better made on the
basis of "concrete units of experience," than on "abstractions on life."
Consequently, it comes as no surprise that Lubarsky's analysis of these six
assumptions leads her to conclude that when "the Jewish sources are thus
considered, it becomes clear that Judaism not only permits abortion for
medical reasons, but also supports abortion for non-medical reasons."[106]
She arrives at this conclusion having systematically argued that the six
normative assumptions, which she highlights, are "not demanded by the
tradition."

This conclusion, however, begs the significant question of what exactly is "demanded by the tradition" in this area. For Lubarsky might be
correct that some of the assumptions she discerns might, at one stage,
not have been an integral part of the tradition. It is, however, an altogether different claim to suggest that Judaism could dispense with some
or all of them – after centuries of adherence – and remain true to what
we understand Judaism to have become. Lubarsky is on solid ground,
for example, when she points out that the assumption that existing human life has precedence over potential human life has deep roots within
the tradition – it is, after all, the normative rabbinic understanding of
Exodus 21:22–23. It is possible, of course, that Exodus 21:22–23 could
have been interpreted differently. The commentators might have decided that the only reason that the fetus mentioned in Exodus 21:22–23
elicited a lesser penalty than the mother is because the probable

---

[105] *Ibid.*   [106] *Ibid.*

experiential life that awaited that particular fetus was judged, vis-à-vis the probable experiential future of its mother, to be less significant. They could have taken this approach, but they did not. Instead, they took the view that the lesser penalty that was applied to the fetus in fact denoted that a non-*nefesh*, a life that was not yet actual, was of lesser standing than existing life. Through the centuries, there has been almost no deviation from this approach. Consequently, over time, there has been virtual unanimity that the assumption of the superiority of existing maternal life over potential fetal life is a hallmark of the Jewish approach to abortion. This is true to such an extent that a strong argument can be made that this understanding in fact connotes what has come to be "demanded by the tradition."

Within a legal framework, therefore, longstanding assumptions are not easily separated from a legal tradition, for in many ways they help to shape a particular tradition and to supply its unique character. It is possible, of course, for these bedrock assumptions to be profoundly transformed and for the new outlook that emerges – based on these reworked assumptions – to be considered an authentic version of Judaism. Indeed, this is precisely what another scholar, Rabbi Rebecca Alpert, calls for within an article that critiques the substantive shifts in Jakobovits' position over the years:

Many lessons can be learned from reading Jakobovits's opinions on abortion. A Jewish conversation about abortion, from traditional or liberal perspectives, must treat women as moral agents. It must not speak in glib language about the use of abortion as a sexual deterrent nor avoid a more complex discussion of sexuality. It must not fail to examine the complexities of the need for abortion in a society with many unwanted children, healthy and unhealthy, and with little concern for how those children (or, for that matter, wanted children) are cared for. And it must not ignore the fact that children are still cared for predominantly by women, often for low wages or at the cost of their own individual and collective development and growth.[107]

Alpert's call to "treat women as moral agents" is reminiscent of Lubarsky's "respecting interiority" argument. Both positions effectively call for the *halakhah* to be remodeled such that a decision as to the appropriateness of a particular abortion is moved away from "moral experts and legislators,"[108] and ceded to the woman concerned.

Clearly, there are opposing views as to the merits of such a change. From a systemic perspective, however, if such a goal is to be achieved

[107] R. Alpert, "Sometimes the Law is Cruel," *Journal of Feminist Studies in Religion*, volume 11, number 2, 1995: 37.
[108] *Ibid.*

within the *halakhah* – as opposed to going outside the *halakhic* structure – only a strong consensus among some Jewish authorities, whose standing is recognized by a substantial subsection of the Jewish people, will produce such an outcome. In essence, that is exactly what happened within the more stringent consensus that emerged in the twentieth century. A number of authorities argued for an explicit connection between abortion and murder, and they succeeded in convincing a substantial section of the Jewish world that this view was consistent with the demands of the tradition and was, therefore, a cogent reading of the law. The Lubarsky and Alpert outlook will need to establish a similar type of consensus if their view is to be considered a viable, coherent Jewish view of abortion. Certainly Lubarsky and Alpert have a vision of how they would like the *halakhic* response to be framed, but it is an open question as to whether their approach will come to be seen as an authentic *halakhic* outlook. Unless mainstream views change considerably, their conceptualizations will continue to be marginalized by the normative consensus positions. Those positions are succinctly encapsulated by Rachel Biale in her study on women within Jewish law: "[t]he Halakhah does not recognize a right of a woman to abort a child because it is unwanted, in order to limit the size of her family, or in order to save herself the pain and suffering which are naturally inherent in giving birth and raising children."[109]

The insights of Greenberg, Lubarsky, and Alpert do, though, add credence to Davis' contention that, should there be an expansion of women's involvement in the *halakhic* process, it *could* ultimately lead to a noteworthy redrawing of the *halakhic* picture. It is appropriate, however, to be cautious about embracing such assessments with undue haste for two reasons. First, by the end of the twentieth century, despite the considerable number of women with knowledge in Jewish law, very few female scholars or rabbis had actually written on the *halakhic* response to abortion. This reality might be explained in different ways, but it may indicate that there was little perception of any urgency to make *halakhic* changes in this area. Second, alongside the more far-reaching views of Greenberg and Lubarsky, there were certainly women who wrote approvingly about the consensus approaches already in place. Thus, for example, Adena Berkowitz, a Jewish ethics scholar, concludes that:

[109] R. Biale, *Women and Jewish Law: The Essential Texts, Their History and Their Relevance for Today*, New York, Schocken Books, 1984, p. 238.

The main line of the Jewish tradition would thus seem to make a much needed contribution to the discussion of abortion. Without sharing the Catholic view that the fetus is from conception fully a person, it stops short of a complete dismissal of the value problem in destroying a fetus. However, whatever value attaches to "potential life," the primary concern lies with the mother. She exists. Her life, no matter how slim her chances of survival, health and well-being come first.[110]

Other female scholars have also written in a similar vein. Judith Antonelli in her feminist commentary on the Torah, while interpreting the law in a lenient direction, states that: "Judaism's view of abortion could, if allowed, provide a much-needed 'middle path' of wisdom in the American debate on the subject and perhaps even break the deadlock between the 'pro-choice' and 'right-to-life' factions."[111] Dr. Judith Hauptman, a Professor of Talmud at the Jewish Theological Seminary, clearly sees the existing Jewish framework as offering an important approach for contemporary women grappling with abortion:

I see the role of Judaism or the rabbi in a case of this sort not as decisor but as alter ego, whose job it is to push the mother to think her decision through with painstaking care, to lay the burden of proof on her shoulders, to help her either justify to herself that abortion is the moral choice in her particular case, or if not, to carry the pregnancy to term.[112]

It is, therefore, by no means clear that the addition of women's voices to the *halakhic* interchange on abortion will reshape the *halakhic* landscape on the subject, though it remains a possibility that cannot be excluded.

THE ROAD AHEAD

Arriving at a single focused response to difficult issues is not the goal of the *halakhic* system. As the scholar Rabbi Daniel Gordis has written,

We ought not confuse Judaism's compromise or ambivalence with apathy. A tradition that both commands abortion in certain cases but that forbids it in many others is not a tradition predicated on a lack of interest; it is a tradition committed to recognizing complexity. Judaism insists that the value of religion ought

---

[110] A. K. Berkowitz, "Thinking about Women in Abortion Controversies," *Sevara*, volume 2, number 2, 1991: 28.
[111] J. S. Antonelli, *In the Image of God: A Feminist Commentary on the Torah*, Northvale, Jason Aaronson Incorporated, 1995, p. 197.
[112] J. Hauptman, "A Matter of Morality," *United Synagogue Review*, Spring, 1990: 18.

not be in providing pithy theological positions that make intricate questions facile. Its real value is in sensitizing human beings and society to the profound intricacies raised by issues such as abortion.[113]

It is not, then, the primary aim of the *halakhah* to dispel differences with dispatch. Acknowledging this reality, it is nevertheless critical to marshal the finest tools to assist in moving towards the best decisions within an area that is replete with so many challenges and considerations. Hence, the question remains: with what we know already, how might the parameters of acceptable abortion *halakhah* best be fashioned in order to respond to the challenges of an uncharted future? Given the separate consensus positions, given the dissolving nexus between fetal non-personhood and maternal suffering in permitting abortion, given the feminist critiques, and given the difficult genetic conundrums that loom on the horizon, what signposts should guide the road ahead?

It would seem that the best answer to this question lies in acknowledging the vital role of three important components that have shaped, and ought to continue to shape, abortion *halakhah*. First, as has been seen, Jewish law pertinent to abortion has consistently conformed to a number of central, though often unstated, principles. The constant employment of these principles inescapably identifies the legal response to abortion as being quintessentially Jewish in nature. Newman details the most fundamental among these principles.[114] First is the notion that human life is sacred, meaning "it possesses intrinsic and infinite value." The second is that, as a consequence of the first principle, "the preservation of life is of the highest moral imperative." The third principle is that "all lives are equal." Fourth is the principle that "our lives are not really our own."[115] Newman writes that these principles were understood by the rabbis to require the centrist position that has come to be so familiar: that while the mother's life must be saved, "the fetus, though not regarded as fully a 'person,' is still alive, and insofar as all human life is sacred, it can be terminated only for the most compelling reason..."[116] Jewish responses to abortion, then, have been built on the underpinning of these distinctively Jewish principles. To be sure, different respondents have interpreted these principles in varying ways, but the function of

[113] D. Gordis, *Does the World Need Jews?*, New York, Scribner, 1997, p. 159.
[114] It is worth noting the striking similarities between the "principles" that Professor Newman offers as worthy of affirmation and the "assumptions" that Lubarsky calls into question. At the end of the twentieth century, despite Lubarsky's objections, these "principles" appeared to be firmly at the core of any approach considered to be broadly representative of Judaism's stance.
[115] Newman, *Past Imperatives*, pp. 107–111.   [116] *Ibid.*, pp. 109–110.

these central tenets as the *sine qua non* of Jewish abortion deliberations remains firm. Any ruling that does not satisfactorily accommodate these principles cannot be said to comport well with the received tradition of Judaism.

The second important component that shapes abortion *halakhah* is the wisdom of the individual *posek*. In the *halakhic* system, rulings are rooted in texts but are applied to particular contexts, so it is the judge who must balance text and context according to the circumstances: as the rabbis teach, *"ein lo la-dayyan ella mah she'einav ro'ot"* (a judge must be guided by what he sees). In actuality, as has been shown by the *teshuvot* on abortion, this is sometimes a more creative process than is generally acknowledged. Rabbi Emanuel Rackman, the former president of Bar-Ilan University, has noted that four myths persist about the practical application of *halakhah*: first, that it is immutable; second, that it is totally objective; third, that it is not influenced by current conditions and circumstances; and fourth, that it never transcends its own rules.[117] Rackman, in explaining these four myths, contends that those who are intellectually honest will agree that not only is the *halakhah* flexible, but it is subject to real change. Indeed, avers Rackman, change must be possible within the *halakhah* for several reasons:

As a matter of fact, there are three factors that play a part in all legal development: One is logic; the second is the sense of justice; and the third concerns the needs of society. All three elements play a part in Jewish law that there's no escaping. This is true of all legal systems and of the *halakhic* system as well.[118]

The evidence of the unfolding history of *halakhah* on abortion offers a strong endorsement of the truth of Rackman's observations. The influence of logic, justice, and societal concerns all figure prominently in the varying epochs. In particular, one can point to the depiction of abortion within Judaism at the close of the twentieth century – a view that presents a substantially different encapsulation from that held by many *poskim* as recently as a century before – as testimony to the impact of these factors. There are, in fact, not many *halakhic* issues for which the responses – at least until the convergent trends of the latter twentieth century – have been as varied as for abortion; there are few areas, consequently, in which the role of the *posek*, who must deal with the peculiarities of each individual case, has been so pivotal.

---

[117] E. Rackman, "Jewish Medical Ethics and Law," in L. Meier (ed.), *Jewish Values in Bioethics*, New York, Human Sciences Press Incorporated, 1986, pp. 150–173.
[118] *Ibid.*, p. 153.

The implication of this reality is that while a *posek*'s ruling must remain bound to the fundamental principles of Judaism, it may be applied with provisions that suit a particular set of conditions. Pregnancy reduction presents a clear example of this truth: had the "rules" stayed the same, abortion for purposes of pregnancy reduction might well have been denied as an act of feticide without maternal suffering. Permission for pregnancy reduction appears to be best accounted for as a "rule change" made in defense of the principle of the preservation of life. While the presumptive power of precedent is great, it is the *posek* who remains the ultimate arbiter of what the law will be in any given situation. *Halakhic* formalism and positivism, therefore, are unlikely to have anything more than temporary suasion over a system that is designed to incorporate human judgment at the center.

The corollary of this second component is that the Jewish approach to abortion is unlikely to become monolithic at any time in the near future. Notwithstanding the two major consensuses that have developed and the body of precedent that may be accumulating, profound differences in ethical orientation, such as those expressed by Waldenberg and Feinstein, will not soon disappear. Indeed, there is a strong likelihood that emerging genetic technologies will provide a continuing stream of complex dilemmas that will occasion further diverse responses from both a lenient and a stringent orientation.

The third important component of abortion *halakhah* is the moral dimension. Sinclair is correct in his conclusion that the history of abortion *halakhah* displays a frequent preoccupation with issues of morality. He is also right in insisting that, in an age in which abortion has become a commonplace occurrence,[119] and in which a host of complex, new abortion questions keep arising, the moral reasoning behind abortion *pesikah* ought to become the subject of explicit scrutiny. To return to Sinclair's example, it is perfectly *halakhically* legitimate – indeed, there exists a compelling *halakhic* logic – for Waldenberg to accede to the abortion of a fetus afflicted with Down's syndrome. However, the essential question of whether such an abortion is in fact morally acceptable represents a central and critical decision. It is a question that must not be evaded and that ought to be a prime factor in arriving at a *halakhic* determination. To do otherwise – to ignore the moral dimension – would be to leave the *halakhah* vulnerable to the charge that a system that is held to be

[119] According to *American Demographics*, December 1996 edition, p. 27, there were one and a half million abortions in the United States in 1992, bringing to an end 27.5 percent of all pregnancies.

the legal embodiment of God's instruction can knowingly allow morally inadequate rulings to stand. The consequence of this neglect would be to permit a focus on *halakhic* methodology to obscure the fundamental Jewish pursuit of *ha-yashar ve-ha-tov*, of that which is "in line" and good.

This is not to suggest that the *halakhah*, of necessity, must conform to some external standard of morality. The more traditional viewpoint that the *halakhah*, God's law from Sinai, is capable of internally yielding the ethically appropriate response when it is extrapolated in the most suitable way need not be discarded. There is a simultaneous duty both to Sinai and to ethics as inseparable requirements for living a coherent, *halakhic* life.[120] As Rabbi Aharon Lichtenstein wrote, "traditional halakhic Judaism demands of the Jew both adherence to Halakha and commitment to an ethical moment that, though different from Halakha, is nevertheless of a piece with it and in its own way fully imperative."[121] But if the "ethical moment" is "fully imperative," then it requires us to go beyond what is *halakhically* plausible and to select the ethically most successful extrapolation of the *halakhah*. Herein lies the problem that the abortion interchange highlights so starkly: how do we know which ruling has rendered the *halakhah* in a way that is ethically most compelling? Can we, for example, definitively establish whether Waldenberg's or Feinstein's *halakhic* response to the Tay-Sachs issue is the more ethically acceptable? Because such a determination involves matters of judgment and perception, the most likely answer is "we cannot."

There is, however, a significant gap between making a definitive ethical pronouncement and making no ethical evaluation at all. If the idea of producing a set of moral governing principles appears to be unrealistic, there may be an alternative strategy for encouraging ethical deliberation. Perhaps a more feasible approach might be to persuade *poskim* to include an ethical analysis of the questions before them as an integral part of their *teshuvot*. Just as an abortion *teshuvah* that fails to cite textual support and *halakhic* precedents would be deemed unsatisfying and incomplete, so an abortion *teshuvah* that fails to provide reasoned moral justification for its conclusions might be regarded similarly. Unlike Sinclair's call for

---

[120] There is a considerable body of literature on the relationship between *halakhah* and ethics. Professor Newman provides a useful list of source materials on this subject. See L. E. Newman, "Ethics as Law, Law as Religion: Reflection on the Problem of Law and Ethics in Judaism," in E. N. Dorff and L. E. Newman (eds.), *Contemporary Jewish Ethics: A Reader*, Oxford, Oxford University Press, 1995, pp. 91–92, n. 1.

[121] A. Lichtenstein, "Does Tradition Recognize an Ethic Independent of Halakha?" in M. Fox (ed.), *Modern Jewish Ethics*, Columbus, Ohio State University Press, 1975, p. 83.

commonly held moral principles, this development would not seek convergence among *poskim* on what is morally acceptable or unacceptable. In fact, different *poskim* might well invoke divergent moral arguments, just as they currently appeal to varying *halakhic* proof-texts and precedents. The proposal, however, would request *poskim* not just to provide rulings that are *halakhically* feasible, but to explain the manner in which a particular ruling is morally defensible as well. Thus, Waldenberg would be asked to include within his Down's syndrome *teshuvah* both the *halakhic* logic that allows him to conclude that the *halakhah* permits the abortion of a fetus afflicted with Down's syndrome, as well as a succinct and cogent *halakhic* argument why such an abortion might also be morally acceptable. Beyond simply discussing the ethical challenges confronted within a given issue, a clear case should be made why the conclusion that the *posek* draws from the texts is the most ethically conducive one. As Professor Newman has written:

[I]f [textual] interpretation is to be more than ad hoc decision-making, it must rest upon a theoretical foundation. And if one wishes to urge others to adopt a particular interpretation, that theory must be stated explicitly and defended. In American jurisprudence, producing a "reasoned opinion" and defending it against competing opinions is standard procedure. Contemporary Jewish ethicists should do no less.[122]

In the future, the *halakhic* enterprise might appropriately become more dependent upon *poskim* issuing their rulings not just as judicial experts, but as Jewish ethicists as well.

A certain amount of ethical deliberation will most probably be an inevitable requirement of the challenge posed by the separation of fetal non-personhood from issues of maternal welfare. If so, it will be a welcome by-product of this reassessment. It is important, though, that these ethical deliberations be pursued across the full range of abortion issues. This is not in any way to suggest that a *shoèl* ought to be free to accept or reject a particular ruling based on the coherence of its ethical reasoning; the ruling of a *posek* should remain binding whether the ethical thinking is convincing or not. But ethical judgments and ethical concerns might, most certainly, become a critical and systematic consideration in *halakhic* evaluations in a way that potentially could lead to ever more refined *halakhic* positions. The notion is not that ethics alone should

---

[122] Newman L. E., "The Problem of Interpretation in Contemporary Jewish Ethics," in E. N. Dorff and L. E. Newman (eds.), *Contemporary Jewish Ethics: A Reader*, Oxford, Oxford University Press, 1995, pp. 155–156.

determine abortion *halakhah*, but that ethical concerns should be explicitly articulated within the *halakhah*. If *poskim* were to accept this direction as their mandate, it would introduce an ethical interchange into the *halakhic* process that would serve to place an explicit focus on ethical concerns, to hone ethical ideas, and to allow for those *poskim* with particular acumen in ethical argumentation to come to the fore.

In Judaism, from the time that Abraham first asked God, "[S]hall not the Judge of the whole universe deal justly?" (Genesis 18:25), legal issues have been indivisible from ethics. It is critical, the Torah teaches, that even though God is the ultimate source of legal instruction, Jews must be ever vigilant to ensure that law conforms to the highest ethical ideals. In the area of abortion, this fundamental goal implies that abortion decisions within Judaism can never be simply about what the law can bear, but must respond to that which leads to the greatest good. This aspiration can continue to be fulfilled provided that the finest characteristics of the abortion *halakhah* of the past are maintained: a commitment to the fundamental principles that characterize the Jewish approach to life-and-death issues, a determination to preserve the prerogative of the individual *posek* to respond with flexibility and wisdom, and an unstinting, overt pursuit of that which is most ethically cogent.

Abortion *halakhah*, it will be recalled, was born in the midst of dispute. Though the original protagonists from that ancient encounter have long since been forgotten, the struggle persists. Indeed, despite the fact that the intense focus upon the abortion debate in the second half of the twentieth century led to the crystallization of initial "Jewish positions" on abortion, the challenges that lie ahead will ensure that contention will remain. But Jewish discussions on abortion will continue to be characterized by distinctive features, for the Jewish interchange has never been one between those for whom the preservation of fetal life is paramount and those for whom the safeguarding of maternal choice is indispensable. Rather, Jewish striving has always been designed to elicit optimum responses to challenging human circumstances, within a world that continues to be imperfect. Awed by the miracle of existence, the Jewish tradition continues to seek a *halakhic* response that balances, with humility and sensitivity, the needs of present life with the call of life in potential. As has been seen, this complex endeavor has continually underscored both how capable and how fallible we human beings are and how remarkable is the power that we have been given by God to discern and to shape the parameters of the gift of life itself.

Glossary

Acharon (pl. *Acharonim*)	A "later" *halakhic* authority who lived from the middle of the fifteenth century to the emancipation of European Jewry at the end of the eighteenth century.
adam	A human being.
aggadah (pl. *aggadot*)	Homiletic, inspirational rabbinic lore.
aggadic	Of or pertaining to *aggadah*.
aliyah	"Going up," either to be called to the reading of the Torah in the synagogue or to live permanently in Israel.
Amora (pl. *Amoraïm*)	A rabbi from the later Talmudic period of the third to the sixth century CE.
Amoraïc	Of or pertaining to the period of the *Amoraïm*.
Ashkenazi (pl. *Ashkenazim*)	Jews of Northern France and German origin, hence primarily European Jews (*Ashkenaz* was the Hebrew name given to Germany).
ason	An injury.
assur	Prohibited by Jewish law.
baʾal tashchit	A legal principle forbidding the wanton destruction of property.
bar kayamah	Viable; a viable human being.
Bavli	The *Talmud Bavli* or Babylonian Talmud. The authoritative Talmud completed in Babylonia in the sixth century CE.
Beit Din	A rabbinic court of law numbering three judges.
brit milah	Circumcision for purposes of entering the covenant of the Jewish people.

chabbalah	Wounding the body.
chakham (pl. *chakhamim*)	A sage.
cherem	A ban.
chiddush (pl. *chiddushim*)	A novel interpretation of Jewish law.
chillul HaShem	The desecration of God's name.
kohen (pl. *kohanim*)	A priest.
dayan (pl. *dayanim*)	A judge.
Eretz Yisrael	The land of Israel.
Gemara	Commentary on and legal expansion of the *Mishnah*, including *halakhic* and *aggadic* discussions of the *Amoraïm*. Together with the *Mishnah*, the *Gemara* forms the Talmud.
Gaon (pl. *Geonim*)	Literally, "genius"; the head of the academy in the post-Talmudic period.
Geonic	Of or pertaining to the period of the Geonim.
goses (pl. *gosesin*)	A person who has been inflicted with a mortal wound and whose death is expected within seventy-two hours.
goses beyedei adam	One whose death is imminent and is dying from some primary injury brought about by human hands.
goses beyedei shamayim	One whose death is imminent and who is dying from a terminal illness brought on by heaven.
gufah acharinah	A separate body.
halakhah	Jewish law applied to life.
halakhic	Of or pertaining to *halakhah*.
Halakhot	Laws.
halakhist	A *halakhic* authority.
ish	A man.
kerodef (pl. *kerodfim*)	Like a *rodef*.
kashrut	Jewish dietary regulations.
kiddush HaShem	The sanctification of God's name.
Knesset	The parliament of the State of Israel.
mamzer (pl. *mamzerim*)	A bastard. The offspring of certain prohibited adulterous or incestuous relationships.
Masekhet	A volume of the Talmud.
Midrash (pl. *Midrashim*)	Rabbinic exegesis or wisdom in the form of homily.
midrashic	Of or pertaining to *Midrash*.

Mishnah	The Oral Law, in six "orders," originally taught orally. Codified and committed into writing during the second century CE, and finally edited by Rabbi Judah HaNasi *c.* 200 CE. Together with the *Gemara*, forming the Talmud.
mishnaic	Of or pertaining to the Mishnah.
Mishneh Torah	Maimonides' Code of Jewish law from the twelfth century.
mitzvah (pl. *mitzvot*)	A Commandment.
mokh	An absorbent material designed to frustrate conception.
mutar	Permitted by Jewish law.
nazir	One who has taken a vow temporarily to forswear certain physical pleasures.
nefel	A baby of doubtful viability.
nefesh (pl. *nefashot*)	A living soul, i.e. a born human being.
Noahide	A non-Jew.
Noahide laws	Seven laws that, according to Jewish law, are required of non-Jews. The rabbis of the Talmud derive these laws from the instructions given to the sons of Noah in Genesis 9.
peshat	The simple or plain meaning of a text.
parshan	A textual commentator.
pesikah	Of or pertaining to the task of a *posek* in deciding questions of Jewish law.
pikuach nefesh	The saving of a life.
pilpul	Theoretical discussion on matter of Jewish law.
posek (pl. *poskim*)	A rabbinic authority who decides questions of Jewish law.
responsum (pl. *responsa*)	A rabbinic legal response that applies the law to a specific inquiry.
Rishon (pl. *Rishonim*)	A *halakhic* authority who lived in the period from the decline of the Babylonian academies in the middle of the eleventh century to the renewal of ordination in the middle of the fifteenth century.
rodef (pl. *rodfim*)	A pursuer; in Jewish law, one who is pursuing another in order to kill the victim.

Sefaradi (pl. *Sefaradim*)	Jews originating in the Iberian peninsula (Spain in Hebrew is *Sefarad*) and in oriental countries.
Shabbat (pl. *Shabbatot*)	The Sabbath.
she̓eilah (pl. *she̓eilot*)	A question put to a *halakhic* authority that had not received a previous reply that could be considered adequate in the current circumstances.
sho̓el	The individual who asks a *she̓eilah*.
Shulchan Arukh	An authoritative code of Jewish law, compiled by Rabbi Yosef Karo in the sixteenth century.
Talmud Bavli	The Babylonian Talmud. The authoritative Talmud completed in Babylonia in the sixth century CE.
Talmud Yerushalmi	The Jerusalem or Land of Israel Talmud. Completed in the fifth century CE.
Talmud	Compendium of rabbinic discourse of *halakhah* and *aggadah*, comprising the *Mishnah* and the *Gemara*, in two versions, the Babylonian Talmud and the Jerusalem (Land of Israel) Talmud.
Talmudic	Of or pertaining to the Talmud.
Tanakh	The Hebrew Bible, comprising three sections, the *Torah, Nevi̓im*, and *Ketuvim* (Torah, Prophets, and Writings).
Tanna (pl. *Tanna̓im*)	A rabbinic scholar and teacher of the early (*mishnaic*) period of the Talmud.
Tanna̓itic	Of or pertaining to the period of the *Tanna̓im*.
tareif	Non-kosher food.
tereifah	One who is suffering from an injury for which there is no cure or hope of recovery.
terumah	A biblically ordained gift offering.
teshuvah (pl. *teshuvot*)	A rabbinic legal response that applies the law to a specific inquiry.
Torah	Specifically, the Five Books of Moses; more generally, a reference to biblical texts, the Talmud, and commentaries thereon.
Tosafists	Rabbinic glossarists of the Talmud, mainly French and German, who during the twelfth

	to the fourteenth centuries composed the *Tosafot* glosses to the Talmud.
Tosafot	Glosses to the Talmud composed by the *Tosafists*.
tractate	A volume of the Talmud.
tumah	The state of ritual impurity.
tzaàrah degufah	Bodily suffering.
tzorekh gadol	A great need.
tzorekh kalush	A small (literally, "thin") need.
ubar	A fetus.
yerekh	A thigh or limb.
Yerushalmi	The *Talmud Yerushalmi*; the Jerusalem or Land of Israel Talmud. Completed in the fifth century CE.
yeshivah (pl. *yeshivot*)	An academy for textual study.
yetzer ha-rah	The evil drive or inclination.
yetzer ha-tov	The good drive or inclination.
Yom Kippur	The day of Atonement.

Bibliography

PRIMARY HEBREW SOURCES

BIBLE AND COMMENTARIES

Tanakh – JPS Hebrew–English Tanakh, Philadelphia, The Jewish Publication Society, 1999.
Mikraot Gedolot, Union City, Gross Brothers Printing Company, 1983, with:
  Rashi.

MIDRASHIM

Horowitz, S. (ed.), *Sifrei Zuta*, Breslau, 1917.
Lauterbach, J. C. (ed.), *Mekilta de-Rabbi Ishmael*, Philadelphia, volume III, *Nezikin*, 1935.
Midrash Shoher Tov, Warsaw, 1893.

TALMUD, COMMENTARIES AND NOVELLAE

Lieberman, S. (ed.) *Tosefta*, New York, 1955 and on.
Mishnah, New York, 1953, with:
  Eger, A., *Tosafot R. Akiva Eger*.
  Lipschutz, I., *Tiferet Yisrael*.
Steinsaltz Talmud, Jerusalem, 1984.
Talmud Bavli, Vilna, 1895, with:
  Rishonim:
    Abulafia, M., *Yad Ramah*, Sloniki, 1798, reprinted Jerusalem, 1971.
    HaMeïri, M., *Beit HaBechirah*, Jerusalem, Avraham Sofer Edition, 1965.
    Rashi – printed in all editions of the Talmud.
    Tosafot – printed in all editions of the Talmud.
  Chiddushim:
    Ramban, Jerusalem, 1928.
    Ran, New York, 1946.
  Acharonim:
    Chajes, Z., *Hagahot Maharitz*.
    Emden, Y., *Hagahot Ya'avetz*.

Talmud Yerushalmi, Vilna, 1922, with:
  Fraenkel, D., *Korban HaEidah*.
  Margolis, M., *Penei Mosheh*.

CODES AND COMMENTARIES

Abraham, A. S., *Nishmat Avraham*, Jerusalem, 1987.
Asher, Y., *Tur*, Jerusalem, 1958.
Babad, J., *Minchat Chinukh*, Vilna, 1912.
Benveniste, C., *Knesset HaGedolah*, reprinted Jerusalem, 1966.
Berlin, N., *HaEmek Sheëilah*, Jerusalem, 1948–53.
Caro, Y., *Shulchan Arukh*, New York, 1966.
Epstein, Y., *Arukh HaShulchan*, Jerusalem, 1969.
Hildesheimer, E. (ed.), *Halakhot Gedolot*, Jerusalem, 1971.
Maimonides, M., *Mishneh Torah*, New York, 1947.
  Abraham ben David, *Hassagot of Ravad*.
  Meltzer, I. Z., *Even HaAzel*, Jerusalem, 1935.
  Soloveitchik, C., *Chiddushei R. Chayim HaLevi*, New York, 1936.
Nachmanides, M., *Torat Ha'Adam, Kitvei HaRamban*, Jerusalem, 1963.
Sefer HaChinukh, Vilna, 1912.
Teomim, J., *Peri Megadim (Mishbetzot Zahav)*, Berlin, 1772.

HALAKHIC COMPENDIUM

Lampronti, Y., *Pachad Yitzchak*, Jerusalem, 1971.

MYSTICAL LITERATURE

Ashlag, Y. (ed.), *Zohar*, Tel-Aviv, 1945–46 to 1964–65.

OTHER PRIMARY SOURCES

Aristotle, *The Politics*, edited by Everson, S., Cambridge, Cambridge University Press, 1988.
Cassuto, U., *A Commentary on the Book of Exodus* (translated by I. Abrahams), Jerusalem, The Magnes Press, 1967.
Jacob, B., *The Second Book of the Bible: Exodus* (translated by W. Jacob), Hoboken, Ktav Publishing House Incorporated, 1992.
Josephus, *The Jewish War* (translated by G. A. Williamson), Penguin Books, 1959.
Midrash Rabbah (translated by H. Freedman and M. Simon), London, The Soncino Press, 1983.
The Works of Philo (new updated edition – translated by C. D. Yonge), Peabody, Hendrickson Publishers, 1993.
Pritchard, J. B., *Ancient Near Eastern Texts Relating to the Old Testament* (3rd edition), Princeton, Princeton University Press, 1969.

The Septuagint Version of the Old Testament and Apocrypha, Grand Rapids, Zondervan Publishing House, 1972.

RESPONSA

Abelson, K., "Prenatal Testing and Abortion," in *Proceedings of the Committee on Jewish Law and Standards of the Conservative Movement 1980–1985*, New York, 1988.

Al-Chakam, Y., *Rav Paʿalim*, Jerusalem, 1905.

Ashkenazi, M., *Panim Meïrut*, volume III, Sulzbach, 1738.

Ayash, Y., *Beit Yehudah*, Leghorn, 1746.

Bacharach, Y., *Chavvot Yaïr*, Lemberg, 1896.

Bakshi-Doron, E., "*Herayon LeShem Hashtalat Rikmot HaUbar LeTzorekh Ripui HaʾAv*," *Techumin*, volume 15, 1995.

Bokser, B. and Abelson, K., "A Statement on the Permissibility of Abortion," in *Proceedings of the Committee on Jewish Law and Standards of the Conservative Movement 1980–1985*, New York, 1988.

Drimer, S., *Beit Shlomoh*, Lemberg, 1878.

Duran, S., *Tashbatz*, volume III, Amsterdam, 1739.

Emden, J., *Sheëilat Yaʿavetz*, Altona, 1739.

Engel, S., *Maharash Engel*, Bardiov, 1926 and on.

Eybeschuetz, Y., *Urim VeTumim*, Karlsruhe, 1755.

Feinstein, M., *Iggerot Mosheh*, New York, 1961 and on.

Feldman, D. M., "Abortion: The Jewish View," in *Proceedings of the Committee on Jewish Law and Standards of the Conservative Movement 1980–1985*, New York, 1988.

Freehof, S., *Today's Reform Responsa*, Cincinnati, The Hebrew Union College Press, 1990.

Gordis, R., "Abortion: Major Wrong or Basic Right?," in *Proceedings of the Committee on Jewish Law and Standards of the Conservative Movement 1980–1985*, New York, 1988.

Grodzinsky, C., *Sheëilot UTeshuvot Achiezer*, volume III, New York, 1946.

Grossnass, A., *Lev Aryeh*, London, 1973.

Halevy, C. D., "*Al Dilul Ubarim VeHaMaʿamad HaHilkhati Shel Ubarim BeMivchana*," in *Sefer Assia*, volume VIII, Jerusalem, 1995.

Hoffman, D., *Melamed LeHoïl*, Frankfurt, 1932.

Horowitz, M. S., *Yedei Mosheh*, Pietrokow, 1898.

Jacob, W., *Contemporary American Reform Responsa*, New York, 1987.
  Questions and Reform Jewish Answers: New American Reform Responsa, New York, 1992.

Jacob, W. (ed.), *American Reform Responsa: Collected Responsa of the Central Conference of American Rabbis 1889–1983*, New York, 1983.

Kaidonover, A., *Emunat Shmuel*, Jerusalem, 1970.

Klein, I., "Abortion and Jewish Tradition," *Conservative Judaism*, volume 24, number 3, 1970.

Kluger, S., *Sefer Tzluta D'Avraham*, Lemberg, 1868.
Landau, E., *Nodah Bi-Yehudah*, Vilna, 1904.
Lifschutz, A., *Aryeh Devei Ilai*, Vishnitz, 1850.
Meislich, D., *Binyan David*, Ohel, 1935.
Mizrachi, M., *Peri Ha-Aretz*, Jerusalem, 1899.
Oelbaum, Y., *Sheeilat Yitzchak*, Prague, 1931.
Oshry, E., *ShuT MiMa'amakim*, New York, 1959.
Ouziel, B., *Mishpetei Ouziel*, Tel Aviv, 1935.
Pallagi, C., *Chayim VeShalom*, Smyrna, 1872.
Perilman, Y., *Or Gadol*, Vilna, 1924.
Plaut, W. G. and Washofsky, M. (eds.), *Teshuvot for the Nineties: Reform Judaism's Answers for Today's Dilemmas*, New York, 1997.
Rozin, Y., *Tzofnat Pa'aneach*, Warsaw, 1935.
Schick, M., *Maharam Schick*, Muncacz, 1881.
Schorr, I., *Koach Shor*, Kolomea, 1888.
Schorr, Y., in *Geonim Batrai*, Turka, 1764.
Schreiber, M., *Chatam Sofer*, Vienna, 1855.
Sperber, D., *Afrekasta D'Anya*, Satmar, 1940.
Teitelbaum, Y., *Avenei Tzedek*, Sziget, 1886.
The Responsa Project, a *ShuT* CD-Rom, Bar-Ilan University, Version 6.0, 1972–98.
Trani, Y., *Maharit*, Lemberg, 1861.
Unterman, I. Y., *"B'Inyan Pikuach Nefesh Shel Ubar,"* *Noam*, volume 6, 1963.
    Shevet MiYehudah, Jerusalem, 1983.
Waldenberg, E., *Tzitz Eliezer*, Jerusalem, 1963 and on.
Weinberg, Y., *"Hapalat HaUbar B'Isha Cholanit,"* *Noam*, volume 9, 1966.
    Seridei Eish, volume III, Jerusalem, 1966.
Winkler, M., *Levushei Mordekhai, Mahadurah Tinyana*, Budapest, 1924.
Yisraeli, S., *Amud HaYemini*, Tel Aviv, 1966.
Yosef, O., *Yabïah Omer*, Jerusalem, 1964.
Zalman, S., *Torat Chesed*, Jerusalem, 1909.
Zand, J. Z., *Birkat Banim*, Jerusalem, 1994.
Zilberstein, Y., *"Dilul Ubarim: ShuT,"* in *Sefer Assia*, volume VIII, Jerusalem, 1995.
Zimra, D., *HaRadbaz*, Venice, 1749.
Zweig, M. Y., *"Al Hapalah Melakhutit,"* *Noam*, volume 7, 1964.

SECONDARY HEBREW SOURCES

Alon, G., *Mechkarim BeToldot Yisrael*, Tel Aviv, 1967.
Arusi, R., *"Halakhah VeHalakhah LeMa'asei BeBitzu'ah Hapalah Melakhutit BeMishpat Ha'Ivri,"* *Dinei Yisrael*, volume 5, 1977.
    "Derakhim BeCheker HaHalakhah UVeVeirurah," *Techumin*, volume 2, 1981.
Drori, M., *"HaHandassah HaGenetit: Iyun Rishoni BeHeibetim HaMishpati-im VeHaHilkhati-im,"* *Techumin*, volume 1, 1980.
Ellinson, E., *"HaUbar BaHalakhah,"* *Sinai*, volume 66, 1969.

Geiger, A., *HaMikrah VeTirgumav*, Jerusalem, 1948.

Sinclair, D. B., "*HaYesod HaMishpati Shel Issur Hapalah BaMishpat HaIvri,*" *Shenaton HaMishpat HaIvri*, volume 5, 1978.

Stern, M., *HaRefuàh L'Or HaHalakhah*, Jerusalem, 1980.

Weinfeld, M., "*Hamitat Ubar: Emdatah Shel Masoret Yisrael BeHashvàah LeEmdat Amim Acherim,*" *Zion*, volume 42, 1977.

OTHER SECONDARY SOURCES

Alpert, R., "Sometimes the Law is Cruel," *Journal of Feminist Studies in Religion*, volume 11, number 2, 1995.

Alpher, J. (editor of English edition), *Encyclopedia of Jewish History: Events and Eras of the Jewish People* (translated by Haya Amir et al.), Ramat Gan, Israel, Massada Publishers, *c.* 1986.

American Demographics, December 1996 edition.

Anderson, B. W., *Understanding the Old Testament* (3rd edition), New Jersey, Prentice-Hall Incorporated, 1975.

Antonelli, J. S., *In the Image of God: A Feminist Commentary on the Torah*, Northvale, Jason Aaronson Incorporated, 1995.

Aptowitzer, V., "Observations on the Criminal Law of the Jews," *The Jewish Quarterly Review*, volume 15, 1924.

Bachi, R., "Abortion in Israel," in Hall, R. E. (ed.), *Abortion in a Changing World*, volume 1, New York, Columbia University Press, 1970.

Belkin, S., *Philo and the Oral Law*, Cambridge, MA, Harvard University Press, 1940.

Berkowitz, A. K., "Thinking About Women in Abortion Controversies," *Sevara*, volume 2, number 2, 1991.

Biale, R., *Women and Jewish Law: The Essential Texts, Their History and Their Relevance for Today*, New York, Schocken Books, 1984.

Bleich, J. D., "Abortion in Halakhic Literature," in *Contemporary Halakhic Problems*, volume 1, New York, Ktav Publishing House Incorporated, 1977.

    Judaism and Healing: Halakhic Perspectives, New York, Ktav Publishing House Incoporated, 1981.

    With Perfect Faith: The Foundations of Jewish Belief, New York, Ktav Publishing House Incorporated, 1983.

    Bioethical Dilemmas: A Jewish Perspective, Hoboken, Ktav Publishing House Incorporated, 1998.

Breitenecker, L. and Breitenecker, R., "Abortion in the German-Speaking Countries of Europe," in Smith, D. T. (ed.), *Abortion And The Law*, Cleveland, The Press of Western Reserve University, 1967.

Brickner, B., "Judaism and Abortion," in Kellner, M. M. (ed.), *Contemporary Jewish Ethics*, New York, Hebrew Publishing Company, 1978.

Callahan, D., "Abortion in a Pluralistic Society: Can Freedom and Moral Probity Coexist?," in Kogan, B. S. (ed.), *A Time to Be Born and a Time to Die: The Ethics of Choice*, New York, Aldine de Gruyter, 1991.

Carmy, S., "Halakhah and Philosophical Approaches to Abortion," *Tradition*, volume 16, number 3, 1977.

Committee for the Investigation of Abortion Prohibitions, "Commission Report: Appendices D and E – *Halakhic* Opinions," *Public Health*, volume 17, number 4, 1974.

Connery, J. R., *Abortion: The Development of the Roman Catholic Perspective*, Loyola University Press, 1977.

Costa, M., *Abortion: A Reference Handbook*, Santa Barbara, ABC-CLIO Incorporated, 1991.

Cytron, B. D. and Schwartz, E., *When Life Is in the Balance*, New York, United Synagogue of America, 1986.

Davis, D. S., "Abortion in Jewish Thought: A Study in Casuistry," *Journal of the American Academy of Religion*, volume 60, number 2, 1992.

Dorland's Illustrated Medical Dictionary (27th edition), W. B. Saunders Company, Harcourt Brace Jovanovich Incorporated, Philadelphia, 1988.

Dorff, E. N., *Matters of Life and Death: A Jewish Approach to Modern Medical Ethics*, Philadelphia, The Jewish Publication Society, 1998.

Elon, M., *Jewish Law: History, Sources, Principles*, Jerusalem, The Jewish Publication Society, 4 volumes, 1994.

Elon, M. (ed.), *The Principles of Jewish Law*, Jerusalem, Keter Publishing House, 1975.

Encyclopaedia Judaica, Jerusalem, Keter Publishing House, 1972–8.

Falk, Z., "The New Abortion Law of Israel," *Israel Law Review*, volume 13, number 1, 1978.

Feldman, D. M., "Abortion and Ethics: the Rabbinic Viewpoint", *Conservative Judaism*, volume 29, number 4, 1975.

"Abortion and a Woman's Right," in Romm, J. L. and Levy, L. (eds.), *Halakhah and the Modern Jew: Essays in Honor of Horace Bier*, Mount Vernon, NY, Union for Traditional Conservative Judaism, 1989.

"This Matter of Abortion," in Dorff, E. N. and Newman, L. E. (eds.), *Contemporary Jewish Ethics and Morality: A Reader*, Oxford, Oxford University Press, 1995.

Birth Control in Jewish Law: Marital Relations, Contraception, and Abortion as Set Forth in the Classic Texts of Jewish Law, Northvale, Jason Aronson Incorporated, 1998.

Fine, M. and Asch, A., "Shared Dreams: A Left Perspective on Disability Rights and Reproductive Rights," in Fine, M. and Asch, A. (eds.), *Women with Disabilities: Essays in Psychology, Culture and Politics*, Philadelphia, Temple University Press, 1988.

Fishbane, M., *Biblical Interpretation in Ancient Israel*, Oxford, Clarendon Press, 1985.

Freund, R., "The Ethics of Abortion in Hellenistic Judaism," *Helios*, volume 10, number 2, 1983.

Friedenwald, H., *The Jews and Medicine*, New York, Ktav Publishing House Incorporated, 1967.

Glendon, M. A., *Abortion and Divorce in Western Law*, Cambridge, MA, Harvard University Press, 1987.

Gold, M., *Does God Belong in the Bedroom?*, Philadelphia, The Jewish Publication Society, 1992.

Goodenough, E. R., *The Jurisprudence of the Jewish Courts in Egypt*, Amsterdam, Philo Press, 1968 (reprint of 1929 edition).

Gordis, D., *Does the World Need Jews?*, New York, Scribner, 1997.

Greenberg, B., "Abortion: A Challenge to Halakhah," *Judaism*, volume 25, 1976.
   On Women and Judaism, Philadelphia, The Jewish Publication Society of America, 1981.

Greenberg, M., "Some Postulates of Biblical Criminal Law," in Haran, M. (ed.), *Sefer HaYovel LeYehezkel Kaufmann*, Jerusalem, Magnes Press, 1960.

Grisez, G., *Abortion: The Myths, the Realities and the Arguments*, New York, Corpus Books, 1970.

Hall, R. E., "Commentary," in Smith, D. T. (ed.), *Abortion and the Law*, Cleveland, The Press of Western Reserve University, 1967.

Hauptman, J., "A Matter of Morality," *United Synagogue Review*, Spring, 1990.

Herring B. F., *Jewish Ethics and Halakhah for Our Time*, New York, Ktav Publishing House Incorporated, 1984.

Israel Yearbook and Almanac 1998, Jerusalem, Israel Business, Research and Technical Translation/Documentation Limited, 1999.

Jacob, B., *Auge um Auge: Eine Untersuchung zum Alten und Neuen Testament*, Berlin, Philo Verlag, 1929.

Jacobs, L., *A Tree of Life: Diversity, Flexibility, and Creativity in Jewish Law*, Oxford, Oxford University Press, 1984.

Jakobovits, I., *Jewish Medical Ethics*, New York, Philosophical Library, 1959.
   "Review of Recent Halakhic Periodical Literature," *Tradition*, volume 5, number 2, 1963.
   "Tay-Sachs Disease and the Jewish Community," *Proceedings of the Association of Orthodox Jewish Scientists*, volumes 3–4, 1976.
   "Jewish Views on Abortion," in Rosner, F. and Bleich, J. D. (eds.), *Jewish Bioethics*, New York, Sanhedrin Press, 1979.

Jones, O. D., "Sex Selection: Regulating Technology Enabling the Predetermination of a Child's Gender," *Harvard Journal of Law and Technology*, volume 6, 1992.

Katz, J., *Shabbes Goy: A Study in Halakhic Flexibility*, Philadelphia, The Jewish Publication Society, 1989.

Kaufman, M., *The Woman in Jewish Law and Tradition*, Northvale, Jason Aronson Incorporated, 1993.

Kelly, B. (medical ed.), *Family Health and Medical Guide*, Dallas, Word Publishing, 1996.

Kirschner, R., "The Halakhic Status of the Fetus with Respect to Abortion", *Conservative Judaism*, volume 34, number 6, 1981.

Lader, L., *Abortion*, New York, Howard W. Sams and Company Incorporated, 1966.

Levin, F., *Halacha, Medical Science and Technology*, New York, Maznaim Publishing
    Corporation, 1987.
Lichtenstein, A., "Does Tradition Recognize an Ethic Independent of
    Halakha?," in Fox, M. (ed.), *Modern Jewish Ethics*, Columbus, Ohio State
    University Press, 1975.
Lindemann, A., "'Do Not Let a Woman Destroy the Unborn Babe in Her
    Belly.' Abortion in Ancient Judaism and Christianity," *Studia Theologica*,
    volume 49, 1995.
Lubarsky, S. B., "Judaism and the Justification of Abortion for Non-Medical
    Reasons," *Journal of Reform Judaism*, volume 31, number 4, 1984.
Margolies, I. R., "A Reform Rabbi's View," in Hall, R. E. (ed.), *Abortion in a
    Changing World*, volume 1, New York, Columbia University Press, 1970.
Meier, L. (ed.), *Jewish Values in Bioethics*, New York, Human Sciences Press
    Incorporated, 1986.
Milner, L. S., "A Brief History of Infanticide," at http://www.infanticide.org/
    history.htm.
Morag-Levine, N., "Imported Problem Definitions, Legal Culture and the Local
    Dynamics of Israeli Abortion Politics," in Cass, F., *Israel, the Dynamics of
    Change and Continuity*, London, 1999.
Newman, L. E., "Ethics as Law, Law as Religion: Reflection on the Prob-
    lem of Law and Ethics in Judaism," in Dorff, E. N. and Newman, L. E.
    (eds.), *Contemporary Jewish Ethics: A Reader*, Oxford, Oxford University Press,
    1995.
    "The Problem of Interpretation in Contemporary Jewish Ethics," in Dorff,
    E. N. and Newman, L. E. (eds.), *Contemporary Jewish Ethics: A Reader*, Oxford,
    Oxford University Press, 1995.
    Past Imperatives: Studies in the History and Theory of Jewish Ethics, Albany, State
    University of New York Press, 1998.
Nitowsky, H., "Abortion and Ethics: Making Informed Decisions," *Conservative
    Judaism*, volume 29, number 4, 1975.
Noonan, J. T. Jr., "An Almost Absolute Value in History," in *The Morality of
    Abortion: Legal and Historical Perspectives*, Cambridge, MA, Harvard University
    Press, 1970.
Novak, D., "A Jewish View of Abortion," in *Law and Theology in Judaism*, New
    York, Ktav Publishing House Incorporated, 1974.
Perry, D. L., "Abortion and Personhood: Historical and Comparative Notes,"
    at http://www.home.earthlink.net/~davidlperry/abortion.htm.
Preuss, J., *Biblical and Talmudic Medicine*, Northvale, Jason Aronson Incorporated,
    1993.
Rackman, E., "Jewish Medical Ethics and Law," in Meier, L. (ed.), *Jewish Values
    in Bioethics*, New York, Human Sciences Press Incorporated, 1986.
Rahman, A., Katzive, L., and Henshaw, S., "A Global Review of Laws on
    Induced Abortion, 1985–1997," *International Family Planning Perspectives*,
    volume 24, number 2, 1998.

Reagan, L. J., *When Abortion Was a Crime: Women, Medicine, and Law in the United States, 1867–1973*, Los Angeles, University of California Press, 1997.

Riddle, J. M., *Contraception and Abortion from the Ancient World to the Renaissance*, Cambridge, MA, Harvard University Press, 1992.

Roberg, N., "Therapeutic Abortion," in Rakover, N. (ed.), *Jewish Law and Current Legal Problems*, Jerusalem, The Library of Jewish Law, 1984.

Rosenbaum, I. J., *The Holocaust and Halakhah*, New York, Ktav Publishing House, Incorporated, 1976.

Rosner, F., *Studies in Torah Judaism: Modern Medicine and Jewish Law*, New York, Yeshiva University Press, 1972.

"Tay-Sachs Disease: To Screen or Not to Screen," *Tradition*, volume 15, number 4, 1976.

Modern Medicine and Jewish Ethics, New York, Yeshiva University Press, and Hoboken, Ktav Publishing House Incorporated, 1986.

Rosner, F. and Tendler, M. D., *Practical Medical Halachah* (3rd edition), Hoboken, Ktav Publishing House Incorporated, 1990.

Roth, J., *The Halakhic Process: A Systemic Analysis*, New York, The Jewish Theological Seminary of America, 1986.

Rudy, K., *Beyond Pro-Life and Pro-Choice: Moral Diversity in the Abortion Debate*, Boston, Beacon Press, 1996.

Sandmel, S., *Philo of Alexandria*, New York, Oxford University Press, 1979.

Sarna, N., *Exploring Exodus: The Heritage of Biblical Israel*, New York, Schocken Books, 1986.

Schiff, D. L., "Developing *Halakhic* Attitudes To Sex Preselection," in Jacob, W. and Zemer, M. (eds.), *The Fetus and Fertility in Jewish Law*, Pittsburgh, Rodef Shalom Press, 1995.

Schiffman, L. H., *From Text to Tradition: A History of Second Temple and Rabbinic Judaism*, Hoboken, Ktav Publishing House Incorporated, 1991.

Reclaiming the Dead Sea Scrolls, Philadelphia, The Jewish Publication Society, 1994.

Schmidt, J. E., *Attorneys' Dictionary of Medicine and Word Finder*, Times Mirror Books, 1991.

Seltzer, R. M., *Jewish People, Jewish Thought: The Jewish Experience in History*, New York, Macmillan Publishing Company, Incorporated, 1980.

Siegel, S., "Abortion: Moral Issues Beyond Legal Ones", *Shema*, volume 8, number 143.

Sinclair, D. B., unpublished chapter provided by the author: "The Interplay of Legal Doctrine and Moral Principle in the Halakhah of Abortion."

"The Legal Basis for the Prohibition on Abortion in Jewish Law," *Israel Law Review*, volume 15, number 1, 1980.

Tradition and the Biological Revolution, Edinburgh, Edinburgh University Press, 1989.

Steinsaltz, A., *The Talmud: The Steinsaltz Edition – A Reference Guide*, New York, Random House, 1989.

Stevens, E. (ed.), *Central Conference of American Rabbis Yearbook*, New York, Central Conference of American Rabbis, volume C, 1991.

Tietze, C., *Induced Abortion: A World Review, 1981* (4th edition), New York, A Population Council Fact Book, 1981.

Urbach, E., *The Sages: Their Concepts and Beliefs* (translated by Israel Abrahams), Jerusalem, Magnes Press of the Hebrew University, 1979.

Van der Tak, J., *Abortion, Fertility, and Changing Legislation: An International Review*, Lexington, Lexington Books, 1974.

Vorspan, A. and Saperstein, D., *Tough Choices: Jewish Perspectives on Social Justice*, New York, Union of American Hebrew Congregations Press, 1992.

Washofsky, M., "Abortion, Halacha and Reform Judaism," *Journal of Reform Judaism*, volume 28, number 4, 1981.

"Morality and Choice: A Response to Daniel Callahan," in Kogan, B. S. (ed.), *A Time to Be Born and a Time to Die: The Ethics of Choice*, New York, Aldine de Gruyter, 1991.

"Abortion and the Halakhic Conversation," in Jacob, W. and Zemer, M. (eds.), *The Fetus and Fertility in Jewish Law*, Pittsburgh, Rodef Shalom Press, 1995.

Westermarck, E., *The Origin and Development of the Moral Ideas*, New York, Macmillan Company, 1906.

Yishai, Y., "Abortion in Israel: Social Demand and Political Responses," in Azmon, Y. and Izraeli, D. N. (eds.), *Women in Israel*, Studies in Israeli Society 6, New Brunswick, Transaction, 1993.

Zemer, M., *Evolving Halakhah: A Progressive Approach to Traditional Jewish Law*, Woodstock, Jewish Lights Publishing, 1999.

Zimmels, H. J., *Magicians, Theologians and Doctors*, Northvale, Jason Aronson Incorporated, 1997.

Index

For EU product safety concerns, contact us at Calle de José Abascal, 56–1°,
28003 Madrid, Spain or eugpsr@cambridge.org.

www.ingramcontent.com/pod-product-compliance
Ingram Content Group UK Ltd.
Pitfield, Milton Keynes, MK11 3LW, UK
UKHW010033140625
459647UK00012BA/1347